Basic Child Psychiatry

Basic Family Therapy
Third Edition
Philip Barker
0–632–03227–8

Basic Behaviour Therapy
Douglas Murdoch & Philip Barker
0–632–02322–8

Basic Forensic Psychiatry
Second Edition
Malcolm Faulk
0–632–03321–5

Basic Child Psychiatry

Sixth Edition

Philip Barker

MB, BS, FRCP(Ed), FRCPsych, FRCP(C)
Professor, Departments of Psychiatry
and Paediatrics, University of Calgary

**Blackwell
Science**

© Philip Barker 1971, 1976, 1979, 1983, 1988, 1995
Blackwell Science Ltd
Editorial Offices:
Osney Mead, Oxford OX2 0EL
25 John Street, London WC1N 2BL
23 Ainslie Place, Edinburgh EH3 6AJ
238 Main Street, Cambridge,
    Massachusetts 02142, USA
54 University Street, Carlton,
    Victoria 3053, Australia

Other Editorial Offices:
Arnette Blackwell SA
1, rue de Lille, 75007 Paris
France

Blackwell Wissenschafts-Verlag GmbH
Kurfürstendamm 57
10707 Berlin, Germany

Blackwell MZV
Feldgasse 13, A-1238 Wien
Austria

First edition published by
    Crosby Lockwood Staples 1971
Reprinted 1973
Second edition published by Granada
    Publishing Ltd in Crosby Lockwood
    Staples 1976
Reprinted 1977
Third edition published 1979
Reprinted by Granada Publishing Ltd 1981
Fourth edition published by Granada
    Publishing Ltd 1983
Reprinted 1984
Reprinted by Collins Professional
    and Technical Books 1985
Fifth edition published by Blackwell
    Scientific Publications 1988
Reprinted 1990, 1992
Sixth edition published by
Blackwell Science Ltd 1995

Set by DP Photosetting, Aylesbury, Bucks
Printed and bound in Great Britain by
the University Press, Cambridge

DISTRIBUTORS
    Marston Book Services Ltd
    PO Box 87
    Oxford OX2 0DT
    (Orders: Tel: 01865 791155
            Fax: 01865 791927
            Telex: 837515)

North America
    Blackwell Science Inc.
    238 Main Street
    Cambridge, MA 02142
    (Orders: Tel: 800 215-1000
            617 876-7000
            Fax: 617 492-5263)

Australia
    Blackwell Science Pty Ltd
    54 University Street,
    Carlton, Victoria 3053
    (Orders: Tel: 03 347-5552)

British Library
Cataloguing in Publication Data
A Catalogue record for this book is available
from the British Library

ISBN 0–632–03772–5

Library of Congress
Cataloging in Publication Data
Barker, Philip.
    Basic child psychiatry/Philip Barker.—
    6th ed.
        p   cm.
    Includes bibliographical references and
    index.
    ISBN 0–632–03772–5
    1. Child psychiatry.   I. Title.
    [DNLM: 1. Child Psychiatry.
    WS 350 B255b   1994]
RJ499.B27   1994
618.92'89—dc20
DNLM/DLC
for Library of Congress   94-1898
                                              CIP

To Thembi and Sibusiso Barker

Contents

Introduction

Like previous editions of *Basic Child Psychiatry*, this one aims to provide a concise, easily read but wide-ranging introductory account of its subject. Since the first edition appeared in 1971, there has been an explosive growth of knowledge in all areas of child psychiatry. There has also been specialization within the field, for example in the areas of infant psychiatry, adolescent psychiatry and the effects of child abuse. Accompanying this growth has been a corresponding increase in the size of each edition of this book. But as the speciality of child psychiatry has grown, several comprehensive textbooks have appeared, none of which was available in 1971. Further books have also appeared on specialized areas such as those mentioned above.

These circumstances, and the urging of my publisher to avoid a steady increase in the size of the book with each new edition, caused me to examine carefully the entire contents to ensure that *Basic Child Psychiatry* remained *basic*. This has led, in this sixth edition, to a renewed emphasis on the more common problems and on general principles. Rare conditions are for the most part dealt with quite briefly, references being cited to enable the reader to obtain additional information when this is required.

The question of how extensively treatment methods should be described and discussed in a book such as this is a moot one. The importance of treatment can hardly be overstated, for a major objective of the study of any area of medicine must be to provide the best possible treatment for those afflicted with the disorders under study. Perhaps only prevention is of comparable importance. Child psychiatric disorders are however complex conditions with, usually, multiple causes. Their treatment is correspondingly complex and it is unrealistic to expect a basic, introductory book such as this to deal with such complexity in a comprehensive way.

This creates a dilemma. On the one hand, readers of this book will undoubtedly seek from it guidance as to how to approach the treatment of the disorders discussed. On the other hand, the sheer complexity of the treatment needs of many children limits what it is possible to include in an introductory text. This dilemma has been addressed in part by the publication of the companion volumes *Basic Family Therapy* (Barker, 1992) and *Basic Behaviour Therapy* (Murdoch & Barker, 1991). Texts are also available on other forms of psychotherapy and on child and adolescent psychopharmacology. In this book I have concentrated on discussing the general principles of treatment. I believe these provide the basic information needed to start developing rational treatment programs. This should be supplemented as necessary by further reading and, especially, by the expert supervision that all those learning the subject must have.

Since the fifth edition of this book appeared, the tenth edition of the World Health Organization's *International Classification of Diseases* (ICD-10) (World Health Organization, 1992) and the fourth edition of the American Psychiatric Association's *Diagnostic and Statistical Manual* (DSM-IV) (American Psychiatric Association (1994)) have been published. The former replaces the previous edition (ICD-9), published in 1977. It incorporates much new knowledge and also provides valuable clinical definitions and descriptions of the various psychiatric disorders of childhood and adolescence. The latter replaces the revised version (DSM-III-R) of American Psychiatric Association's *Diagnostic and Statistical Manual* (APA, 1987). These two revised classification schemes are used throughout this book.

Primarily to assist readers who do not have a medical background, each previous edition included a glossary of terms. In this edition, in response to suggestions received, I have instead provided brief explanations of such terms when they first appear in the text. This should make for easier reading and means that readers will not have to refer to another part of the book whenever an unfamiliar term is encountered. In addition I have redoubled my efforts to avoid unnecessary jargon and to explain everything, as far as possible, in simple, straightforward English.

I hope that *Basic Child Psychiatry* will continue to provide the newcomer to the field with the basic information needed to get started on the study of the emotional and behavioural problems of children and adolescents.

Philip Barker
Calgary, 1994

Acknowledgements

Once again it is a pleasure to acknowledge the help and encouragement I have received from many people in the writing of this, as of previous editions of this book. Many years ago now, Dr Philip Connell taught me the basics of child psychiatry. Since then I have learned much both from the many colleagues with whom I have worked – now too numerous to list – and from the children and families who, over the years, have come to me with a wide variety of problems.

During the last 14 years my colleagues in the Department of Psychiatry and the Mental Health Program at Alberta Children's Hospital, Calgary, have taught me much. I am particularly grateful to Dr Douglas Murdoch, who read and commented most helpfully on the section on psychological tests in Chapter 5.

The task of writing this book, and especially that of obtaining and checking the many references it contains, has been enormously lightened by the help always freely given by Barbara Hatt, librarian at Alberta Children's Hospital, and her assistant, Elisabeth Neilson. Their unfailing willingness to meet my requests, and to hunt out elusive references and material, goes well beyond the line of duty.

As usual, Richard Miles, my publisher, has been helpful and supportive. We now have a long history of working together, on this and other books, from the days when *Basic Child Psychiatry* was published by Crosby Lockwood Staples, through a period with Collins Professional and Technical Books, to our present home with Blackwell Science Ltd. I am happy also to acknowledge the help of Sue Moore, Senior Editor at Blackwell. She and copy editor Judith Murray have contributed much to the final presentation of this edition.

Author's note

Throughout this book it has been necessary to refer repeatedly to the principal diagnostic systems used in classifying child psychiatric disorders, namely the tenth edition of the *International Classification of Diseases*

(World Health Organization, 1992) and the fourth edition of the *Diagnostic and Statistical Manual of Mental Disorders* (DSM-IV) (American Psychiatric Association, 1994). To avoid needless repetition, and to save space, I have not cited the reference each time one of these diagnostic schemes is mentioned. Instead, I have simply referred to them as ICD-10 and DSM-IV. Similarly the earlier version of the WHO diagnostic system (World Health Organization, 1977a) is referred to as ICD-9, and those of the American Psychiatric Association (1980 and 1987) as DSM-III and DSM-III-R, respectively.

The full references to each of the above appear in the list at the end of the text.

Chapter 1

Developmental Considerations

The psychiatric assessment of children requires a sound knowledge of normal child development. Many behaviours are normal at certain ages but not at others, and many of the problems with which child psychiatrists deal are primarily manifestations of disordered development. While some child psychiatric disorders are syndromes with characteristic features – childhood schizophrenia, obsessive-compulsive disorders and Tourette's syndrome are examples – in many others, the essence of the problem is that development in one or more areas of function is not proceeding normally. This applies not only to conditions generally regarded as 'developmental' – for example, mental retardation, developmental language disorders and functional encopresis – but also to that very large group of child psychiatric disorders, the 'conduct' and 'oppositional defiant' disorders. These are probably best understood as disorders of the process of socialization. For whatever reason – and usually several factors combine to produce the problem behaviours – children with antisocial behaviours have not learned to abide by society's norms. But more of that in Chapter 6.

Learning about normal development

The best way to learn how children develop is to be with them as they develop. You can do this in both formal and informal settings. The most informal setting is your own family – if there are children in it. It is important to remember, though, that the lives of children in the relatively affluent, middle class families of most health professionals may differ significantly from those in other sections of society – to say nothing of the many other cultures that exist throughout the world. These differences have their implications for child development.

The more formal observation of children may be done in daycare centres, nursery schools, schools for older children or indeed anywhere where children of different ages may be found. Supervision of your learning by experienced child health professionals should be a part of this experience. They can draw your attention to points of importance.

The newcomer to work with children should also study the descriptions of child development which have been written by authors of various theoretical persuasions.

Reading materials

Many aspects of child development have been studied, including the development of cognitive skills, emotional responses, relationship skills and social behaviour. In addition, children develop within their social settings, which also invite study.

Aside from children raised in institutional settings – and these are nowadays few in western society – the family is the most important part of the developing child's environment. But the family needs to develop and change as its children grow. Understanding the changing context of the developing child – or the lack of adequate change that we sometimes observe – is therefore essential if we are to come to have a good understanding of child development. Normal family functioning and development are outlined in *Basic Family Therapy* (Barker, 1992) and fuller accounts are those of Duvall & Miller (1985) and McGoldrick & Carter (1982).

Among the many who have studied aspects of child development are Sigmund Freud (1905), Erik Erikson (1965, 1968), Jean Piaget (whose theories have been well summarized by Flavell (1963) and reviewed critically by Hobson (1985)), Anna Freud (1966) and Melanie Klein (1948). Also relevant is the work of Bowlby (1969; 1979) and of Ainsworth and her colleagues (1978) on attachment and the process of 'bonding' between children and those caring for them. While it is useful to consult these sources, books are available which bring together the work of the different schools and cover development from a variety of perspectives. A useful one is *Encounters With Children* (Dixon & Stein, 1992).

Among the many published studies of child development, the New York Longitudinal Study (Thomas & Chess, 1977; Chess & Thomas, 1984) stands out. It followed a cohort of children from infancy to early life and the results, reported in a series of books and articles, contain much of importance to child psychiatry.

Developmental stages

Space considerations allow mention only of the main points of that complex process we call child development. It is well to remember that the division of development into different stages is artificial and in reality the process is a continuous one; the transition from one 'stage' to the next is not usually abrupt but takes place over a period of time.

The first year of life

This is a period of rapid change. Its main features are:

● The development of *basic trust* (Erikson, 1965), the child coming to experience the world as a place that is nurturing, reliable and trustworthy. This is considered to be the basis for developing the capacity for intimacy.

● Great advances in social behaviour and responsiveness. Smiling, at first a reflex activity (the *endogenous smile*), becomes selective by two to three months (the *social smile*).

● Associated with the above, the ability to distinguish between familiar and unfamiliar people. This appears at six to eight months of age, and with it there are signs of anxiety in the presence of strangers, and 'separation anxiety' when the child is parted from the mother or other significant caretaker, especially if in an unfamiliar place or with unfamiliar people.

● *Bonding* between the child and the familiar caretaking figures. Features of attachment behaviour normally evident in the first year include crying, calling, and the stranger anxiety and separation anxiety mentioned above.

● The rapid development of motor function. By about one year of age the child is walking.

● Rapid intellectual development. The first year is Piaget's *sensorimotor period*. Children learn that objects exist apart from themselves and continue to exist when they can no longer see them; they learn simple cause-and-effect relationships and start to understand spatial relationships; and they acquire an idea of how one thing may symbolize another.

The second year of life

This is characterized by:

● What Erikson (1965) calls *autonomy* – a sense of being in control of oneself, as opposed to entertaining feelings of shame and doubt.

● The further acquisition of social skills. As the ability to walk and explore is acquired, the behaviour permitted is restricted and the child learns what is permissible and what is not. The child also learns to live as a member of the family group, and may have experience outside the family in daycare, nursery school or play group situations. Toilet training may commence in the second year.

● Rapid development of motor skills, including the ability to walk, climb and manipulate objects.

● The acquisition of a limited verbal vocabulary.

● Resistance to the caretakers' behavioural restrictions, expressed as temper tantrums and through other behaviours.

● Continuing evidence of attachment behaviour.

● Further rapid advances in cognitive functioning. The middle of the second year sees the start of Piaget's 'concrete operations of classes, relations and numbers'. The first part of this is the *pre-conceptual stage* in which the child starts to become able to represent one thing by another, using language symbols and drawing for this purpose. In their second year children still feel at the centre of the world and remain closely dependent on their parents.

The pre-school period (roughly from two to five years)

This is a period of great change. Its main features are:

● The acquisition of Erikson's (1965) sense of 'initiative' – the feeling of being able to do many exciting, even almost magical things, as opposed to feeling frightened and guilty about taking the initiative. Normally developing children emerge from this stage confident in their abilities but with their impulses under adequate control.

● The development of a rich fantasy life, perhaps with imaginary friends; and, often, the use of *transitional objects*. The latter may be almost any object (an old blanket, a teddy bear, a toy) to which the child develops a special attachment, and may use as a source of security in stressful situations (Shafii, 1986; Hong, 1978).

● A further big advance in socialization, the child acquiring many more of the skills required to live as a member of the family group.

● Identification with the parents and the resulting development of the motivation to do certain things and be a certain kind of person.

● The beginnings of conscience formation. This is closely related to the process of identification with the parents.

● Rapid progress in the development of the child's sexual identity. Psychoanalysts call this the *genital stage* because of the importance that has been attributed to sexual development during this period.

● Further development of intellectual functions and cognitive skills. The processes initiated at the start of Piaget's 'pre-conceptual stage' are continued, as the ability to represent one thing by another develops further. The child stills feels at the centre of the world and considers inanimate objects to have feelings and opinions.

● A rapid increase in the complexity of language used and understood.

● The establishment of a pattern of *mental defence mechanisms*. These will be discussed further in the following chapter.

● The development of patterns of behaviour towards the world outside the family.

Middle childhood

This is the period from the start of school at 5 or 6 to about age 10. Its main features are:

● Learning what Erikson (1965) called 'the fundamentals of technology'. As this happens, children gain the satisfaction that comes from doing the things they learn – which vary from culture to culture. This is the period during which formal schooling comes to occupy a large part of children's lives. The normally developing child comes to enjoy the resulting personal satisfaction, recognition and opportunities to relate to other people. In calling this the stage of 'industry versus inferiority', Erikson (1965) also drew attention to the danger that children may fail to learn what they need to at this time of life and thus develop feelings of inferiority and failure. The teaching of children is not confined to school but occurs in the family and in many other situations, for example Cub Scouts, Brownies, youth groups and clubs, Sunday School and other organized youth activities.

● Continuing psychosexual development, though this may be less obvious (indeed psychoanalysts have called this the period of *latency*). While in western society sexual interests may be concealed, sex play and masturbation (the latter more frequent in boys than girls) are common during this period of life.

● Continued development of a pattern of *defence mechanisms*. This is discussed further in the next chapter, but by this time the normally developing child has a well developed conscience. The personality attributes the child has now acquired tend to persist into adult life.

● Further refinement of cognitive skills. Piaget's 'intuitive substage,' in which children can give reasons for their actions and beliefs, though their thinking is still 'pre-operational' – that is based on immediate perceptions rather than on mental representation of concepts – gives way to the 'sub-period of concrete operations', in which children can internalize the properties of objects and their thinking becomes less egocentric. Objects can be put in order, or classified, by size, shape or colour, without being physically compared with each other. This period also sees a great advance in the capacity for cooperative play.

Adolescence

This starts with the onset of puberty. This is marked physically by the onset of menstruation in girls and of seminal emissions in boys. These changes usually occur between 11 and 13 in girls and between 13 and 17 in boys, though the range of normal is wider. The Group for the Advancement of Psychiatry (1968) suggested that the principal developmental tasks to be completed by the end of adolescence are:

● changing from being nurtured and cared for to being able to nurture and care for others;
● learning to work and acquiring the skills to become materially self-supporting;
● accepting and becoming proficient in the adult sexual role, and coping with heterosexual relationships;
● moving out of the family of origin to form a new family of procreation.

Other features of normal adolescent development are:

● The achievement of a firm sense of one's identity, which Erikson (1965) contrasts with 'role confusion.' The healthy young adult knows who he or she is and is confident in making this identity known to the world. This personal identity becomes the basis of the individual's relationships. On the other hand, those who are in a state of role confusion do not know who they are or where they want to go in life. Identity formation has started long before adolescence, of course, but should be complete in its main essentials by the end of the teen years.

● Acquiring a more flexible cognitive style. Piaget called adolescence the period of 'formal operations.' Its main features are:

- the ability to accept assumptions for the sake of argument and to formulate hypotheses and set up propositions to test them;

- the ability to look for general properties and laws in symbolic, especially verbal, material and so to invent imaginary systems and conceive things beyond what is tangible, finite and familiar;
    — becoming aware of one's own thinking and using it to justify the judgments one makes;
    — becoming able to deal with such complex ideas as proportionality and correlation.

The Group for the Advancement of Psychiatry (1968) summarized the resolution of adolescence as comprising:

- the attainment of separation and independence from parents;
- the establishment of a sexual identity;
- the commitment to work;
- the development of a personal moral system;
- the capacity for lasting relationships, and for both tender and genital sexual love in heterosexual relationships; and
- a return to the parents in a new relationship based on a relative equality.

The above is but an outline of child and adolescent development. It does not take into account the many cultural differences which have their effects on aspects of development. Also, the developmental pathways that lead to some alternative lifestyles, such as homosexual ones, differ in certain respects from those I have outlined.

The development of self-esteem

The acquisition of a sense of self-worth is a major developmental task of childhood. Problems in this area are common in children presented for psychiatric assessment and treatment. It therefore merits a section of its own.

The development of one's sense of self-esteem is a continuing process which starts in infancy and continues throughout childhood and adolescence. Indeed it does not stop even when a person enters adulthood.

Since there is no absolute standard by which an individual's worth can be judged, for practical purposes we are what we believe we are, and this depends very much on our childhood experiences.

Cotton (1983) reviewed the process whereby self-esteem develops. It starts in infancy with 'relationships with empathic others,' and the child's emerging capacity to accomplish tasks successfully. The 'basic trust' described by Erikson (1965) develops in the context of an empathic parent-child relationship, ideally one in which the parents' and the child's temperamental characteristics are well matched. The development of the toddler's self-esteem continues to depend on parental attitudes, opinions and behaviour, combined with the child's experience of mastery of the environment.

As toddlers learn to walk, explore their environment, play, throw things, talk and engage in all kinds of social interactions, they look to their parents and other adults for their reactions. In healthy families these are affirming and supportive, even when limits have to be set on the child's behaviour. The parents also need to set realistic expectations for their child.

A similar process continues in middle childhood but children's social circles widen, so that their self-esteem comes to be influenced by a wider range of people. How much effect the attitudes and expressed opinions of others have also depends upon how highly such people are valued by the child. A mother's reaction can be expected to have a more telling effect than a stranger's. Important, too, are children's successes and failures. Those with handicaps may compare themselves unfavourably with others, so that it may be more difficult for them to obtain that sense of mastery over their environment that is an important ingredient of self-esteem.

Coopersmith (1967), on the basis of a study of pre-adolescent, white and 'normal' (that is free of symptoms of stress and/or emotional disorder) boys, concluded that self-esteem is likely to develop in conditions of:

- 'total or nearly total acceptance of the children by their parents';
- 'clearly defined and enforced limits';
- respect and latitude for the individual's actions, within defined limits.

As the years pass, children's feelings about their worth and capabilities increasingly become internalized, that is, they are less dependent upon the immediate response of the environment. By the time they reach adolescence, their self-images have become part of their personality structures, or what Erikson (1968) calls their 'ego-identity', though they are still subject to modification. Changing a person's self-image, however, becomes a bigger task as the years succeed one another.

Development in adulthood

Erikson (1965) described three more 'ages of man'. These are the stages of development through which children's parents and grandparents pass.

The first is that of 'intimacy versus isolation'. The young adult, having completed her or his search for identity, is now ready for intimacy with others, in close relationships including sexual union. Failure at this stage results in isolation. Instead of developing close relationships the person may isolate, or even destroy, forces and people that appear threatening in some way.

The next stage is that of 'generativity versus stagnation'. The essence of generativity is the establishing and guiding of the next generation. This is achieved not only, nor even necessarily, by parenthood. For many people, though, becoming parents is a central feature of this process. Failure to achieve generativity leads to a sense of stagnation and personal impoverishment.

The final stage is that of 'ego integrity versus despair'. Ego integrity is the mature integration of one's life's experiences, people and things taken care of, triumphs and disappointments accepted. It is the feeling of things accomplished and a life lived satisfactorily. Failure to achieve ego integrity results in despair, a characteristic of which is fear of death due to the feeling that time is now too short to live another life.

Family development

As we have seen, most children's development occurs within the family unit. In western society this is usually primarily the *nuclear family*. Traditionally this consists of two parents and their offspring but nowadays such family units are a minority in many sections of western society. One parent families are common and so are *blended* families in which there is a couple one or both of whom have been married or have borne children previously – children which they have brought into the new union. In many parts of the world the *extended family* plays as big as, or a bigger, role than the nuclear family. On the traditional African homestead, for example, a *collective* consisting of grandparents, aunts, uncles, older siblings and more distant or even unrelated adults care for the children. In practice the distinction between siblings and cousins is often slight and is not regarded as important by those concerned. (This arrangement is fortunate as there are not usually any 'child welfare' services to care for children whose parents are, for any reason, unable to care for them.)

In western society, child rearing is usually the responsibility of either one or two parents with relatively little help and support from the extended family. There are exceptions to this, of course, especially in smaller communities; but in many instances it is the state, through its child welfare and other related agencies that steps in and tries to assist when things are not going well in a family.

The challenges facing the contemporary family, whether it is a blended family, or a single parent family, or a traditional nuclear family, are considerable. One of these is adapting to change as children are born into it and develop through childhood into adolescence and then adulthood.

Family development has been the subject of much study and various stages have been identified. A useful scheme is that proposed by McGoldrick & Carter(1982). They distinguish six stages:

(1)   *The unattached young adult*. This is a person between families. Such an individual should have achieved separation from his or her family of origin, a sense of self differentiated from the family of origin, the capacity to develop intimate relations with peers, and a suitable place in the workforce.

(2)   *The joining of families through marriage*. Nowadays this may not be legally formalized, but it involves commitment of the two partners to each other, with the formation of a new marital system. At the same time adjustments must be made in the couple's relationships with extended family and friends.

(3)   *The family with young children*. The arrival of the first child necessitates great changes in the family system. To the marital system is added a new parental system. The new generation must be accepted into the family system and there is further change in the family's relationships with the extended family. The grandparents may assume significant and important roles in relation to the family.

(4)   *The family with adolescents*. This stages sees a gradual but substantial change in parent-child relationships. The children become increasingly independent and for a time the adolescent may move in and out of the family, the boundaries of which become more flexible. At the same time the parents turn their attention again to marital, as opposed to parental, issues. Some parents, usually mothers, who have stayed at home to rear their children return to the workforce or seek new careers or social activities.

(5)   *Launching children and moving on*. This is a relatively new stage, since until the last few decades most parents were engaged in raising their children throughout their adult lives. The low birth rate in many western societies, and the longer life span, have changed this and many couples live for many years after their children have left home. During this period different family members may enter or leave the family. The parents may become ill or frail and thus dependent on *their* children. A new

relationship develops with the children who have left home, one based on adult-to-adult equality. Then, as the children marry and start their own new families, the role of grandparent develops. During this stage the family may have to deal with illness or deaths in the older generation.

(6)   *The family in later life.* The parental generation has now become the grandparental generation, and the grandparents may now be on their own. They may need to acquire new interests and a new social circle. The middle generation comes to play a more central role in the affairs of the family, perhaps looking after the older one, rather than the reverse. It may, and ideally it probably should, also make room for, and use, the wisdom and experience of the older generation.

This scheme is but one way of conceptualizing and simplifying a complex process. Many things may happen which modify or interrupt the above sequence of events. These include separation and divorce, remarriage, serious illness or deaths in family members, the late arrival of a child, the separation of parents because of vocational demands or imprisonment, financial disaster, the loss of the family home by fire or foreclosure, and any of the other vicissitudes of life.

Families are liable to get into difficulties when faced with transition from one phase of development to the next. Barnhill & Longo (1978) defined nine 'transitions points', based on a scheme of family development proposed by Duvall & Miller (1985). They suggest that families are especially subject to stress when one of the transitions has not been successfully achieved. This is discussed more fully in Chapter 2 of *Basic Family Therapy* (Barker, 1992).

Consideration of the family's developmental stage, and whether it has had or is having difficulty in accomplishing some of its developmental tasks, is essential when children are undergoing psychiatric assessment, since many child problems are related to family developmental ones.

Normal families and their development are discussed more fully in *Basic Family Therapy* (Barker, 1992). Other helpful books are *Marriage and Family Development* (Duvall & Miller, 1985) and *The Family Life Cycle* (Carter & McGoldrick, 1980).

Chapter 2

Causes of Child Psychiatric Disorders

The behavioural and emotional disorders of children need to be considered in their developmental contexts. While further emotional and personality development is possible at any age, in adult psychiatry one is usually dealing with disorders in subjects whose personality is relatively fixed, even though there is scope for further development. In children this is not so. Their development is still unfolding and many of the physical and psychosocial causative factors we identify operate by interfering in some way with the child's normal developmental course. Children have not reached the relatively *steady state* of development of most adults.

The following four groups of factors may contribute to a child's psychiatric problems:

- constitutional, including genetic factors;
- physical disease and injury;
- temperamental factors;
- environmental, including family factors.

Constitutional factors

Constitutional factors, that is those which operate from the time of birth, may be divided as follows:

- genetic factors;
- the effects of chromosome abnormalities;
- the consequences of intrauterine injury;
- the results of birth injury.

Genetic factors

Few child psychiatric disorders are due to specific single genetic factors, though such factors are responsible for certain forms of mental retardation. The most common of these is phenylketonuria (PKU). This is an inborn error of metabolism which is inherited as a Mendelian recessive trait. Untreated, it leads to severe mental retardation. Many more people are carriers of the gene than have PKU, but when two carriers of the gene have children each child has a one in four chance of suffering from PKU. Fortunately, treatment by means of a diet low in phenylalanine is effective (see Chapter 19).

The above is an example of *monogenic inheritance*, that is, a pattern of inheritance that involves a single gene. In child psychiatry, *polygenic inheritance* is believed to be more important. This term refers to the process whereby a characteristic is coded for by two or more genes located at two or more loci which, acting additively, increase the likelihood that a particular trait will be manifest. In many cases environmental factors also play a part in determining whether the trait appears. When this is the case, inheritance is said to be *multifactorial*. Polygenic influences, combined with environmental factors, are believed to play significant roles in the causation of many child psychiatric disorders, as well as in determining intelligence levels.

Twin and adoption studies can tell us how much polygenic factors contribute to the development of particular traits. Monozygotic (MZ) twins have identical genes, so that if genetic factors were wholly responsible for a trait the correlation between MZ twins for that trait would be 1.0.

In practice it is never that high, and has been found to be usually in the range of 0.75 to 0.85, the higher figure being for monozygotic twins reared together, the latter for those reared apart. Dizygotic twins and full siblings of the same sex have half of their genes in common, so that the correlations between their intelligence levels tends to be lower.

Summarizing the findings of family, twin and adoptions studies, Scott (1994) concludes that about 50% (± 20%) of the variation of intelligence 'in a given population' is genetically transmitted, and that this is due almost entirely to polygenic mechanisms rather than to conditions due to individual genes. Thus the contribution of the environment is substantial.

The term *heritability* is used to describe the degree to which a trait is attributable to genetic factors. It consists of the variance due to genetic factors divided by the total variance observed in the subjects. Sometimes the variation due to environmental factors is referred to by the unhappy term *environmentality* (Simonoff, *et al.*, 1994). It is only meaningful when applied to populations, since certain individuals may have particularly unfavourable (or favourable) environmental experiences. The former might cause a great lowering of intelligence (if that were the trait being studied), regardless of the person's genetically determined potential.

Recent years have seen great advances in genetics. These have made it even clearer that it is the interaction of the effects of genes and of the environment that results in the personalities, temperaments, reactions to stress – indeed virtually every characteristic that we observe in ourselves and others. Our genes do not generally determine how we develop. They play only a part in that process. Even when a condition – phenylketonuria is an example (see also Chapter 19) – is due to a single gene modification, the environment can have major effects. In the case of phenylketonuria, a diet low in phenylalanine usually prevents the symptoms of the condition appearing.

The complex interactions of genes and environment are described and discussed at greater length by Simonoff, *et al.* (1994).

Chromosome abnormalities

Observable abnormalities of the chromosomes may cause physical abnormalities, many of which are severe or fatal; they may affect intelligence; and they may contribute to other psychological problems. In trisomy 21, or Down's syndrome (discussed further in Chapter 19), affected individuals have three of the chromosomes numbered 21, instead of the normal two.

The Prader-Willi syndrome (see Chapter 19) is associated with a deletion of the short arm of chromosome 15. The other known abnormalities of the autosomes (the non-sex chromosomes) are of rather small practical importance in child psychiatry. Many are incompatible with life and lead to abortions or stillbirths.

Sex chromosome abnormalities generally have less severe effects. About one in every 4000 girls has Turner's syndrome, a condition in which there is only one X chromosome instead of the normal two. These girls' total complement of chromosomes is thus 45, rather than 46 (45, XO). They tend to have difficulty dealing with spatial information, in the 'organization of disparate elements into synthetic wholes' and in 'perceiving, visualizing and remembering spatial configurations' (Walzer, 1985). Consequently they have depressed performance IQ scores, and trouble acquiring mathematical and scientific skills. Though they tend to be small and immature as children, most do not show evidence of psychiatric disorder.

Girls with extra X chromosomes tend to be of below average intelligence, mildly so in the case of the triple X condition (27,XXX). Mental retardation is more severe in those rare cases in which there are more than three X chromosomes. Girls with 47,XXX find the auditory processing of information difficult and they have impaired receptive and expressive language difficulties, especially the latter. Thus an extra X chromosome seems to be associated with poor verbal skills, while the lack of an X chromosome adversely affects non-verbal skills.

In Klinefelter's syndrome the individual is phenotypically a male but may have some feminine characteristics and has the chromosome complement 47,XXY. These boys tend to be taller than controls and to be awkward with mild neuromotor deficits. This condition is associated, in about half of these boys, with impaired language development, particularly expressive language. Auditory processing, auditory memory, language, reading and spelling may all be affected (Walzer, 1985). Otherwise children with Klinefelter's syndrome probably do not have a higher incidence of psychiatric disorders than children generally. There seems to be an increase in social adjustment problems in adolescence but most do not have any definable psychiatric problems (Ratcliffe, *et al.*, 1982; Robinson, *et al.*, 1990).

About one in every 1000 boys born has a 47,XYY complement. Such boys tend to be taller than the average for their age but the association which was at one time thought to exist with aggressive or criminal behaviour is open to question. These boys are typically of normal intelligence though their intelligence level is usually lower than that of their siblings. They may however have a somewhat increased incidence of emotional disorders and their language development and progress in reading tend to be delayed (Ratcliffe, *et al.*, 1990; Robinson, *et al.*, 1991).

The 'fragile X' syndrome, also known as 'X-linked mental retardation', is characterized by an abnormality near the end of the long arm of a proportion of the X chromosomes. At least 20% of males are unaffected by this abnormality but they can pass the trait on to their daughters who are also asymptomatic. However members of the next generation often show mental impairment. This suggests that the fragile X mutation must pass through the female germ line before it is expressed clinically (Davies, 1991). Fragile X is the most common inherited form of mental retardation and affects 1 in 2500 males and 1 in 2000 females. Girls with the condition are generally more mildly affected but often have learning problems (Chudley, 1991).

Physical abnormalities associated with the fragile X chromosome include a high forehead, low-set protruding ears and a protruding jaw. After puberty the testicles may be enlarged. Speech patterns may be altered and it has been suggested, indeed at times strongly asserted, that there is an association between this condition and autism. Recent research has cast doubt on this, though some autistic features such as gaze avoidance, hand flapping and hand biting are found in many of these children (Hagerman & Sobesky, 1989).

Children and Young Adults with Sex Chromosome Aneuploidy (Evans, *et al.*, 1991) provides much additional information about sex chormosome abnormalities and their associations.

Intrauterine damage or disease

The fetus may be adversely affected in various ways during pregnancy. Infections such as rubella, toxoplasmosis, syphilis and acquired immune deficiency syndrome (AIDS) may be transferred from the mother to the fetus. Fetal damage or retarded development may also be caused by placental insufficiency or anything else which leads to an impaired supply of oxygen.

In recent decades a common, tragic cause of fetal damage seems to have been on the increase, namely the abuse of drugs, including alcohol, by pregnant women. The 'fetal alcohol syndrome' may follow severe alcohol abuse during pregnancy. It comprises growth deficiency, mental retardation, short palpebral fissure, a thin upper lip and abnormalities of the nose, eyes, ears and heart (Little & Streissgath, 1981). It may affect 0.4 to 3.1 per 1000 live born children, but among the children of alcoholic mothers its incidence probably ranges from 24 to 690 per 1000, depending on the severity of the mother's alcohol abuse (Cooper, 1987). Heavy smoking during pregnancy also affects adversely the development of the fetus and is associated with lower birth weight and poorer adjustment at age 7 (Davie, et al., 1972). Parental smoking, drug abuse and alcoholism tend, however, to be associated with personality problems and a variety of family difficulties. Children in such families are thus faced with a variety of adversities and it can be hard to sort out the relative effects of these.

Premature birth and injury at birth

While many premature babies develop normally, especially when neonatal care of high quality is available, they are at some risk. Driscoll, et al. (1982) reported on 45 infants weighing 1000 grams or less at birth treated in a neonatal intensive care unit. Twenty-eight died. Of the 23 followed up, 19 (83%) were neurologically normal but the overall complication rate, including mental retardation was 30%. Babies who are small for their gestational age at birth tend to be less developmentally advanced and to show behavioural differences when compared with children of normal birth weight (Parkinson, et al., 1986).

Many of the factors mentioned above have as a main effect the lowering of intelligence. While severe mental retardation is a serious condition in its own right, many individuals whose intellectual functioning has been affected nevertheless lead full lives without showing evidence of psychiatric problems.

Physical disease and injury

Brain disease and injury may produce impairment of intelligence, loss of particular motor or sensory functions, epilepsy or (probably) specific forms of abnormal behaviour such as motor hyperactivity. Less specific effects may also result. In the Isle of Wight epidemiological study, children with definite evidence of brain damage were found to have psychiatric disorders five times as often as the general child population, and three times as often as children with chronic physical handicaps not involving the brain (Rutter, *et al.*, 1970a).

Brain damage may be caused by injury, infections, metabolic disorders, tumours, a wide variety of degenerative disorders, and severe malnutrition in early life. 'Non-accidental injury' (see Chapter 20) may also cause brain injury and it may be accompanied by poor nutrition and other forms of neglect.

Head injuries are common in childhood (Goodman, 1994) and many brain injured children are later found to have behavioural or emotional problems. This is due in part to the tendency of such children to suffer head injuries more often than other children. Head injuries are also more likely to occur in the children of poorly functioning families. Such families are inclined to be less effective in safeguarding their children from injury. Nevertheless, even when potentially confounding factors are taken into account, evidence is that severe head injuries lead to cognitive impairments, disinhibited and socially inappropriate behaviour, and other psychiatric problems (Goodman, 1994).

Physical diseases not affecting the brain can have psychological repercussions. They may act through the physical handicap they impose, or the anxiety or guilt child, parents or the whole family may experience (Barker, 1993a). Much can be done to help children with severe handicaps such as cerebral palsy or blindness lead full lives. They need not develop complicating emotional problems. This requires special skill and patience in those caring for and educating them. Other chronic conditions such as diabetes, asthma, congenital heart disease and the various forms of dwarfism may cause emotional problems through their physically handicapping effects, the restrictions they impose on children's social lives, the anxiety and fear of death they may provoke, and their effects on the attitudes of family friends and teachers (Barker, 1993a).

Injuries, especially serious ones like severe burns, can have similar effects. They may give rise to guilt feelings in children or parents, any or all of whom may blame themselves for the injury.

Temperamental factors

Children's temperaments vary, probably as much as their physical characteristics. Children's temperaments were studied by Thomas and Chess in their course of their New York Longitudinal Study (NYLS) of 133 children from infancy into early adult life. They have summarized their 25 years' work in a book (Chess & Thomas, 1984). They identified nine categories of temperament in the course of their study:

'(1)   Activity level: the motor component present in a given child's functioning and the diurnal proportion of active and inactive periods.

(2)   Rhythmicity (regularity): the predictability and/or unpredictability in time of any biological function.

(3)   Approach or withdrawal: the nature of the initial response to a new stimulus, be it a food, toy, place, person, etc. Approach responses are positive, whether displayed by mood expression (smiling, verbalizations, etc.) or motor activity (swallowing a new food, reaching for a new toy, active play, etc.). Withdrawal reactions are negative, whether displayed by mood expression (crying, fussing, grimacing, verbalizations, etc.) or motor activity (moving away, spitting new food out, pushing a new toy away, etc.).

(4)   Adaptability: responses to new or altered situations. One is not concerned with the nature of the initial responses, but with the ease with which they are modified in desired directions.

(5)   Threshold of responsiveness: the intensity of stimulation that is necessary to evoke a discernible response, irrespective of the specific form the response may take, or the sensory modality affected.

(6)   Intensity of reaction: the energy level of response, irrespective of its quality or direction.

(7)   Quality of mood: the amount of pleasant, joyful and friendly behaviour; as contrasted with unpleasant, crying and unfriendly behaviour.

(8)   Distractibility: the effectiveness of extraneous environmental stimuli in interfering with or altering the direction of the ongoing behaviour.

(9)   Attention span and persistence: two categories which are related. Attention span concerns the length of time a particular activity is pursued by the child. Persistence refers to the continuation of an activity direction in the face of obstacles to its continuation.'

(The list shown above is reproduced from Chess & Thomas (1984) *Origins and Evolution of Behaviour Disorders from Infancy to Early Adult Life*, pages 42–43, and quoted with kind permission of Brunner/Mazel Inc., the publishers.)

Analysis of the data obtained in the study revealed three main 'temperamental constellations'. The first group, about 40% of the NYLS sample, were characterized by:

- regularity;
- positive approach responses to new stimuli;
- high adaptability to change;
- mild or moderate mood intensity which is predominantly positive.

These were the 'easy children'. They quickly fall into regular sleep and feeding schedules, and take readily to new foods, strangers, new schools and the rules of new games, as well as accepting frustration without much fuss.

By contrast, the 'difficult child' – about 10 per cent of the sample – showed:

- irregularity of biological functions;
- negative withdrawal responses to new stimuli;
- non-adaptability or slow adaptability to change;
- intense mood expressions which are frequently negative.

These children sleep and demand food irregularly, and adjust with difficulty to new foods, routines, people and situations. They cry and laugh loudly, are easily frustrated and often have tantrums.

The third group – about 15% – show:

- negative responses of mild intensity to new stimuli, with slow adaptability after repeated contact;
- mild intensity of reactions generally;
- less irregularity of biological functioning than the 'difficult' children.

These children have been categorized as 'slow-to-warm-up'.

The remaining 35% of the children did not fit into any of these categories, but had a variety of other combinations of temperamental traits.

The above descriptions are simply of behavioural styles. The nine categories and their variations, and the three commonly met with constellations, are the temperamental equivalents of the variations in body build, or eye or hair colour, observed in any population. How children with particular temperamental styles fare depends also upon other factors, especially environmental ones. There is also evidence that parents' characteristics can affect children's temperamental styles over time (Cameron, 1977). A study of pre-term infants at 3, 6 and 12 months of age, found significantly more 'difficult' children in the sample than in a comparable series of full-term infants. These traits seem to be related to the features of the mother-child interaction, rather than to the severity of perinatal or post-natal complications.

Environmental factors

A child's personality and adjustment in society are the result of the interaction between genetic inheritance and biological make-up on the one hand, and the environment on the other. The family is the most important feature of a child's environment with the obvious exception of those unfortunate children who do not grow up in a family setting. The family should provide a sheltered training ground in which the child learns to live as a member of a society. Families are miniature societies in which children make their first attempts at adapting to others, and in which they learn patterns of social behaviour which tend to persist throughout life.

The family should facilitate development from infantile dependence to adult independence. As children grow up they should be expected progressively to assume more self-control and responsibility for their actions. At each age neither too little nor too much should be done for them. If too much is done, the process of growing up and becoming independent may be retarded; if too little, the child's level of anxiety may become intolerably great and a psychiatric disorder may develop.

Poor early adjustment to family life is often followed by poor adjustment in society at large. Attitudes towards parents may become generalized, and later may be applied to a wider circle of people. As a background for the transfer of responsibility from parents to child, a secure and stable family setting, with reasonably consistent and constant parent figures is second to nothing. 'Secure and stable' does not mean that there must never be disagreements or arguments, or that members of the family will not sometimes be angry with one another. On the contrary, children need to be exposed to a range of emotions and situations, as they will be throughout their lives. They also need to witness these emotions being displayed in appropriate ways and conflicts being resolved constructively.

Children who are deprived of a stable family group in which to grow up suffer a serious handicap. Changes of family or caretakers, as when children are repeatedly placed in and out of the care of child welfare agencies, or are moved frequently from one home to another, can be damaging and impair seriously the process of personality development. Some children survive such changes relatively well. They may have innate personality strengths and often seem to be helped by positive factors in their environments, such as a continuing healthy relationship with a stable adult figure. Many, however, are burdened by problems such as feelings of insecurity, poor self-esteem, unresolved anger, and difficulty in engaging in trusting, loving relationships with others.

Various schemes have been devised for understanding families and how they function. Descriptions of these are more appropriate to texts on family therapy and are to be found in *Basic Family Therapy* (Barker, 1992) and other family therapy texts. What is basically needed is a stable, ordered, consistent family environment. There should be appropriate boundaries between the different parts of the family, and in particular between the generations, and also between the family and the world outside the family, including the extended family. Not only do parents and other adult figures involved in the rearing of children need to be good role models, they need also to encourage (the technical behavioural term is *reinforce*) desired behaviour, and to discourage antisocial behaviour.

Factors such as the stability of the family and the role its structure requires the child to play in it can help determine whether the child develops psychiatric problems – and, if so, what sort of problems. Even more important in many cases are the drastic disruptions in children's lives caused by such things as the loss of a parent by death; prolonged care in a hospital or other institutions (Tizard & Hodges, 1978); parental depression (Wolkind, 1981); and the separation or divorce of their parents. In the case of divorce, however, the prolonged family or marital strife that has sometimes existed for many years previously may be a more important factor than the actual divorce (Hetherington *et al.*, 1982). Many children cope quite well with the stress of divorce, and some even seem to benefit as a result of having no longer to live as witnesses of severe marital or family strife or violence. The outcome of divorce for the children depends on many factors, including their previous experiences in the family, whether the divorce is amicable or characterized by conflict, and the resources of the custodial parent. Wallerstein (1983) discusses the tasks children whose parents have been divorced face:

- acknowledging the marital disruption;
- regaining a sense of direction and freedom to pursue customary activities;
- dealing with loss and feelings of rejection;
- forgiving the parents;
- accepting the permanence of the divorce and relinquishing longings for the restoration of the pre-divorce family.

Children's subsequent adjustment depends largely upon how well they accomplish the above tasks. Divorce and its consequences are discussed further by Wallerstein & Corbin (1991).

School influences
These are important factors in the development of children. Just how important emerged in a study of secondary schools in London (Rutter, *et*

al., 1979; Rutter, 1980a). The progress of a large group of children entering secondary schools was studied. The children had been assessed before entering secondary school and the extent to which they were at risk of developing the problems with which the research was concerned had been determined. Large differences in the children's academic progress and behaviour were found in the different secondary schools – even taking into account differences in the children admitted to the various schools. Much proved to depend on the characteristics of the schools as social institutions. Favourable factors were:

(1)   A reasonable balance between intellectually able and less able children.
(2)   The ample use of rewards, praise and appreciation by teachers.
(3)   A pleasant, comfortable and attractive school environment.
(4)   Plenty of opportunity for children to be responsible for and participate in the running of the school.
(5)   An appropriate emphasis on academic matters.
(6)   Good models of behaviour provided by teachers.
(7)   The use of appropriate group management skills in classrooms.
(8)   Firm leadership in the school, combined with a decision-making process involving all staff and leading to a cohesive approach in which staff members support each other.

The wider social environment
This is also important. Living in a neighbourhood in which there is a high incidence of crime and much drug abuse and violence, for example, increases the risk that a child will get involved in such activities.

The higher urban rates of psychiatric disorder apply to boys and girls, men and women, and to crime, delinquency, depression and emotional disorders. It seems that various aspects of the ecology of cities, including the schools, contribute to the causation of these disorders. While some of the factors, such as those operating in schools, affect children directly, many seem to have their effects through families. The greatest effect is apparently on 'early onset, chronic disorders in children which are associated with severe family pathology' (Rutter, 1981).

Other considerations

Goodness of fit
Chess & Thomas (1984) emphasize the importance of the goodness, or poorness, of the 'fit' between child and environment. In Chapter 22 of their book they give examples of children from the New York Long-

itudinal Study in whom there were various degrees of fit, and describe how these affected the children's development. They make it clear that there is no universal *optimal* temperamental style, nor is there one ideal environment for children's development.

As an illustration of the above point, Chess & Thomas (1984, pages 289–90) mention a study by de Vries of 47 infants, aged 2 to 4 months, of the Masai tribe in Kenya. Ratings of temperament were obtained just as a severe drought was beginning, and the ten infants with the easiest temperaments and the ten with the most difficult, were identified. Five months later, de Vries returned to the area and was able to discover what had happened to seven of the *easy* babies and six of the *difficult* ones. The other families had moved to escape the drought. Five of the easy babies had died but all six of the difficult ones had survived. The adaptive value of any particular temperamental style depends on the fit between it and environmental circumstances. Of especial significance, it seems, is the fit between the temperaments of the parents and those of their children.

Self-esteem

Though it is hard to define, self-esteem is important in determining people's behaviour, how they relate to others, and whether they develop psychiatric disorders. We have seen that the acquisition of good feelings about oneself is one of the major developmental tasks of childhood. Such feelings develop as children have the experience of mastering the environment in ways which provide feelings of satisfaction and appropriate, affirming feedback from the environment. 'Unfavourable experiences with social functioning and task mastery, together with confusing, contradictory, and inappropriate environmental feedback, will ... foster the development of negative self-esteem' (Chess & Thomas, 1984, page 280).

Mack & Ablon (1983, page xiii) point out that:

'The quest for a sense of personal worth, so critical to small children, remains of central importance for human beings throughout their lives. It motivates much of our activity in seeking personal attachments and meaningful work ... Nothing is more important for the maintenance of well-being. Conversely, no experience is more obviously distressing, or more intimately linked to emotional disturbances of many kinds and, in psychiatry, to various types of psychopathology, than is a diminished sense of worth or a low opinion of oneself.'

For many disturbed children, a low measure of self-esteem is a central problem. This can be self-perpetuating or even self-reinforcing. As children act out their feelings of being 'bad' people, others in their environments may react by making critical remarks or labelling them, in one way or another, as inferior individuals.

So while we must look carefully at the background factors which have led to the situations we encounter when we assess disturbed children, we need also to consider the children's current views of themselves. We should strive to understand how these are being reinforced, or modified, by their environments, in order to devise suitable treatment plans.

Coopersmith (1967, page 4) pointed out that:

'... in children domination, rejection, and severe punishment result in lowered self-esteem. Under such conditions [children] have fewer experiences of love and success and tend to become generally submissive and withdrawn (although occasionally veering to the opposite extreme of aggression and domination). Children reared under such crippling circumstances are unlikely to be realistic and effective in their everyday functioning and are more likely to manifest deviant behaviour patterns.'

In summary
The etiology of most child psychiatric disorders is multifactorial, factors in the child – genetic, biological or psychological – interacting with all the many environmental influences, to produce the clinical pictures we observe in our work. We should not stop searching and thinking when we come across one possible or probable cause. If we do, we will make many mistakes. *Linear thinking* – which understands one thing as leading directly to another – is generally to be avoided. *Circular* or *systems* thinking – which is based on the concept that many things are interacting in complex, dynamic ways – is more useful in clinical work with both children and families.

Chapter 3

The Classification of Child Psychiatric Disorders

Establishing a satisfactory scheme for the classification of child psychiatric disorders has proved a difficult task. Over the last 20 years, however, it has become generally accepted that, to be useful, a diagnostic system should have certain characteristics (see Cantwell & Rutter, 1994):

(1) It should be multiaxial.
(2) It should be based on data, rather than on concepts or theories of psychopathology.
(3) It should use cross-sectional behaviour patterns. Age and mode of onset, the presence of particular symptoms, pervasiveness across various situations and the results of special investigations, may all need to be taken into account.
(4) The various categories should be operationally defined.
(5) Developmental issues should be addressed.
(6) Patterns of co-morbidity should be taken into account.

Multiaxial classifications consider different aspects of a patient's disorder and classify the disorder according to the different parameters, or axes, considered. Many axes are possible. Theoretically, at least, a disorder might be classified along any or all of the following axes:

● clinical psychiatric syndrome present,
● intellectual level,
● specific delays in development,
● medical conditions,
● temperamental style,
● personality variables,
● abnormal psychosocial situations,
● the degree of psychosocial stress the patient faces,
● a global assessment of functioning.

Most, though not all, of the above have been used in multiaxial schemes but no existing scheme includes more than five axes. More might place an undue burden on the busy clinician.

Currently diagnostic schemes are derived from two sources – the World Health Organization (WHO) and the American Psychiatric Association (APA).

The WHO Diagnostic Schemes

The 9th edition of the *International Classification of Diseases* (ICD-9) (WHO, 1977a) was adapted for multiaxial use by Rutter *et al.* (1975b). The latest revision (ICD-10) (WHO, 1992) supersedes ICD-9 but as this is written only the volume dealing with 'clinical descriptions and diagnostic guidelines' has appeared. While we are promised texts on diagnostic guidelines for researchers, a multiaxial presentation and 'crosswalks' – which will allow cross-referencing between corresponding terms in ICD-10, ICD-9 and ICD-8, these are not available as this book goes to press.

Mental and behavioural disorders are listed and described in Chapter V(F) of ICD-10. The final three 'blocks' in this scheme are those most specifically concerned with children although, as in DSM-IV, categories in the other blocks may be used for children when appropriate.

Block F70–79 consists of four categories of mental retardation, mild, moderate, severe and profound, together with 'other' and 'unspecified' categories.

The block F80 – F89 comprises 'disorders of psychological development'. The main groupings are:

- specific developmental disorders of speech and language,
- specific developmental disorders of scholastic skills,
- specific developmental disorder of motor function,
- mixed specific developmental disorders,
- pervasive developmental disorders,
- other disorders of psychological development,
- unspecified disorder of psychological development.

The block F90–F98 covers 'behavioural and emotional disorders with onset usually occurring in childhood and adolescence'.

The main categories are:

- hyperkinetic disorders,
- conduct disorders,
- mixed disorders of conduct and emotions,
- emotional disorders with onset specific to childhood,

- disorders of social functioning with onset specific to childhood and adolescence,
- tic disorders,
- other behavioural and emotional disorders with onset usually occurring in childhood and adolescence.

While the multiaxial version of ICD-10 is not currently available, it is easy to see that the F90–98 block and most of the earlier block dealing with primarily adult disorders might make up Axis I, while block 80–89 might make up Axis II and block 70–79 might be Axis III. This would be a similar arrangement to that proposed by Rutter *et al.* (1975b). Associated physical conditions might be classified in Axis IV.

The APA Diagnostic Scheme

The APA's *Diagnostic and Statistical Manual, Fourth Edition* (DSM-IV) (American Psychiatric Association, 1994) has recently succeeded DSM-III-R, especially in North America.

DSM-IV is designed as a multiaxial system. Its five axes are:

- Axis I: Clinical disorders.
            Other conditions that may be a focus of clinical attention.
- Axis II: Personality disorders
            Mental retardation.
- Axis III: General medical conditions.
- Axis IV: Psychosocial and environmental problems.
- Axis V: Global assessment of functioning.

Axis I: Clinical disorders
    Other conditions that may be a focus of clinical attention
This axis covers the great majority of psychiatric disorders, together with 'other conditions that may be the focus of clinical attention'. Several of the latter are of particular interest to those working with children, especially 'relational problems' (including parent–child and sibling–sibling problems) and problems related to the various forms of child abuse and neglect.

Axis I includes a list of 'disorders usually first diagnosed in infancy, childhood or adolescence'. The main categories listed are:

- Learning disorders.
- Motor skills disorders.
- Communication disorders.
- Pervasive developmental disorders.

- Attention-deficit and disruptive behaviour disorders.
- Feeding and eating disorders of infancy and early childhood.
- Tic disorders.
- Elimination disorders.
- Other disorders of infancy, childhood or adolescence.

Axis I contains many other disorders which may afflict children and adolescents, but which are presumably not included in the above list because they do not 'usually' have their onset during these periods of life. These are:

- Substance-related disorders
- Schizophrenia and other psychotic disorders.
- Mood disorders.
- Anxiety disorders.
- Somatoform disorders.
- Dissociative disorders.
- Sexual and gender identity disorders.
- Eating disorders.
- Sleep disorders.
- Impulse-control disorders not elsewhere classified.
- Adjustment disorders.

There are also categories for delirium, dementia, other cognitive disorders and mental conditions which are 'due to a general medical condition not elsewhere classified'.

Excluded from this axis is mental retardation, which is included in Axis II.

Axis II: Personality disorders
        Mental retardation

In DSM-IV only personality disorders and mental retardation are included in this axis, whereas in DSM-III-R the various specific and pervasive developmental disorders were listed in this axis.

Personality disorders are discussed in Chapter 15 and mental retardation in Chapter 19.

Axis III: General medical conditions

These are to be classified using a modification of ICD-9 known as ICD-9-CM.

Axis IV: Psychosocial and environmental problems

This is for the reporting of 'psychosocial and environmental problems that may affect diagnosis, treatment and prognosis of mental disorders'. It is an advance on the Axis IV of DSM-III-R in that the latter addressed itself primarily to the 'severity of psychosocial stressors', rather than to their nature. In DMS-IV, problems are grouped as follows:

- Problems with primary support group.
- Problems related to the social environment.
- Educational problems.
- Occupational problems.
- Housing problems.
- Economic problems.
- Problems with access to health care services.
- Problems with relation to the legal system/crime.
- Other psychosocial and environmental problems.

DSM-IV does not require the diagnostician to rate the severity of any stressors patients may face.

Axis V: Global assessment of functioning
It is abbreviated as the 'GAF scale'. It is little changed from the scale of the same name in DSM-III-R. Functioning is rated on a scale from 1 to 100, with 100 being superior functioning and 1 severely impaired functioning.

DSM-IV provides operational definitions for all the diagnostic categories listed.

The relative merits of the different classification schemes

Classification of psychiatric disorders is needed so that meaningful communication can occur between those who work in the field. Devising a valid and generally acceptable scheme for child psychiatric disorders has proved difficult, largely because many of these 'disorders' are not discrete, well-defined entities, but are rather varied reactions to a multiplicity of factors. Devising a diagnostic scheme involves difficult choices. On the one hand is the Scylla of defining disorders in broad, clinical terms which may lack precision and be subject to widely differing interpretations; on the other is the Charybdis of trying to define in precise, scientifically objective terms conditions which in reality are not distinct, clearcut entities, even though they have properties in common. ICD-9 tended towards the first of these alternatives, while DSM-III and its modification, DSM-III-R, inclined towards the second. Both ICD-10 and DSM-IV seek a middle ground.

Reconciling the needs of clinicians and researchers presents a challenge. The latter generally require more tightly defined categories than clinicians need. The WHO's intention to provide for ICD-10 different operational definitions, those for researchers being tighter and more precise than those for clinicians, may help resolve this dilemma.

An interesting, and for child psychiatrists, useful aspect of DSM-III and DSM-III-R was the inclusion of the 'V' codes. This section has been further refined in DSM-IV so that it now covers a range of relationship and interactional problems, as well as the effects of the various forms of child abuse and neglect, and such issues as bereavement, occupational and academic problems, religious and spiritual problems and acculturation problems.

It is rather unfortunate that there have existed two different, but both widely used, systems for classifying psychiatric disorders. It does seem, however, that the two are coming closer, though ICD-10 and DSM-IV still differ significantly. The existence of the two schemes does illustrate that any scheme is in reality an arbitrary construct depending, as it must, on the particular focus chosen by those devising.

The practising psychiatrist will ordinarily use the system of diagnosis that is favoured by the hospital, clinic or other institutions in which he or she works. Each of the above schemes has merit and each has drawbacks. It is important to be familiar with one, but to recognize its limitations.

Chapter 4

The Epidemiology of Child Psychiatric Disorders

In 1965 a major study of children's disorders in a defined population – that of the Isle of Wight, an island off the south coast of England – was carried out (Rutter, *et al.*, 1970b). The study was well planned and comprehensive and the research team managed to get excellent compliance, so that almost all the children in the age ranges targeted were covered. While there have since been many further studies with different populations, and using a variety of methods, the Isle of Wight researchers set a high standard for such studies and their findings remain of interest and value.

The Isle of Wight study was a cross sectional one, taking as its subjects all the 10- and 11-year-old children in the island. Screening questionnaires of known reliability and validity were first completed by parents and teachers. These gave a preliminary indication of the number of children with psychiatric disorders (and also of other disorders since the study was not confined to psychiatric conditions). The responses to the questionnaires provided an indication of the prevalence of the conditions being studied. Randomly selected samples of both those tentatively identified as disturbed and those who appeared, from the questionnaire results, to be free of psychiatric disorders were then individually assessed by psychiatrists. These assessments involved the children and their parents. This enabled corrected prevalence figures to be calculated. Psychiatric disorder was considered to be present if 'abnormalities of behaviour or relationships were sufficiently marked and sufficiently prolonged to be causing persistent suffering or handicap in the child ... or distress or disturbance in the family or community'.

Rutter, *et al.* (1975a) found a prevalence of psychiatric disorders, defined as above, of 6.8%. There were nearly twice as many boys as girls with psychiatric disorder.

The Isle of Wight is mainly rural with a few small towns and the prevalence of psychiatric disorders tends to be higher in large urban areas. A subsequent survey, using similar methods, in an inner London borough found a rate of disturbance about double that in the Isle of Wight (Rutter, *et al.*, 1975a). Prevalence rates also vary depending on the age range studied.

The biggest single group of disorders identified in the Isle of Wight study was that of conduct disorders. Nearly two-thirds of the children with psychiatric problems were found to have conduct disorders (see Chapter 6). Including children with mixed conduct and emotional disorders (who were considered by the researchers to have more in common with the 'pure' conduct disordered children than with the children with pure emotional disorders) the prevalence of conduct disorders was 4%. This contrasts with a prevalence of 2.5% for 'emotional' disorders, leaving only 0.3% of the children with other psychiatric disorders. 'Monosymptomatic' disorders, however, were not included in these totals.

The Ontario Child Health Study (Boyle, et al., 1987; Offord, et al., 1987) examined a large sample of children in the Canadian province of Ontario. A representative sample of households from various parts of the province was selected using census data, and 91.1% of these agreed to participate. The households of native North Americans living on Indian Reserves were not included, nor were children living in institutions. All children aged from 4 to 16 in the household selected were studied, so that a broader age range was covered than in the Isle of Wight study. The percentage prevalence rates are set out in Table 4.1.

Somatization refers to the presence of somatic symptoms without evident physical cause. The Ontario prevalence rates are considerably higher than those found in the Isle of Wight. The difference is probably due to a variety of factors. The age range of the children, the study methods, and the definitions of disorder used were all different, and the studies were conducted on different continents some 20 years apart. It is not surprising, therefore, that the prevalence rates emerging from the two studies are different. Yet another major difference is that there are no large

Table 4.1   Prevalence of disorders by age and sex (percentages): Ontario Child Health Study (Offord *et al.*, 1987).

Age	Sex	One or more disorders	Conduct disorder	Type of Disorder Hyperactivity	Emotional disorder	Somatization
4–1	Boys	19.5	6.5	10.1	10.2	–
4–11	Girls	13.5	1.8	3.3	10.7	–
12–16	Boys	18.8	10.4	7.3	4.9	4.5
12–16	Girls	21.8	4.1	3.4	13.6	10.7
4–16	Boys	19.2	8.1	8.9	7.9	–
4–16	Girls	16.9	2.7	3.3	11.9	–

urban areas on the Isle of Wight, while many of the children in the Ontario study did live in such areas.

These differences also illustrate the important point that it is not possible to state precise, universally applicable figures for the prevalence of psychiatric disorders. Much depends on the context and the definitions and methods used. There have therefore been many estimates of prevalence rates.

Gould, *et al.* (1980) surveyed 25 prevalence studies carried out in the United States between 1928 and 1975. Based on this survey, these authors concluded that the prevalence of 'clinical maladjustment' among US children was 11.8%. Brandenburg, *et al.*, (1990) reported a survey of eight prevalence studies reported from five countries during the 1980s – Australia, the Netherlands, New Zealand, Canada and the United States. Some of these distinguished between *severe* cases and those in which the disorders were considered to be of only *moderate* severity. Overall prevalence rates ranged from 5.0 to 26.0%. The paper by Brandenburg, *et al.* (1990) is useful, both in providing a summary of recent research findings and in its discussion of the issues to be considered in conducting epidemiological studies, and in interpreting the results.

One of the points that repeatedly emerges from epidemiological studies is that the results obtained depend, to a large extent, on who you ask. Thus the reports of parents and those of teachers often differ, and if assessed prevalence figures are based only on interviews with the children themselves the results are different again. These differences are due in part to the established fact that children's behaviour is to a con-siderable extent context dependent. Many children *do* display different behaviours at home than those they display at school. Many childhood problems are not simply a function of the characteristics of the children concerned but are the result of complex interactions between the children and their environments.

The most recently published epidemiological study of psychiatric problems in childhood and adolescence is that reported in papers by Cohen, *et al.* (1993a and b). These authors report the results of a study of a sample of children and adolescents in the age range 10 to 20 living in two counties in New York State. Most of these had been the subjects of a study of children in the 1- to 10-year-old age range in 975 families carried out in 1975. The assessments were carried out by pairs of interviewers who interviewed child and parents simultaneously. With a few exceptions (4% of the sample interviewed in 1983 could not be contacted in 1985–86), the interviews were repeated 2½ years after the first assessment. Full diag-nostic information for 734 children was available in both of the assess-ments.

This study not only provides prevalence figures for different disorders at different ages and for each sex, but also provides information about the persistence of disorders.

As the authors of the first of the above quoted papers point out, this study bridged the period between childhood, in which behaviour problems in boys tend to make the greatest demands on mental health services, to adulthood, when depression and anxiety in women tend to predominate. The two papers contain valuable analyses of the changing patterns of disorders over the age range studied. For most diagnoses, one-third or more of those diagnosed at ages 9 to 18, received the same diagnosis 2½ years later. The main exceptions were those diagnosed as having major depressive disorders, which tend to follow an episodic course. It appears therefore that many of the psychiatric disorders encountered in this age range are not just transient disruptions of development, but have more serious implications.

Chapter 5

Assessing Children and their Families

A flexible approach to the assessment of children and families is necessary. What will yield the best results depends on the age of the child(ren) involved, the nature of the problems, the context in which the assessment is being carried out and whether the assessment is being done by an individual or a team.

Some psychiatrists like to interview child and parents separately, while others like to start by seeing the whole family. If the parents are seen first the child may feel, perhaps with justification, that the parents have been reporting unfavourably on him or her. This may make it more difficult than it otherwise would have been to gain the child's confidence. If the child is seen first, the interviewer may lack adequate information about the nature of the presenting problems. With younger children the merits of the two approaches are generally quite evenly balanced but adolescents are usually best interviewed first unless they are seen in company with their parents.

The problem of deciding who to see first is avoided if one starts by seeing all family members together. Family members can then hear what everyone else says and they can dispute others' statements or offer differing views. In addition, the interviewer has an opportunity to learn much about how the family functions and the members interact with each other. While some needed information, for example about a child's developmental history, may not emerge during the family interview, this can be obtained later in interviews with the parents.

The option of interviewing the whole family is not always available, for example in the emergency departments of hospitals and in residential institutions. One then must work with whoever is available.

Family interviews

Several models for the assessment of families, and a practical scheme for interviewing families, are described in *Basic Family Therapy* (Barker, 1992). What follows is a shortened version of that scheme.

The assessment of a family should proceed through the following stages, which may overlap:

(1) the initial contact;
(2) joining the family and establishing rapport;
(3) defining the desired outcome;
(4) reviewing the family's history, determining its present developmental stage and constructing a genogram; and
(5) assessing the current functioning of the family.

The initial contact

If the family members are to be interviewed as a group as part of the initial assessment they should be told, when the appointment is set up, that all family members in the household should attend. (Whether you will want non-family members who may be living in the household to attend will depend on the circumstances.) If the family question the necessity of this, they can be told that knowing the family in which a child lives makes it easier to understand that child's problems. Other points that may be made are that the behaviour of every family member inevitably affects the other members; and that other family members can often be part of the solution to the presenting problems, and can be of assistance to the interviewer. It is generally unwise to suggest that they are part of the problem.

It is usually easy to persuade parents that they are important to their children, but they may be reluctant to bring siblings they consider to be well adjusted and problem-free. In that case the point can be made that the children who are functioning well in the family may be of help to those who are not.

Joining the family and establishing rapport

The establishment of rapport is an essential first step in any interview. Rapport is best described as a state of understanding, harmony and accord. People in rapport feel warmly about each other. Time spent establishing and enhancing rapport is never wasted. Precipitate attempts to obtain information before adequate rapport is established are short-sighted and tend to be unproductive.

Establishing rapport has been given other names, such as 'joining' the family (Minuchin, 1974), or 'building working alliances' (Karpel & Strauss, 1983). As it develops, the participants become increasingly involved with each other. Hypnotherapists have long recognized the importance of rapport and know that failure to induce an hypnotic trance is more often due to the lack of sufficient rapport than to any other cause. In this connection Milton Erickson and his colleagues (1961, page 66) described rapport as:

> ... that peculiar relationship, existing between subject and operator, wherein, since it [hypnosis] is a cooperative endeavour, the subject's attention is directed to the operator, and the operator's attention is directed to the subject. Hence, the subject tends to pay no attention to externals or the environmental situation.' (Erickson *et al.*, 1961, page 66.)

When rapport is well developed the therapist can say almost anything without the client becoming upset. Even remarks which could be construed as insulting are likely to be taken as meant jokingly, or at least not seriously.

Rapport may be fostered by both verbal and non-verbal means but the non-verbal ones are probably the more important.

It is desirable that both our verbal and non-verbal behaviours are such as will promote the development of rapport from our very first contact with those who are coming to see us, even if this is a telephone conversation. One's tone of voice and manner of speaking, whether on the telephone or face to face, convey powerful messages. A warm, friendly tone of voice and a respectful, interested and accepting approach are important. I like to greet each family that comes to see me personally in the waiting room and to address each member by name, if I know their names. I shake hands with all family members except for very small children.

Comfortable physical surroundings are desirable, though it is possible to establish rapport in prison cells, school classrooms, public parks or hospital emergency rooms. When the family includes young children, it is usually desirable to have a few toys, appropriate to the children's ages, in the interview room. If there are only adolescents this is not usually necessary. Your dress should conform to cultural norms, though clothes which are too formal can lead some children to feel ill at ease; the same applies to the white 'lab coats' so beloved of many doctors and other hospital staff.

Most important of all is the interviewer's behaviour. Rapport is promoted by matching or 'pacing' the behaviour of those who you are interviewing. You can do this by matching their body postures and movements, respiratory rhythm, speed of talking, and voice tone and volume. You can also 'mirror' their movements, moving, for example, your left arm or leg in response to similar movements of your client's arm or leg. You can also move another part of your body, for example moving your hand or finger in response to similar rhythmic movements of the client's foot. Examples of movement which may be matched are crossing and uncrossing the legs, tilting the head to one side or the other, and leaning forward or settling back.

Pacing should be done sensitively and unobtrusively and it is not necessary to match all aspects of the client's behaviour. If these guidelines are followed, clients do not become consciously aware that you are matching their behaviours. When interviewing a family, or any other group, it is usually best to pace the person you are addressing at each moment and, when the family members are talking, to pace them as they address you.

The developers of 'neuro-linguistic programming' (NLP) have paid much attention to rapport building which they describe as leading to:

'a kind of synchrony [that] can serve to reduce greatly resistance between you and the people with whom you are communicating. The strongest form of synchrony is the continuous presentation of your communication in sequences which perfectly parallel the unconscious processes of the person you are communicating with – such communication approaches the ... goal of irresistibility.' (Dilts, *et al.*, 1980, pages 115–116.)

The content of one's verbal communications is also important. Rapport is promoted when your predicates – words which say something descriptive about the subject of a sentence – match those of your clients. There are visual ('I see what you mean'); auditory ('that sounds terrible'); kinesthetic ('that's a big weight off my shoulders'); olfactory ('this business smells fishy to me') and gustatory ('it leaves a bad taste in my mouth') predicates. Most people have a preference – which is quite unconscious – for using one sensory channel for processing information, usually either the visual, the auditory or the kinesthetic (Bandler & Grinder, 1979). Noting which one a person uses, and matching that person's predicates with those you use, can greatly enhance rapport. It does not help, for example, to respond to 'That sounds good', with 'I see what you mean'. A better response would be, 'I hear what you're saying'.

As well as matching predicates, it is also helpful to listen carefully to the vocabularies of those you are interviewing, noting the words and expressions they use. Few things impede the establishment of rapport as much as repeatedly using words or expressions with which those with whom you are speaking are unfamiliar. This applies with particular force when we are speaking with children whose vocabularies are in varying degrees limited, though it applies also to adults.

Other ways one may promote rapport include:

- accepting the views of those you are interviewing without initially challenging these;

- adopting a 'one-down' position;
- talking of experiences and interests you have in common.

The 'one-down' position might be adopted, for example, when one is faced with parents who have strong views about the nature of their child's problems. You may disagree with these but it is often best initially to accept them rather than risk becoming embroiled in an argument. It may be better to say that, while you do not yet understand the situation, you are grateful to them for their suggested explanation, which is helpful.

Some people, especially children, tend to be overawed or to feel intimidated by physicians and other health professionals. For them a one-down approach might involve something as simple as asking them how to spell their names or to tell you about something in which they have expertise and you do not – perhaps video games or skateboarding – or, for older adolescents or adults, their job.

Common experiences might be having lived in the same city, country, province, county or state as the family has in the past. Hobbies, sports and pastimes you have in common with family members may be used in similar ways.

Defining the desired outcome

Almost invariably, children are brought for psychiatric consultation because someone wants some change to occur, whether this be in the child's behaviour, emotional state, school performance, relationships with others, or mental or physical development. Defining, and if necessary clarifying, the changes sought is important for several reasons:

- it formally acknowledges the family's concerns;
- it defines your involvement as therapeutic and oriented towards promoting change;
- it helps avoid misunderstandings about the purpose of the child's or the family's attendance;
- it provides an opportunity for the family members to clarify their thoughts, and if necessary to consider the outcome they want, rather than just complaining about the current situation;
- it can inspire hope by having the family look forward to a better future, rather than dwelling on the past;
- if all, or even several, members of the family are present it offers an opportunity for them to discover whether they all have the same objectives;
- there is no way the success of the help you provide can be assessed if no desired outcome has been defined.

The goals of a consultation should be defined in positive rather than negative terms. It is not enough for parents to say that they want their child's temper tantrums to cease. They should be asked also to define the behaviour they would like the child to display in those situations in which the tantrums have been occurring. Other points to consider are:

- What consequences will follow once the goals have been achieved?
- Are there any drawbacks which may be associated with these consequences?
- Under what circumstances are the changes desired? Most behaviours have value in some situations.
- What has stood in the way of change in spite of the attempts which have so far been made to bring it about?
- How quickly should the changes desired come about? Too rapid change can be stressful to those concerned and adjusting to new situations can take time. (Embedded in this question there is also the idea that change *will* occur, attention being focused instead on its time frame.)

Reviewing the family's history, determining its developmental stage and constructing a genogram

These tasks can conveniently be tackled together with all family members present. The parents can first be asked where they were born and brought up, what kinds of families they were raised in, how they got along at school and what they did when they left school. As they answer these questions they will probably speak of their parents and siblings. They can next be asked how they met and courted, and invited to outline the course of their married life to date.

Enquiry may next be made about the births of the children in the family and their development to date. It will be clear by now what stage in its life cycle the family has reached. There may also have emerged evidence of any difficulty the family is having in passing from one developmental stage to the next.

The construction of a genogram (sometimes called a geneogram) – which, when speaking with the family, may be referred to using the less jargonistic term *family tree* – is much to be desired as the family's history is being discussed. The genogram provides a concise, graphic summary of the family's current composition. It should also show the extended family network, the ages of the family members, the dates of the parents' marriage, and of any previous marriages, divorces or separations, and it indicates how the family members are related. It can also show who is the identified patient although I prefer to omit this when I am working on a genogram with family members. The geographical locations of the family members can be indicated. Brief summaries of the salient points concerning each family member – occupation, school grade, health, past illnesses, accidents, losses, incarcerations and so on – may also be noted.

Some therapists prepare the genogram later, using the information they have obtained from the family members during the meetings they have had with them, but I prefer to do it with the active participation of the family.

Figure 5.1 shows an example of a genogram. In this family, the parents of the identified patient, Brad (distinguished by a double boundary), cohabited in a 'common law' relationship from 1965 to 1969, when they got married. They separated in 1973 and were legally divorced in 1980. Carmen, Brad's mother, lived with Eric from 1973 to 1976 and they had two daughters, Jane and Holly. Carmen commenced living with Ken in 1978 and they were married in 1982. Her two children by Eric, and one by Ken, make up their present family unit. Brad and his father, Dave, live with Katrina and her 10-year-old daughter by her former husband, Len. Katrina also had a previous pregnancy which ended in a miscarriage in 1974. Carmen is an only child and both her parents are dead. Dave is the fourth in a family of one girl and four boys.

A major advantage of a genogram, as opposed to a narrative account, is the quick, visually explicit view it gives of the family. During its construction information may be volunteered, often by children, which might not otherwise emerge (like, 'Uncle George – he's always drunk', as one girl exclaimed while I was constructing a genogram; until this moment the history of alcoholism in the extended family had been concealed by the adults in the family). Genograms are discussed more fully in *Basic Family Therapy* (Barker, 1992), and *Genograms in Family Assessment* (McGoldrick & Gerson, 1985) provides extensive information on their construction, interpretation and clinical uses.

Assessing the current functioning of the family

You will learn more about how a family functions from the experience of interacting with it, than by asking the members how they believe they function. Information about family relationships may be obtained during interviews in various ways:

- by the experience of interacting with the family;
- by observing the interactions between the members, and studying carefully the family's responses, both verbal and non-verbal.

In addition to these methods there are various standardized tests and

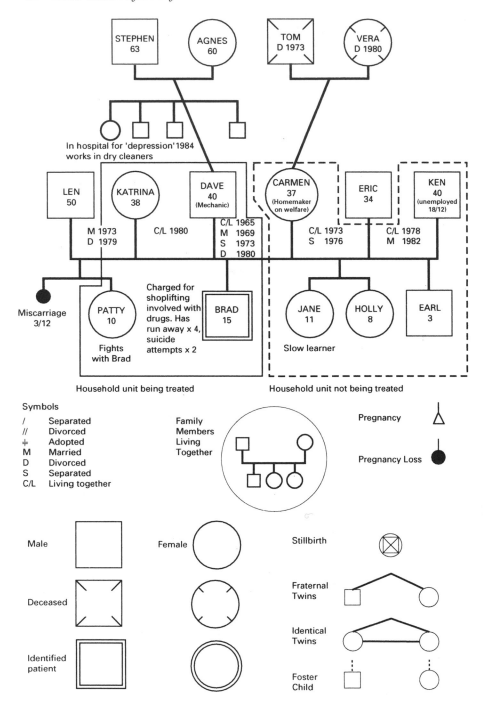

Fig. 5.1   The Green family genogram, 1985.

questionnaires that can provide assessments of family functioning. Details are to be found in family therapy texts such as *Basic Family Therapy* (Barker, 1992).

Families have difficulty describing how they function. While they may describe the formal organizational structure, this says little about how the members and subgroups in the family habitually interact, nor about how the family system as a whole functions. This is not because the family wish to deceive the interviewer but because they are too intimately involved in the family's interactions to be able to view them objectively. The most effective questions are therefore those which reveal this indirectly.

There are many ways of interviewing families. The Milan group of therapists (Palazzoli, *et al.*, 1980) suggested that the interviewer, or team (they preferred to work as a team) should first develop some hypotheses, based on the available information, and should then test these hypotheses during the interview with the family. They describe an active process in which the therapist asks questions to explore the family members' relationships with each other and, usually to a lesser extent, with others outside the immediate family group. The therapist is to be a mover rather than an observer. If the therapist behaves in a passive manner the family, 'conforming to its own linear hypothesis, would impose its own script, dedicated exclusively to the designation of who is 'crazy' and who is 'guilty', resulting in zero information for the therapist' (Palazzoli, *et al.*, 1980, page 5).

Hypotheses should be systemic, that is they should concern the family system as a whole. The objective of the family interview is to come to understand the relationships between the family members, rather than to explore the mental states of the individual members.

The Milan group also describe 'circular interviewing'. The therapist responds to information the family gives about relationships by formulating more questions, to which the family then responds again, and so on. The questions, too, are framed in a circular way, one member of the family being asked to describe the interactions between two others, for example. This has been called 'triadic interviewing'.

Triadic theory, the idea that two people (or groups or agencies – even nations) in conflict tend to involve a third person or group in the conflict, has been described as 'one of the cornerstones of many models of family therapy' (Coppersmith, 1985). The process of bringing in a third person is sometimes referred to as 'triangulation', and the ability to think in terms of triads (or triangles, which are essentially the same thing) is an important skill for the family therapist. The questions asked of family members, or groups of members, are often about differences between the behaviours or responses of two other members or groups of members.

The emphasis is on relationships between people rather than on the behaviour of individuals.

Other practical points about interviewing families suggested by the work of the Milan group are:

● It is better to ask questions about specific behaviours than about how people feel about situations, or how they interpret or understand them. For example, one might ask one of the children in a family:

'What does your father do when Billy loses his temper and swears at your mother?' Then, when the father's reaction has been described: 'And what does your mother do then? And if your big sister is around, what would she be doing?'

● Differences may be revealed by asking people to rank the family members in terms of specific behaviours. Thus the members of a family in which one child has been physically aggressive to a younger one might be asked:

'When Chad hits Dorothy, who is most likely to step in and try to stop him? And who is next most likely to do this? And then? . . .' (And so on, until it is determined who is least likely to intervene.)

● Questions concerning changes in the patterns of relationships are often revealing, for example those following specific events. Members of a family which has recently moved, or in which there has been a marital separation, a remarriage, an illness or accident affecting a family member, or a child's entry into school or departure to university, might be asked about differences in the behaviours of members relative to one another before and after the event.

● Questions may be asked about how behaviours or relationships vary in differing circumstances, real or hypothetical:

'Who would be most upset if Eric was seriously ill?'
'Do Frances and Gillian fight more when Dad is at home than when he is not?'
'What does Mummy do when Harry misbehaves? Does she react differently when Dad is at home?'

The Milan group also stressed the importance of *neutrality*. By this they mean that the interviewer must be careful not to become allied with any family member or members. Nor should the therapist accept a particular family member's view of the family's situation. Some of the questions above might seem to ally the therapist with the person being questioned, but the alliance shifts when the questioning moves to another family member, involving everyone in turn. 'The end result of the successive alliances is that the therapist is allied with everyone and no one at the same time' (Palazzoli, *et al.*, 1980). The interview should also avoid declaring any judgements, whether implicit or explicit, while meeting with the family.

While the above principles are sound and their application can greatly facilitate the process of gaining understanding of how families function, there is much more to the effective interviewing of families. Further information is in the family therapy literature (for example, *Basic Family Therapy* (Barker, 1992) and *Family Evaluation* (Karpel & Strauss, 1983)). Useful as books can be, however, there is no substitute for properly supervised practice, preferably using one-way screens or video cameras and recordings, to enable an experienced interviewer to give feedback.

Taking the history

At some stage during the assessment a history of the child's problems and development should be obtained. If possible, both parents should be interviewed. It is important that both are concerned with the study and treatment of the child from the outset, so both should be asked to come to the assessment. If only one comes, I ask to see the other later. This applies to the parents with whom the child is living, even if one is a step-parent or they are unmarried. It also applies to foster and adoptive parents. When the parents are permanently separated or divorced, involvement of the non-custodial parent at some stage is usually helpful but I do not usually ask that parent to come to the initial interview. Sometimes they show up anyway, which in itself provides important information.

It is best to let the parents start by talking freely about the child's problems. They should be allowed to explain the situation as they see it, in their own way and with a minimum of prompting. When they have finished speaking of one issue or problem they can be asked if there are any others and, if so, again asked to explain them in their own words. During this process information is often obtained about the nature of the relationship between the parents.

I prefer to discuss symptoms in terms of the changes the parents seek. If they complain of their child's mealtime behaviour, I ask them to describe how they would like the child to behave. If they want a certain behaviour to stop, for example hitting a sibling, I ask them to tell me how they would like the child to behave in circumstances in which the hitting currently occurs. How would they like to see their children interact?

The development of symptoms, their duration and frequency, whether they are getting better or worse or have remained much the same for a while, and how the parents have attempted to deal with them – and with what success – all need to be explored.

The next step is to enquire about any of the following areas which have not so far been covered:

(1) *The digestive system:* Eating habits, nausea, vomiting, abdominal pain, constipation, diarrhoea, faecal soiling, pica.
(2) *The urinary system:* Bedwetting, wetting by day, over-frequent or painful micturition.
(3) *Sleep:* Problems over going to bed, problems in sleeping, night-mares, sleepwalking, night terrors, excessive sleepiness.
(4) *The circulatory and respiratory systems:* Breathlessness, cough, palpitations.
(5) *The motor system:* Restlessness, overactivity, underactivity, clumsiness, tics, abnormal gait, motor weakness, whether right- or left-handed.
(6) *Habitual manipulations of the body:* Nail biting, thumb sucking, head banging, rocking and other repetitive habits.
(7) *Speech:* Over-talkativeness, mutism, faulty speech of any type, including late development of speech and stuttering, comprehension of what is said.
(8) *Thought processes:* Poor concentration, distractibility, disordered thinking, day dreaming, delusional ideas.
(9) *Vision and hearing:* Any defects, evidence suggesting hallucinations.
(10) *Temperamental traits:* See the section on 'temperamental factors' in Chapter 2.
(11) *Behaviour:* Follower or leader, relationships with siblings, teachers, friends. Fearfulness, sensitiveness, tearfulness, sulking, irritability, temper tantrums. Obedience/disobedience, cooperativeness/negativism, constructiveness/destructiveness, truthfulness/untruthfulness, stealing, wandering away from home, staying out late, group or gang membership, smoking, drinking or drug-taking. Involvement with police, court appearances, probation, or placement away from home. Involvement of social agencies.
(12) *Affective state (mood):* Is the mood appropriate or is the child depressed, elated, anxious, fearful, or showing evidence of other mood disturbance? Does mood vary a lot? If so, is this related to environmental circumstances, or does it appear to be independent of them? Has there been any evidence of suicidal ideation? Have there been any attempts at suicide?
(13) *Fantasy life and play:* The types of games the child plays. Content of play. Does he/she have much, or little, imagination? Fantasy

friends, transitional objects. Content of fantasy as expressed in play, drawing, painting, conversation or dreams.

(14) *Sexual issues:* Sex instruction given, child's reaction to it, sexual attitudes, masturbation, heterosexual or homosexual experiences, onset of menstruation, dysmenorrhoea, any history of sexual abuse?

(15) *Attack disorders.* Epilepsy, fainting, other alterations of consciousness, breath-holding attacks.

(16) *School:* Attitudes to school, behaviour at school, school class or grade, progress in school, social adjustment in school.

(17) *Physical abuse or neglect:* Is there any history of past maltreatment?

The amount of detail which needs to be sought in each of the above areas will depend on the circumstances. Sometimes a general enquiry about whether the child has had any physical health problems, rather than detailed questioning about each bodily system will be sufficient, but in other cases a detailed history of the child's physical health will be indicated.

Although the above list consists largely of possible problems, it is important also to enquire about strengths and areas of healthy functioning. It is as important to know that a child does well at school, or has musical talent, or gets along well with siblings or friends, or has an easy temperament, as it is to know about the problem areas.

Enquiry should be made about the duration, frequency and degree of both problem behaviours and strengths. The way parents describe their children's symptoms is significant. They may make light of a child's problems, or describe them in over-dramatic terms, or even be highly critical of behaviours which are scarcely outside the range of normal.

In obtaining the above information, an active, structured approach, used sensitively and with the interviewer alert for clues to the presence of unusual symptoms, usually works best. It is often important to establish the absence of symptoms, as well as those that are reported – hence the merits of going through the above list.

In eliciting feelings, as opposed to facts, a more non-directive approach, with direct requests for the expression of feelings, but otherwise with less talk, usually yields best results.

The developmental history

An account of the child's developmental history from conception to the date of the interview should be obtained. This should cover:

- The course of the pregnancy, any complications, whether the mother used drugs or alcohol and, if so, how heavily.
- The child's birth and neonatal condition.
- The subsequent progress of the child's development – motor, speech, feeding, toilet training, social behaviour and adjustment, progress in school and so on.
- Any previous illnesses, injuries or emotional problems.

It is helpful to obtain a description of how the child was as a baby, a toddler, over the period of starting school, and so on up to the present time.

Examining the child

It is not possible to specify a set, generally applicable routine for the psychiatric examination of children. Much depends on the child's age, language skills, willingness to talk and personality. Contact with children below the age of five has to be largely through the medium of play, though even pre-school children can sometimes reveal a remarkable amount of information in conversation. Older children, and especially adolescents, can often be approached much as adult patients are. In the intermediate age range, a mixture of play and conversation usually works best, the proportion of each depending on the child's interests and reactions.

It is seldom the presenting child who is complaining of symptoms. Usually the concerns expressed are those of one or more adults, either parents or teachers, or both. The adults are either expressing concerns on the child's behalf or they are objecting to some aspect of the child's behaviour. For this reason it is usually a mistake to start the interview by discussing the presenting complaints. Indeed to do so can prove to be a serious error as it can lead the child to identify the interviewer with disapproving adults, and thus to become guarded or suspicious. A trusting relationship with the child may therefore become more difficult to establish.

The first step, as in any interview, is to establish rapport. Ascertaining facts can wait until the child's confidence has been obtained and rapport is well established. The principles set out above for establishing rapport apply as much to children as to adults. There are, however, some special points to bear in mind when one is dealing with children.

Children, like adults, need to feel that they and their points of view are respected and valued. The atmosphere should be relaxed and friendly but not condescending. Toys, play materials, and painting and drawing materials, appropriate to the child's age, should be available and in view. Younger children are best seen in a playroom. It is advisable not to have a desk between child and interviewer; to do so tends to distance child and interviewer emotionally as well as physically. It should be made clear to young children that the toys and materials are there for their use. If they do not wish to talk this should be accepted and they should be allowed to play for a while. It may be possible to start a conversation later, when the child is playing.

It is usually best to start talking with children about topics well removed from the symptom areas, unless they bring those topics up themselves. You may start by discussing how they travelled to the clinic or office, their interests and hobbies, games they like to play, toys they have at home, any recent birthday, school (unless this is known to be an area of difficulty), friends, siblings, and their ambitions for the future. If Christmas, Easter, Thanksgiving, or some other such occasion has occurred recently, it may be discussed.

The presenting problems may come up as the interview proceeds. If they do not, they can be broached once adequate rapport seems to have been established. It is especially important to tread cautiously with children who have been engaging in antisocial acts such as stealing. There is little point in asking questions such as, 'Did you steal such-and-such?' If the question is answered at all, the child may say yes or no. If yes, the interviewer is usually none the wiser for the question is only likely to be asked if it is known that the child is thought to have stolen. If no, the child has been forced into the position of withholding information – unless, of course, the allegation is false. Such questions are inclined to lead to situations in which the children are manoeuvered into withholding information. This may damage the developing relationship between interviewer and child. Even more unhelpful are questions such as, 'Why did you steal something?' Such a question is futile, since children scarcely ever have the understanding of their behaviour to give a useful answer. What it *is* likely to do is to place the interviewer in the same category, in the child's mind, as other critical, punitive, lecturing authority figures. While one wishes to understand what is behind the child's stealing, it is naive to suppose that this can be learned simply by asking the child.

The early part of the first interview, occasionally the whole of it, should be spent gaining the child's confidence. Once this has been achieved, it is justifiable to ask, in a general way, what has brought the child to the clinic, office or hospital. An accurate reply is often given, but if it is not, the subject should not be pressed.

Once rapport has been established, particular areas of the child's life may be explored. This should be done gently, using words and in a manner appropriate to the child's age and personality – of which, by this time, you will have acquired at least a beginning impression. Asking a series of direct questions is not usually the best approach. It is more a matter of saying, 'Lots of people have dreams when they are asleep at night ... I wonder if you do?' The child who admits to having dreams can then be invited to recount one, and perhaps asked whether the dreams are mostly nice ones or nasty ones. The child who denies remembering any dreams may be told, 'Often when people who don't have dreams come to see us, they like to make up a dream ... to pretend they've had one ... I wonder if you would like to do that?'

This is one way of exploring children's fantasy lives. Another is to ask them to imagine they can have three 'magic' wishes and that whatever they wish will come true; what would they then wish to happen? (The question can be modified to omit the magic part for adolescents, many of whom prove to be quite willing to wish for three things to happen.) Children often take their wishes very seriously. The interviewer can then go on to say something like, 'Now I'd like you to pretend you were all alone on an uninhabited (or desert) island (or in a boat) and you could choose one person to be with you ... anyone in the whole world but just one person ... I wonder who you would choose?' The child may then be asked to select a second person, then a third.

You can enquire in similar ways for fears, worries, and somatic and other symptoms. Conversation about family, friends (whom the child can be asked to name and describe), and school should also be encouraged. Throughout all of this the interviewer must respond appropriately, trying to share the child's sorrow at the loss of a pet, or pleasure at being a member of a winning sports team. Above all, it is important to convey both interest in, and respect for, the child's point of view. This does not, of course, necessarily imply approval of, or agreement with, what the child says.

Children who have not reached adolescence should be invited to draw, paint and/or play with some of the toys that are available. This enables you to observe their powers of concentration, attention span, distractibility and motor dexterity. The content of children's play, and their artistic productions, often provides useful information about them and their world. I usually ask any child I see to draw a picture, preferably of his or her family, and if possible of the family doing something – this tends to give more information that just asking for a series of figures. The appearance of the different family members, their respective sizes and relative positions, what they are doing, and even who is included and who is left out, can be revealing.

It can also be useful to invite the child to draw a person and then discuss the person the child has drawn (let us assume it is a male figure), asking questions like, 'What makes him happy?' 'What makes him sad?' 'What makes him laugh?' 'How many friends does he have?' 'Does he make friends easily?' 'Do people like him?'... and so on. The answers may reveal much about the child's view of himself or herself and of the world.

Much can be learned from children's drawings and paintings. Some pictures bristle with aggression. Guns are firing, people are being hurled over cliffs or otherwise killed, and all sorts of violence is depicted. Others portray sadness, with people depicted looking unhappy or crying; or the subjects may be represented as feeling ill or even being about to die. Yet other pictures show happy scenes, or illustrate fulfilment of the artist's ambitions ('This is me in a space ship'). Children's drawings and paintings should be kept as part of their clinical records. What they say as they draw or paint or make models should also be recorded, together with any comments they may have on the finished productions.

What children draw, paint or model, like everything else they tell us, must be interpreted in the light of the total clinical picture. *Interpreting Children's Drawings* (DiLeo, 1983) is one of number of books which can be helpful in understanding children's artistic productions. Adolescents may not wish to paint or draw, but it is usually possible to judge whether it is appropriate to suggest this. As well as drawing I invite children – except for very young ones – to write something, for example their name and address on the picture they have drawn, providing me with a rough estimate of their writing skills.

Clinical Interviews with Children and Adolescents (Barker, 1990) gives further practical guidance and suggests various approaches to the interviewing of particular groups of children.

When the interviews described above are complete, an assessment of the child along the following lines should be made:

(1) *General appearance and behaviour:* Are there any obvious physical abnormalities? Bruises, cuts or grazes? Mode of dress? Is it appropriate for the season and current weather? Does the child look happy or unhappy, tearful or worried? Attitude to the examiner and the assessment procedure?

(2) *Motor function:* Is the child overactive, normal or underactive? Clumsy or dexterous? Any abnormal movements such as tics? Right- or left-handed? Can the child distinguish left from right? Is the gait normal? If not, what is the abnormality? Can the child write, draw and paint, and if so, how well?

(3) *Speech and language:* Articulation, vocabulary and use of language? Are non-verbal communications congruent with verbal ones? How much does the child talk? Ability to read and write?

(4)   *Content of talk and thought:* What does the child talk about? How easy is it to steer the conversation towards particular topics? Are any subjects avoided? Does the stream of thought flow logically from one thing to the next? Is there any abnormal use of words or expressions? Evidence of hallucinations or delusions?

(5)   *Intellectual function:* It is helpful to make a rough estimate of the child's level of intellectual functioning, based on general knowledge, content of conversation, level of play, and knowledge of time, day, date, year, place and people's identity, taking into account the child's age.

(6)   *Mood and emotional state (additional to what is observed under 'general appearance):* Happy, elated, unhappy, frankly depressed, anxious, hostile, resentful, suspicious, upset by separation from parents? Level of rapport which has been established. Has the child ever wanted to run away, or to hide, wished to be dead or contemplated suicide? Does the child cry, and if so how often and in what circumstances? Specific fears? How are they dealt with? Appropriateness of emotional state to subject being discussed?

(7)   *Attitudes to family:* Indications during conversation or play.

(8)   *Attitudes to school:* Does the child like school? Attitudes towards school work, teachers and other staff, other pupils, play and games.

(9)   *Fantasy life:* The child's three magic wishes. The three most desired companions on an uninhabited island. What dreams are reported or made up? What is the worst thing – and the best thing – that could happen to the child? Ambitions in life? What fantasy material is expressed in play, drawing, painting, modelling or conversation?

(10)   *Sleep:* Does the child report any difficult in sleeping? Fear of going to bed or to sleep? Fear of the dark, nightmares, night terrors (see Chapter 17), pleasant dreams?

(11)   *Behaviour problems:* Does the child reveal anything about behaviour problems, delinquent activities, illicit drug use, running away, sexual problems, trouble with police or school authorities, or appearance in court?

(12)   *Placement away from home:* Has the child been placed, or lived away from home at any time? If so, where, when, for how long and what is the child's understanding of the reason for this? Reaction to the experience?

(13)   *Attitude to referral:* How does the child view the referral and the reasons for it? Is he or she aware of a problem, and if so, what?

(14)   *Indications of social adjustment:* Number of reported friends, hobbies,

interests, games played, youth organizations belonged to, leisure time activities? Does the child feel a follower or a leader, or bullied, teased or picked on? If so, by whom?

(15) *Other problems:* Worries, pains, headaches, other somatic symptoms, relationship difficulties?

(16) *Play:* A general description should be provided of the child's play. What is played with and how? To what extent is play symbolic? Content of play? Concentration, distractibility and constructiveness?

(17) *Self image:* This has usually to be inferred from the sum total of what the child does and says, the ambitions and fantasy ideas expressed, and the child's estimate of what others think of him or her.

Children's behaviour should be described as objectively as possible. Savicki & Brown (1981) provide helpful guidelines on how to do this.

In many instances it is not possible to obtain all the information above in a first interview. Assessment should be regarded as on ongoing process. It is unrealistic to expect to discover everything about a child in one session, and it must also be remembered that children's emotional states and behaviour are very much context dependent and are liable to change over quite short periods of time.

The psychiatric state of non-speaking children is assessed by making all the observations that do not require spoken replies from the child, supplemented by collateral information from the adults in their lives – as with other children. The fact that a child does not speak, whether because of inability or refusal to do so, is itself an important piece of clinical information.

Clinical Interviews with Children and Adolescents (Barker, 1990) contains additional information about interview techniques for use with children of different ages, together with sections on how to approach interviewing certain special groups, such as mentally retarded children, children who may have been abused, and suicidal children.

The physical examination

Unless the child's physical state has already been assessed or is being investigated by a colleague, a physical examination by a medical collea- gue should be a part of the assessment. Some psychiatrists prefer to arrange for the physical examination to be carried out by another physician, believing that if they carry out the procedure this may impede the development of a psychotherapeutic relationship.

Other sources of information

Useful information is often available from other sources, such as the staff of the child's school. It is advisable to ask the parents for consent to obtain information from the school of every child of school age, whether problems in school are reported or not. The fact that a child is functioning well in school, despite having problems in other situations, is a significant piece of diagnostic information in itself. Written reports from school are useful but talking with teachers, ideally face to face but even on the telephone, is often better, especially when there are complaints about a child's behaviour, adjustment or progress in school. A joint meeting involving school staff, parents and other involved adults, and perhaps the child also, can be therapeutic as well as providing diagnostic information.

Aponte (1976), a family therapist, recommended that when the main problems are at school, the first face to face contact should be a family-school interview. This has much merit, especially when the initiative for the referral comes from the school.

The following may also supply valuable information:

- schools the child has attended in the past;
- physicians or other professionals who have assessed or treated the child in the past;
- any other professionals who are currently involved with child or family;
- any social agencies that have been involved with the child or the family, for example child protection and child welfare agencies and probation services;
- hospitals and institutions in which the child has been treated or has received care;
- foster parents and others who have cared for the child.

Permission to contact any of the above must always be obtained. It may be advisable to obtain the written permission of both parents, when there are two parents involved.

Psychological tests

Psychological tests can add to the information obtained in clinical interviews. Many require special training and should be administered and interpreted by psychologists trained in their use. They can be used at all stages of the assessment and treatment process, in measuring outcome, and in follow-up. They can be especially useful when the assessment procedures have not produced a clear understanding of the child's case difficulties; when a child or adolescent has been unwilling or unable to cooperate fully in the assessment; in resolving conflicting and confusing data; and when decisions which may have especially serious consequences have to be made, such as whether criminal prosecution is appropriate, or when the discharge from hospital of patients who may be suicidal or homicidal is being considered.

The main groups of tests available for use with children are:

- Intelligence tests,
- tests of academic attainment,
- personality tests,
- behaviour checklists,
- tests designed to assess specific psychological conditions, such as anxiety, depression, self-esteem and sustained attention.

Intelligence tests

These are designed to assess children's abilities in performing various cognitive tasks compared with those of other children of the same age. Many intelligence tests are composed of numbers of subtests, allowing separate estimates of specific areas of functioning in addition to a global estimate of intelligence.

Originally, intelligence was measured as a 'mental age'. A child displaying similar ability to others of the same age had a mental age that was the same as the chronological age. If more ability was shown, then the mental age was higher than the chronological age, and if less, then the mental age was lower. The intelligence quotient or IQ was calculated as a ratio of the child's mental age divided by the chronological age, multiplied by 100:

$$IQ = \frac{\text{mental age}}{\text{chronological age}} \times 100$$

The concept of mental age is rarely used nowadays as it is considered misleading. We know that a normal child aged 8 and a 12-year-old with a mental age of 8 are very different. Principally for this reason, most IQ scores are reported as standard scores.

Nowadays intelligence tests are standardized on large populations in order to determine how the average child functions and how variable the test scores are. In interpreting the results, however, it is important to be aware of the population on which the test has been standardized. Applying a test standardized on, for example, British children, to children living in other cultures, for example in Africa, cannot be considered valid unless it has been shown empirically that the same norms apply. Similar considerations apply even in a single country where there is significant sociocultural diversity. Thus norms derived from Caucasian Canadian children may not be applicable for use with native Canadians.

The intelligence tests most commonly used with both pre-school children and school-age children are:

- The Wechsler Preschool and Primary Scales of Intelligence – Revised (WPPSI-R).
- The Wechsler Intelligence Scale for Children – 3rd Edition (WISC-III).
- The Stanford-Binet Intelligence Scale – 4th Edition.
- The Kaufman Assessment Battery for Children (K-ABC).
- The McArthy Scales.

The two Wechsler Scales listed above both provide a global or full scale IQ, a verbal IQ and a performance IQ. The verbal IQ is derived from a set of subtests that tap the ability to understand and use language, whereas the performance IQ is a measure of the child's abilities in subtests that require visual analysis and a motor response. Each IQ scale has a mean of 100 and a standard deviation of 15. This means that 66% of all children in the population will have IQ scores between 85 and 115. Two standard deviations (IQ 70–130) will cover about 95% of the population and three (IQ 55–145) will cover over 99%.

The other tests of intelligence listed have similar goals, and even subscales, but each is constructed somewhat differently. There are circumstances in which one intelligence test is preferred over the others. This is an area where the specialized knowledge of the psychologist is valuable.

There are also tests for specific populations:

- The Bayley Infant Scales of Mental and Motor Development.
- The Merrill-Palmer Scales.
- The Gesell Developmental Schedule.
- The Leiter Scales – for language and hearing impaired children, an entirely non-verbal test.

The Peabody Picture Vocabulary Test is an easily administered test of verbal skills.

Intelligence tests are not infallible and various factors can affect the results. Many psychologists prefer to report the IQ as a range (average, low average, superior, etc.) rather than as a numerical score. A statement of the psychologist's confidence in the result is usually included, together with any relevant observations regarding circumstances that might have affected the results, such as the child's approach to the test, or state of health, or any apparent fatigue. The psychologist's observations of the child's behaviour during testing may be as important as the actual scores obtained. Intelligence tests were originally intended to be predictors of school performance and to identify those children requiring special educational services. They subsequently came to be overvalued and were sometimes attached to children like labels. We can only say that on a particular date, on a specified test, the child achieved a score in a particular range. It is important to bear in mind that any test can only sample some abilities. Thus none of the tests mentioned above measures creativity, which many consider an important aspect of intelligence.

Despite the above reservations, intelligence tests can be invaluable. They can help identify children who are underfunctioning, that is to say not making full use of their intellectual potential; and also those of whom more is being demanded than is appropriate in light of their current cognitive functioning. They can also help in the identification of learning disabilities which sometimes underlie conduct or other problems. They can identify areas of strength on which parents, teachers and therapists can capitalize. They are also the cornerstone of neuropsychological assessment – a highly specialized type of investigation of specific aspects of cognitive functioning that can pinpoint areas of difficulty, and even on occasion uncover previously unrecognized neurological problems.

Tests of educational attainment

These are available to assess children's current level of achievement in basic school subjects. Like intelligence tests, attainment tests are standardized on large populations, so that they can be used to discover how children are performing in relation to the population at large. Tests of reading, arithmetic and spelling are available and, if desired reading, arithmetic and spelling ages, and grade equivalents, can be calculated using the same principles as are used in calculating mental ages. There is however a strong trend towards the use of standard scores for these tests also. If intelligence testing is carried out at the same time as attainment testing, it is possible to compare academic achievement with academic potential, at least as assessed by the test used.

Children's educational attainments and problems are of interest to the psychiatrist for several reasons. In many instances difficulties in school play important roles in the genesis of both behaviour and emotional disorders. Some children experience stress because they are struggling to achieve in areas in which they have specific weaknesses. Testing can help determine what their special educational needs are. There is also a strong association between behaviour problems and poor reading skills. Finally, some intellectually gifted children run into difficulties because they are not being adequately challenged and stimulated in regular school programs, and require appropriately modified schooling.

Both intelligence and academic attainments can be assessed using *group tests*. These are often used in schools. Groups of children write answers to questions and/or instructions on forms which are often constructed using a multiple choice format. These tests can be of practical value, especially in assessing group performance on the tasks. The test scores obtained for individual children should be treated with caution, however, since it is harder to detect the child who is not cooperating, perhaps because of sickness, fatigue or hostility. These tests also have the limitation that they are predominantly verbal.

Personality tests

These can sometimes be of great help in contributing to the clinical assessment and diagnosis. The assessment of personality is more difficult than the estimation of intelligence or academic attainment. It is easier to define average intelligence or average reading attainment, than it is to define average personality, but projective tests can provide much information on how people think and feel and about their attitudes in many areas of their lives. For these reasons they can usefully supplement the information obtained at the more free-flowing clinical interviews described earlier.

Projective tests involve the presentation of ambiguous material to the subject being tested, with the aim of eliciting responses which may reflect the person's personality and mental state. The oldest and best known projective test is the Rorschach Test. The subject is presented with a series of printed shapes, originally derived from ink blots, and asked to say what they resemble. The blots themselves have no designed meaning, so any response must be a projection. Interpretation is difficult and requires special training.

In testing children, the Children's Apperception Test (CAT) is probably used more frequently than the Rorschach Test. It consists of somewhat ambiguous pictures about each of which the child is asked to tell a story. A newer test, the Roberts Test for Children, has some advantages over the CAT and is growing in popularity. The Thematic Apperception Test (TAT) was designed for adults and has more realistic pictures than the CAT. Other widely used tests are the Kinetic Family Drawing, the Draw-a-Person Test and the House-Tree-Person Test. In each of these the child is asked to draw the items mentioned and the results can be examined and scored to give information about the child's personality and emotional state.

Many other personality tests and questionnaires are available designed to assess different aspects of children's functioning, social adjustment and social maturity. One of the most widely used is the Child Behaviour Checklist (Achenbach & Edelbrock, 1983) which consists of a list of questions to which the child's parents or other caregivers are asked to check off the appropriate answers. It has been extensively tested on clinical and non-clinical populations. It yields a number of scores which give information that can be helpful in assessing a child's behavioural, emotional and mental state. It has been widely used in research.

EEGs, X-rays and laboratory tests

If there are no symptoms suggesting organic disease and physical examination reveals no relevant abnormality, it is not usually necessary to arrange any further investigations of the child's physical state. On the other hand, when there is suggestive evidence of a physical disorder, investigations may be indicated, and it may be appropriate to request the opinion of another specialist, for example a paediatric neurologist.

The electroencepahlogram (EEG) is a useful aid – though no more than that – in the diagnosis and management of epilepsy (see Chapter 15). It can also assist in the diagnosis of other diseases of the brain and is a valuable research tool. Abnormalities in the EEG have been reported in various groups of disturbed children, including autistic children and some with severe behaviour disorders. Their significance remains unclear and they are at present of little or no value in the management of such children.

Recent years have seen the development of new methods of brain imaging, which have supplemented, and in some cases replaced, earlier radiological techniques. These include computerized axial tomography (the CAT scan procedure), magnetic resonance imaging (MRI) and positron emission tomography (the PET scan). These techniques make possible more accurate and less invasive investigation of brain structure and function. They promise to reveal much about the function of the brain in psychiatric disorders but their use in child psychiatry – as opposed to child neurology – has so far been limited mainly to research.

Laboratory tests such as blood counts and biochemical tests have little role to play in the routine study of child psychiatric patients, unless there is reason to suspect an associated physical disorder. A study of laboratory tests carried out on a population of 100 adolescent inpatients by Gabel & Hsu (1986) showed that the results contributed little or nothing to the management of these patients.

The formulation

When the assessment of child and family is complete, a formulation of the case should be developed. If a team has been involved in the assessment, the formulation is usually worked out at a meeting of the team. The practitioner working alone should carry out a similar procedure.

The formulation is a concise summary of the case, setting out the understanding of the problems presented in the light of the information that the assessment procedure has revealed. It is an essential part of the assessment and should be the basis of the management and treatment plan that emerges from the assessment. It may be developed by considering the following factors:

(a) *Predisposing:* What pre-existing factors contributed to the development of the disorder? Constitutional, temperamental, physical and environmental factors should all be considered.
(b) *Precipitating:* Have any possible precipitating factors come to light? Why did the problem(s) appear at the particular time reported? Again, it is helpful to think in terms of constitutional, temperamental, physical and environmental factors.
(c) *Perpetuating:* What is maintaining the condition? The four sets of factors should again be considered.
(d) *Protective:* What are the child's and the family's strengths? What factors are limiting the severity of the disorder and promoting healthy functioning?

The grid in Fig. 5.2 may be used as an aid to the development of the formulation, but it must be remembered that a formulation is not just a list of causative, contributing or associated factors but also a description of their interplay and relative importance.

	Constitutional	Temperamental	Physical	Environmental
Predisposing				
Precipitating				
Perpetuating				
Protective				

Fig. 5.2   Formulation grid of contributing factors.

Based on the information in the grid, if one is used, the formulation should be a clearly written, logical, dynamic explanation of how the case is understood, leading to a plan of management, treatment and, if required, further investigation. Strengths as well as weaknesses should be included and the expected outcome should be stated. If a *problem-oriented* or *goal-orientated* system of clinical recording is used, the formulation should be the basis of the problem and strength lists.

The formulation should be updated from time to time during treatment, since new information usually comes to light as treatment or investigation of the case proceed, and as the child's circumstances in family, school or elsewhere change.

Recording clinical information

In child psychiatry, as in other branches of medicine, good clinical records are essential. An assessment summary, preferably typed, should be prepared following the initial consultation. The subheadings used in this chapter make a convenient framework for this and may prevent points of information being overlooked. The summary may take the form of a letter to the referring physician or other professional. Children's drawings and paintings should be preserved as part of the clinical record. Records should be safely stored, access to them being limited to those having legitimate reasons to examine them.

Chapter 6

Conduct and Oppositional Disorders

Definition and classification

In this chapter we consider disorders characterized by antisocial behaviour. Their essence is an established pattern of oppositional or antisocial behaviour. Children with these disorders have failed to learn those patterns of social behaviour that are expected of people in the society in which they are growing up.

ICD-10 defines six subgroups of 'conduct disorders'. These are:

(1) Conduct disorder confined to the family.
(2) Unsocialized conduct disorder.
(3) Socialized conduct disorder.
(4) Oppositional defiant disorder.
(5) Other conduct disorders.
(6) Conduct disorder, unspecified.

DSM-IV considers conduct disorders, oppositional defiant disorders and 'attention-deficit/hyperactivity' disorders in a section entitled 'Attention deficit and disruptive behaviour disorders'. On the other hand, ICD-10 has a separate category for 'hyperkinetic disorders'. DSM-IV further distinguishes two types of conduct disorder: those with childhood onset and those with adolescent onset. It also requires 'severity specifiers', indicating whether they are mild, moderate or severe.

In reality these diagnostic groupings are attempts to describe, and bring some order into, a very mixed bag of social-emotional disorders affecting children. What these conditions have in common is that the course of the social development of those with them has deviated, to a serious degree, from that considered normal, or at least acceptable, in their community. In most cases a complex set of interacting causes is responsible, and there is an almost infinite variety of ways in which the failure to conform to society's social norms may be manifested. Any classification scheme is therefore inevitably somewhat arbitrary. Yet these disorders are the most common of all child psychiatric disorders and they vary widely in their presentation. Therefore some form of subdivision, even if arbitrary, is desirable.

ICD-10 defines conduct disorders as being characterized 'by a repetitive and persistent pattern of dissocial, aggressive or defiant conduct'. It involves 'major violations of age-appropriate social expectations, and is therefore more severe than ordinary childish mischief or adolescent rebelliousness'. ICD-10 also states that 'isolated dissocial or criminal acts are not in themselves grounds for the diagnosis'.

The above quotations hint broadly at one of the problems with which clinicians are faced when they deal with children displaying antisocial behaviour – that of distinguishing between 'childish mischief' and more serious disorders. While sometimes the distinction is easy, in others it is not and the borderline is both arbitrary and, often, vague. Moreover research has shown that what may appear as relatively mild behaviour problems in young children, even toddlers, may presage serious problems later.

Prevalence

In the Isle of Wight study (Rutter, *et al.*, 1970b) nearly two-thirds of the 10- and 11-year-old children who were found to have psychiatric disorders had conduct disorders. Including children with mixed neurotic and conduct disorders, the prevalence of conduct problems was 4%. In a London borough studied later it was 12% (Rutter, *et al.*, 1975a). Conduct disorders have repeatedly been shown to be more common in boys than in girls.

The percentage prevalence rates for conduct disorders found in the Ontario Child Health Study (Offord, *et al.*, 1987) were:

Boys aged	4–11:	6.5	Girls aged	4–11:	1.8
	12–16:	10.4		12–16:	4.1
	4–16:	8.1		4–16:	2.8

In the Ontario study the urban and rural rates were quite similar at 5.6% and 5.2% respectively.

Causes

There is probably no better illustration of the biopsychosocial nature of child psychiatric disorders than that provided by conduct disorders. Seldom, if ever, is it possible to pinpoint one specific cause for a child's antisocial behaviour. The reasons why children fail to adopt society's norms for behaviour as their own are exceedingly complex. Factors in any or all of the categories discussed in Chapter 2 may be involved.

(1) Constitutional factors

(a) Genetic factors
It is unlikely that conduct disorders themselves are hereditary, but genetic factors – probably polygenic ones – may contribute to the development of a predisposing personality and temperamental characteristics. Both twin and adoption studies suggest a genetic predisposition to adult criminality, though the evidence is less strong in the case of children (Vandenberg, *et al.*, 1986, Chapter 10).

(b) Chromosome abnormalities
The possession of an extra Y chromosome is no longer believed to predispose to antisocial behaviour (Ratcliffe, *et al.*, 1990). Chromosome abnormalities associated with impairment of cognitive functioning (see Chapter 2) may indirectly contribute, as a result of the learning difficulties and problems in social adaptation such children may experience.

(c) Intrauterine disease or damage
The various hazards the fetus may face were discussed in Chapter 2. Resulting brain damage may contribute to the development of antisocial behaviour. It has long been known that psychiatric disorders generally are more common in children with neurological disorders than in children without such disorders (Rutter, *et al.*, 1970a).

(d) Birth injury and prematurity
These may predispose to antisocial behaviour just as damage during pregnancy may do. A confounding, but possible additional risk factor is the separation of baby and parents that may occur when the child is of very low birth weight or very ill in the neonatal period, requiring intensive care in hospital. This may affect adversely the developing relationship between parents and baby, with difficulties in the bonding process.

(2) Physical disease and injury

Physical damage to the brain occurring after birth, like that occurring prenatally, is associated with an increased risk of the development of antisocial behaviour. Research studies have shown that adverse medical histories are more common in delinquent children than in matched controls. Evidence of trauma to the central nervous system (CNS) has been found to be particularly common among aggressive young people, including juvenile murderers (Lewis, *et al.*, 1988a).

How does brain damage or disease lead to conduct disordered behaviour? We do not have a precise answer to this question but Lewis (1991) suggests that severe medical problems affecting the CNS may contribute to hyperactivity, lability of mood and impulsivity, which in turn may predispose to conduct disorder. It is clear that socially acceptable behaviour has to be taught, or modelled, by those among whom children grow up and impairment of brain function may impede this process, as it may impede the learning of other things, including the academic material taught at school. There may be an association between epilepsy, especially when this arises from a focus in the temporal lobe, and aggressive behaviour (Lewis, *et al.*, 1988b) but how often epilepsy is a significant factor in the aetiology of conduct disorder remains a matter of dispute. It is clear, though, that many epileptic children do not suffer from conduct disorders or, indeed, any other psychiatric disorder.

Lewis and her collaborators have also described an association between severe behaviour problems in young people, specifically delinquent youths incarcerated for major crimes, and psychotic symptoms such as 'paranoid ideation' and auditory or visual hallucinations. Lewis (1991) also cites the association between conduct disordered behaviour, on the one hand, and depression, suicidal ideation and attempts, and drug and alcohol abuse on the other. One study revealed that 60% of a sample of delinquents incarcerated in secure settings had histories of incarceration in psychiatric hospitals or residential treatment centres earlier in their lives (Lewis & Shanok, 1980). In fact there is evidence that the origins of many conduct disorders can be discerned very early in life, even at the toddler stage.

Other mechanisms may operate in children who have organic diseases, whether neurological or not. The presence of handicap or disease may provoke rejecting, fatalistic or other unhelpful attitudes in parents and others. These may be associated with adverse rearing practices and may affect the child's self-esteem.

(3) Other biological factors

A number of reports in recent years have suggested that various biochemical factors may play a part in the genesis of conduct disorders (Lewis, 1991), but research in this area is at an early stage.

(4) Temperamental factors

We have seen, in Chapter 2, how temperament varies from child to child and how some children have constellations of temperamental character-istics that are considered *difficult*. It seems clear that some children are more difficult to rear than others and that those who are more difficult are at greater risk of developing antisocial behaviour. Whether they do so seems to depend in part on the goodness of fit between the tempera-mental style of the child and the temperaments and responses of the parents. A clash of temperaments may be the basis of difficulties that become serious and longlasting. On the other hand, some parents manage to rear successfully children with strikingly difficult temperaments.

(4) Environmental factors

(a) The family
In most industrialized western cultures it is the nuclear family's task to rear and socialize its children. In other cultures, for example many traditional African ones, responsibility for the rearing of children is spread among the extended family, with grandparents – especially grandmothers – playing a major role. In western society, on the other hand, many children are reared by single parents, most often mothers. While it is certainly possible for single parents to raise their children successfully, the task is a more challenging one than that facing a stable parental couple.

Children who lack a permanent family group in which to grow up are liable to suffer grave disadvantage. Fortunately the days of the large impersonal orphanage are past, at least in most western societies. This is not the case, though, in other parts of the world, as was so graphically illu-strated when conditions in Romanian orphanages came to light after the end of the communist regime. Many children deprived of a normal family life, however, experience repeated moves from one home to another. Those most likely to do so may be those who are most vulnerable because of their difficult temperaments or other biological factors. Frequent moves deprive the child of the consistent learning experiences needed for the process of socialization. The emotional attachment to care-givers, which is so important as a basis for development, is likely to be impaired when consistent parent figures are not available. Children who are moved frequently from care-giver to care-giver also lack consistent, permanent and stable figures with whom to identify. Children who have been in care earlier in childhood have been found to show significantly more deviant, especially antisocial, behaviour later (Wolkind & Rutter, 1973).

Living in a permanent family group, even one containing both natural parents, does not guarantee a childhood free of antisocial behaviour or other problems. Not only may temperamental and biological factors be operating to make the child's adjustment in society more difficult, but precisely what happens in the family is crucial. There is widespread agreement that children develop best in a stable and consistent environment in which there is acceptance, affirmation of their worth as individuals, and proper social training. The latter is provided by parental precept and example, and through the consistent setting of rules and expectations, rewards and consequences being used as needed. In the setting of a happy home characterized by warm, loving relationships between family members, the responses may need to be no more than a smile or a word of encouragement, or a frown or minor reproof. Such family environments help promote children's sense of emotional security and self-esteem and facilitate the process of socialization.

What should parents avoid in rearing their children? According to Patterson (1982) antisocial behaviour is associated with:

- Lack of 'house' *rules* – that is, no set routines for meals and other activities, and a lack of clarity about what the children may or may not do or how they are expected to behave.
- Failure by the parents to monitor children's behaviour, and to know what they have been doing and how they feel.
- Lack of effective contingencies – that is, inconsistent responses to undesired behaviour, with failure to follow through with threatened consequences or with rewards for desired behaviour.
- Lack of techniques with which to deal with crises or problems in the family, so that tensions and disputes arise but are not satisfactorily resolved.

Wilson (1980), in a study of delinquents, found weak parental supervision to be the factor most strongly associated with delinquency, among the factors she investigated. Poorly supervised children roam the streets without their parents knowing where they are; they do not know when they are supposed to be home; and they engage in many activities independently of their families. The conclusions of these two investigators are thus quite similar.

Family dysfunction may take many forms, not all of which are incompatible with successful child rearing. Some, however, involve the adoption by children of idiosyncratic roles, such as that of the *family scapegoat*, which may require them to be the 'bad' child. As a general rule, families which fail to provide satisfactory social training for their children often have many of the problem-solving, communication, role behaviour, affective involvement, control and other difficulties described by family therapists, and discussed in *Basic Family Therapy* (Barker, 1992, especially Chapters 5 and 10).

(b) Extrafamilial factors

These comprise the school, the wider social setting of family and school, and the child's peer group. We have seen, in Chapter 2, how important a child's school can be in influencing both academic progress and behaviour. These findings are supported by clinical experience. Dramatic changes in children's behaviour and progress, for better or for worse, may follow a change of school or, sometimes, even a change of teacher or class.

Several studies have found a higher prevalence of conduct disorders in urban than in rural areas. Prevalence is particularly high in the more run-down and deprived areas of big cities. This cannot be entirely explained by the migration to cities of poorly functioning families or the mentally ill (Rutter, 1981). It seems that, generally speaking, cities are less healthy places to rear children than rural settings, though the prevalence of problems can vary a lot in different areas of the same city. The effects of city life may operate more at the family level than on individual children, but at present they are far from being understood. Close supervision of children tends to be more difficult in large urban areas than in villages and rural areas. In the country everyone tends to know everyone else's business. This may have its disadvantages but it does tend to mean that children can get away with less without being caught, and that if they are not where they are supposed to be, their parents are more likely to hear about it!

Adolescents in particular are often greatly influenced by their peer groups. How great a role group pressures and dynamics play in the genesis of antisocial behaviour is however unclear. Many serious antisocial activities are carried out in the company of others, rather than alone. This has been found to apply to girls even more that it does to boys (Emler, *et al.*, 1987). Possible explanations for these findings are that involvement with the group is a causal factor; or that delinquent youths choose to associate with one another but do not become more delinquent as a result; or that young people tend to do things together and that this applies no more to delinquent than to other activities. On the whole it seems likely that there is a causal connection.

(5) The interaction of factors

The causative factors discussed above are not independent of each other. Temperament, for example, is in part genetically determined but may be modified by environmental factors. The same applies to many aspects of cognitive functioning. Physical disease may lead to adverse parental attitudes in addition to its more direct effects on children. The *goodness of fit* between child and environment may be a crucial issue ... and so on. The antisocial behaviour we observe in children is usually the outcome of the interplay of many forces. Some of these may be difficult or impossible to modify but there are always some that are open to intervention.

Description

Children with conduct disorders display what ICD-10 describes as 'a repetitive and persistent pattern of dissocial, aggressive, or defiant conduct'. These disorders involve major violations of age-appropriate social expectations. Typical behaviours are bullying and fighting; severe destructiveness to property; firesetting; excessive levels of disobedience, rudeness, uncooperativeness, and resistance to authority; severe tantrums and uncontrolled rages; and cruelty to animals and to other children. Older children may engage in extortion and violent assault. The behaviour may or may not be confined to specific situations such as home, school or community.

The following are the main features of the categories of conduct disorders proposed in ICD-10:

(a) Conduct disorder confined to the family context

In many cases conduct disorder symptoms first become evident within the family group. Behavioural difficulties are often evident long before the child's behaviour patterns are sufficiently disturbed to meet the criteria for conduct or oppositional defiant disorder. On the other hand, not all 'naughty' behaviour in young children presages serious behaviour problems later. Yet the origins of later problems can often be traced back many years – to the pre-school or even the toddler period.

For the ICD-10 criteria for 'conduct disorder confined to the family context' to be met, the features mentioned above must be present and the abnormal behaviour must be entirely, or almost entirely, confined to the home or to interactions with the immediate family. In practice, though, such clinical pictures do not suddenly emerge in their complete form. Some of these children have had difficult temperaments from early in life and the process of teaching them 'prosocial' behaviour has proved difficult. Oppositional behaviour, disobedience, or aggressive behaviour, lying and stealing may have been problems long before the criteria for conduct disorder are met.

(b) Unsocialized conduct disorder

Both ICD-10 and DSM-III-R have made a distinction between socialized and unsocialized conduct disorders. In DSM-IV, this distinction is not drawn. According to ICD-10 a diagnosis of unsocialized conduct disorder is appropriate when there is 'persistent dissocial or aggressive behaviour ... with a significant pervasive abnormality in the individual's relationships with other children'. The general criteria for conduct disorders have to be met. The offences are usually, but not invariably, carried out by the subject alone.

(c) Socialized conduct disorder

This involves behaviours similar to those seen in unsocialized disorders, the main distinction being that these children are generally well integrated into their peer group. They have adequate, lasting friendships with other children, usually but not invariably of about the same age. This does not preclude their bullying or being aggressive to others. Relationships with adult authority figures tend to be poor. As the disorder progresses, the antisocial behaviours may be manifest in an increasingly wide range of situations. Truancy from school, staying out late, running away from home and acts of vandalism may be followed by progression to criminal activities such as shoplifting, stealing from cars, and breaking into, and stealing from, houses.

Sometimes the behaviour problems first appear in school. They may coincide with a deterioration in the quality of school work, as the child's hostile attitudes are expressed as defiance of the teachers' instructions. In yet other cases, particularly when conduct disorders first develop in adolescence, the problem behaviours are first manifest in the wider community. Careful enquiry may however reveal evidence of co-existing problems at home and/or in school.

(d) Oppositional defiant disorders

DSM-IV describes these disorders as distinct from conduct disorders, although they are grouped with conduct disorders under the heading 'disruptive behaviour disorders'. ICD-10, on the other hand, classifies them as a subgroup of conduct disorders but states that they are 'characteristically seen in children below the age of 9 or 10 years'. Oppositional defiant disorder (ODD) is defined 'by the *presence* of markedly defiant, disobedient, provocative behaviour and by the *absence* of more severe dissocial or aggressive acts that violate the law or the rights of others' as ICD-10 puts it. The overall features of conduct disorders, set out above, need to be present, but children with these disorders do not violate the rights of others by such behaviours as theft, cruelty, bullying, assault and destructiveness.

DSM-IV, while describing ODD in similar terms, makes a clearer distinction between ODD and CD. It states that if the criteria for CD are met the diagnosis of ODD should not be made.

Whether there is a qualitative difference between ODD and other conduct disorders (CD), or whether the difference is one of degree is unclear. According to ICD-10 conduct disorders in older children are 'usually accompanied by dissocial or aggressive behaviour that goes beyond defiance, disobedience or disruptiveness'. Children with such disorders may have previously displayed the symptoms of oppositional defiant disorders.

Specific symptoms

Stealing is common in CD. Virtually every child has stolen something at some time and stealing only becomes abnormal when it is severe and persistent and fails to respond to commonsense measures instituted by parents or others. Persistent failure to respect others' property is a sign of deviant development. It may be associated with rejecting, inconsistent or indifferent parental attitudes.

Aggressive behaviour is a common cause of referral. It may present as temper tantrums, verbal threats or physical attacks on others, often occurring with little apparent provocation.

Truancy from school is one of the features of conduct disorder listed in both ICD-10 and DSM-IV. It is the wilful and unjustifiable avoidance of attendance at school by a child who is supposed to be there. It differs from school refusal, sometimes known as 'school phobia', which is a condition in which the child stays away from school because of overwhelming anxiety associated with the idea of going to school. The truant, by contrast, fails to attend because of a greater desire to do something else, be it play in the park, attend the video arcade or sit at home watching television. These children may leave home and return there at the appropriate times, but without having gone to school. The parents may think they are at school, while the school staff assume there is a legitimate reason, such as illness, for their absence. It is remarkable how long this situation sometimes continues. If there is no parent at home during the day the child may sit at home, failing to answer the doorbell and destroying any letters that may come from the school. Some forge notes, ostensibly from their parents, excusing them from attendance. Others get their friends to impersonate their parents in telephone calls to the school.

Truancy is seldom purely the child's problem. These are often poorly supervised children whose parents may take little interest in their schooling and may not rate education highly. Some even actively encourage or excuse truancy in order to have the child at home to babysit for younger children or help with housework. Truants, unlike most children with school refusal, tend to have poor academic records and the consequent lack of satisfaction they get at school may be an additional factor discouraging attendance. Many truants come from materially and culturally deprived homes, though some are rebellious children from affluent families.

Factors in school may contribute to truancy. Other things being equal, a child is more likely to attend a school if it provides an enjoyable, rewarding and affirming experience, and its staff are willing and able to help the child with any learning, personal, or family problems that may exist.

Like most children's behaviour problems, the causes of truancy are complex. An excellent, concise summary is that of Reid (1986). Other useful sources are Reid (1985) and Berg (1985).

Vandalism, the wanton damaging or destruction of property, is often a group activity of adolescents. Whether it is carried out by a group or an individual, however, it seems usually to be a means whereby the vandals are expressing hostile, aggressive feelings. Such feelings may arise from disturbed relationship with parents, but the choices which young people make to select schools or churches for their attentions suggest that other feelings may sometimes play their part. In healthily developing children, aggressive drives are channelled into constructive activities – that is, they are 'sublimated'. Failure of sublimation may be due to faulty relationships and identifications. Social factors may operate also. The absence of suitable facilities for sports and recreational programs, together with pressures from antisocially inclined peers may be contributing factors. Closely related to vandalism is the raising of false alarms, for example sending ambulances or the fire brigade to non-existent emergencies.

Firesetting is a relatively uncommon – compared to other conduct disorder symptoms – but serious symptom. Many children go through a stage of playing with matches and lighting fires, but this usually responds to parental training and precept. Children who instead go on to set fires deliberately are often expressing severe, deep-seated aggressive feelings, arising from profoundly disturbed family relationships.

Some 2 to 3% of children referred for child psychiatric help have set fires (Jacobson, 1985a). In many cases this is but one of a number of conduct disorder symptoms but a small group are referred specifically because they have set fires (Jacobson, 1985b).

Jacobson (1985a) reviewed the cases of 104 firesetters seen in an inner London clinic, comparing them with 'age-, sex- and class-matched non-firesetters with equivalent diagnoses'. Most were diagnosed as having conduct disorders. Specific reading retardation was more common in the fire-setters than in the non-firesetting controls, and the former were also found to show 'marked antisocial and aggressive behaviour'. Family discord was 50% more frequent in the firesetters who comprised 5.5% of the children with conduct disorders. The boy:girl ratio was 5:1 for the fire setters, compared with the overall clinic ratio of 1:82 and that for all conduct disorders of 1:82. In firesetters under 11 it was 13:1, with only four girls among a total of 61. Over the age of 11 the ratio was 2.3:1. There were age peaks at 8 and 13 (Jacobson, 1985b).

Bradford & Dimock (1986) studied 46 adolescent arsonists, 39 (85%) boys and 7 (15%) girls, referred for forensic psychiatric examination and compared them with a group of 57 adult arsonists similarly referred. The juveniles had backgrounds characterized by parental alcoholism and major psychiatric illness, physical abuse and father absence (the latter in 40% of cases). Seven (15%) were mentally retarded. There was a history of significantly more violent behaviour in the juvenile group. Half of both groups set their own homes alight, most commonly in acts of revenge.

Gaynor & Hatch (1987) provide a comprehensive review of child fire-setting. Emphasizing the scale of the problem they point out that 48% of all those arrested for firesetting in the USA in 1984 were under 18 years of age; and that children under 13 constituted 17.1% of arson arrests in 1977. They suggest that it is important how children's natural curiosity about fire is handled. Upon this depends whether they develop 'fire-safe' or 'fire-risk' behaviour. They summarize the factors associated with fire-setting as follows. Firesetters:

- are mainly boys ten years or older;
- are usually of normal intelligence, though they may have learning disabilities;
- experience overwhelming anger and express aggression inappropriately;
- may have been previously diagnosed as having conduct or personality disorders;
- have unsatisfactory relationships with peers;
- behave and achieve poorly at school;
- have not been well handled when they have displayed previous firesetting behaviour and other behavioural problems;
- often belong to single-parent families and have parents who are distant and uninvolved;
- have families in which there is much aggressive behaviour and a high frequency of stressful events such as repeated geographical moves.

Drug abuse is common among children with conduct disorders, especially adolescents, though younger children are not immune. The latter may sniff glue, solvents, benzine or petrol (gasoline), often in the context of severe emotional deprivation (O'Connor, 1979). Children addicted to inhalants are commonly found among the deprived urban populations of Third World countries, and in deprived subgroups of more developed countries. The abuse of other drugs more often commences in adolescence. It is discussed further in Chapter 18.

Deviant sexual behaviour is a feature of some conduct disorders. It may take the form of intercourse at unacceptably early age. Some behaviourally disturbed children sexually victimize other, often younger, children. Although rape and other sexual offences may be part of a general pattern of antisocial behaviours, especially in teenagers with severe conduct disorders, they sometimes occur as isolated symptoms in young people who are otherwise socially conforming. In such cases the psychopathology is mainly in the area of psychosexual development. Many of these children have themselves been previously sexually abused.

Juvenile delinquency

Juvenile delinquency is more a legal term than a clinical one. It is usually applied to the commission of offences that are against the law. Whether a young person is defined as a delinquent depends on many factors including luck (whether the police are nearby at the time of an offence); the effectiveness of the police in tracking down and prosecuting offenders; local policy concerning the prosecution of juveniles (many are let off with warnings); whether the accused has a lawyer and how skilled the lawyer is; the witnesses the police produce; and the age of the child (in most jurisdiction there is a minimum age of legal responsibility – usually about 10 to 12 – below which a person cannot be charged).

Although it is partly fortuitous whether a child becomes a legally defined delinquent, those who do so tend to be more seriously disturbed than those with conduct disorders who do not.

Associated disorders

There is considerable overlap between conduct disorders and *attention-deficit/hyperactivity disorder* (ADDH) (DSM-IV) and *hyperkinetic disorders* (ICD-10). The features of both may co-exist and DSM-IV permits the making of both diagnoses in the same patient. It also acknowledges their close relationship by listing both under the same heading. In the ICD-10 diagnostic scheme, hyperkinetic disorder is 'diagnosed with priority over conduct disorder' when its criteria are met, but ICD-10 also has a category of 'hyperkinetic conduct disorder' for use when both the overall criteria for hyperkinetic disorders and those for conduct disorders are met. This seems to be an acknowledgement that this is often the case. ADDH and hyperkinetic disorders are discussed further in Chapter 7.

Reading disability

This is commonly associated with conduct disorders. Epidemiological studies have found that about one-third of children with conduct disorders are retarded in reading and one third of those with reading retardation have conduct disorders (Rutter, *et al.*, 1970b; Rutter, *et al.*, 1975b). It seems more likely that common factors contribute to both problems rather than one being the *cause* of the other. Follow-up studies suggest that the combination of reading retardation and behavioural problems often leads to serious difficulties later (Maughan, *et al.*, 1985).

Depression

This may also be associated with conduct disorders. Puig-Antich (1982) reported that 37% of pre-pubertal boys with major depression also met the DSM-III criteria for conduct disorder, and that behaviour improved when the depression responded to treatment, relapsing again when depression recurred.

Marriage, *et al.* (1986) reported that 11 of 33 children with affective disorders (33%) also met DSM-III criteria for conduct disorder. Ten had dysthymic disorders (see Chapter 10) and one major depression.

Treatment

Since children with the disorders described in this chapter have failed to learn and/or apply some of the rules and customs of the society of which they are part, treatment should aim to correct the learning process and promote prosocial as opposed to antisocial behaviour. In order to do this a careful assessment of child and family, and of the wider environment, particularly the child's situation in school, is necessary. This assessment, and the formulation arising from it, should point to the factors that have led to the failure in the socialization process. This information then makes it possible to develop a rational treatment plan.

Some causative factors are more susceptible to therapeutic intervention than others. Environmental, as opposed to biological, including temperamental ones, are generally easier to modify.

Constitutional factors

These do not generally lend themselves to ready modification, though there is probably much scope for prevention in this area. High quality antenatal care and the better nutrition and stimulation of infants are likely to pay dividends in the long term. The consequences of some biological disorders may be also be addressed. An example is the dietary treatment of phenylketonuria which can prevent those with this condition becoming mentally retarded. Also, it can be helpful to explain to parents and other care-givers that certain problem behaviours are related to the child's temperamental style, for which biological factors are principally responsible, rather than to the way the child has been reared. This can help both by reducing parental guilt feelings and by framing the problem as being that of a child requiring specially skilled parenting rather than one who is being wilfully naughty. The situation is thus presented as a challenge to be met, rather than as the result of parental failures.

Physical diseases, injuries and handicaps

These cannot always be completely rectified. Children who have problems with reading or other specific learning problems can usually be helped by appropriate special educational measures. Treatments of various kinds – occupational therapy and physical therapy – can also help children with motor coordination problems or more severe physical disabilities.

Temperamental factors and *goodness of fit* often need to be addressed. While there are few research data about how we may improve the *fit* between the temperaments of children and those of their parents, it is usually helpful to make the *lack of fit* explicit and discuss with all family members what modifications each of them needs to make to rectify the situation. The principles of learning theory, described in Chapter 21, can be helpful here, but simply clarifying what the problem is can itself be valuable.

Environmental factors

There are often the ones that are most susceptible to change. The family environment is of crucial importance. Patterson (1982) suggests that parents may need to learn:

- to develop and apply well defined house rules, with clearly set expectations concerning meals and other activities;
- to monitor consistently the behaviour of their children, so that they know what their children are doing and how they are feeling;

- to apply effective contingencies, that is consistent responses to the children's behaviour, following through with appropriate rewards and consequences when these are needed;
- effective techniques for dealing with crises or problems in the family, so that tensions and disputes are resolved before they get out of hand.

There are various means whereby the above may be achieved. Any of the following may be indicated.

(a) Parental counselling

This may be done with parental couples (or single parents) seen on their own, or in group settings. The teaching of the principles of behaviour modification (see Chapter 21 and also Murdoch & Barker, 1991) is often a good basis for this work.

(b) Family therapy

There are often major problems in the families of children with conduct disorders. When this is so, changes in the way the family functions may be necessary before there can be substantial change in the children's behaviour. In the more seriously dysfunctional families, it is not usually sufficient to tell the parents to make the kinds of changes listed in the previous section. A certain level of family stability may be needed before they can do this and problems like parental alcoholism and the abuse of other drugs may need to be tackled as a first priority.

Family therapy is discussed further in Chapter 21 and in more detail in *Basic Family Therapy* (Barker, 1992).

(c) Behaviour therapy

Well planned behaviour therapy programs, instituted with attention to detail, seem to be the most effective direct means of treating conduct disorders. As mentioned above, they may be used as a basis for the counselling of parents, and they may be used directly with children in schools, treatment centres, residential institutions and in the home. Behaviour therapy is discussed further in Chapter 21.

Other therapeutic options

The school environment

This often requires attention. Changes in the way children are dealt with in school, including the rational use of behaviour therapy techniques, may be indicated. While we are not usually in a position to bring about radical changes in the social structures of schools, contacts with teachers, school counsellors and school psychologists can be very productive. They may provide school staff with a better understanding of the needs of the child and the family, and suggest alternative management techniques when those they have been using have proved unsuccessful. It is also important that there be good relationships and close cooperation between family and school. When children have been playing truant from school, it is essential that parents and school staff are agreed on how to ensure that any failure to attend school without due cause is promptly detected and dealt with in a planned and rational way.

Berg (1985) provides an excellent account of an approach to the management of truancy used in the UK. A successful approach for less disturbed truants seems to be the *adjournment procedure*. The case is taken to court which simply adjourns it for a few weeks to give time for school attendance to be re-established. A few adjournments two to four weeks apart may be enough to restore satisfactory attendance. Berg (1985) also suggests that this may reduce delinquent behaviour.

In some cases a change of school or teacher can be helpful. The question of *goodness of fit* between child and teacher is probably relevant. Clinical experience suggests that some teachers find certain children, for example, those with *difficult* temperaments particularly hard to deal with, whereas another teacher may fare better with the same child. We know also that the social climates in schools vary (Rutter, *et al.*, 1979), which probably explains why a change of school can sometimes have a salutary effect, occasionally even marking a turning point in the progress of a child who seemed headed for behavioural disaster.

Individual psychotherapy

This has a rather small part to play in the treatment of children with conduct disorders, except when these are associated with past abuse, especially sexual abuse. Unfortunately many of these children have little or no motivation to engage in psychotherapy. It is rarely they who are complaining about the problems with which they are presented for treatment, and indeed they may sometimes get some vicarious satisfaction from their defiant or antisocial behaviour. Nevertheless, in that minority of children who have a high level of consciously felt anxiety, which includes some abused children, and those who have a strong conscious desire to change their way of life, individual therapy has a place. Many children displaying antisocial behaviour have low levels of self-esteem and in this area also individual therapy can be of value.

Group psychotherapy

This suffers from some of the same disadvantages as individual therapy. Nevertheless, groups which enhance the young person's self-esteem, or provide these children with opportunities to learn new social or vocational skills – for example, drama, dance, martial arts, ceramics, gymnastics, carpentry or metalworking – can provide significant help. For abused children, participation in a group with other children who have had similar experiences can be powerfully therapeutic.

Residential treatment

This has often been advocated for children with severe conduct disorders but its results have been generally disappointing. The best results seem to be those of centres using well planned and intensive behaviour therapy methods. It is relatively easy to achieve improvement in the behaviour of children with conduct disorders if they are placed in a highly structured residential setting with strict behavioural controls – that is consistently applied rewards and sanctions. This is of little value, however, if the improved behaviour is not generalized to other situations. Indeed it often happens that children who appear to have done well while in residential settings, revert to their old behaviour on return to the community from which they have come. The best way to avoid this unfortunate turn of events seems to be to involve the parents actively while the child is in residential treatment. They need to learn, and then to use, the behavioural management techniques used by the treatment staff and to continue doing so after their child is discharged home. The outcome depends very much on how willing and able they are to do this.

Day treatment

This is an alternative to residential treatment. It has the advantage of not separating the young person from the family full-time. When the child is at home in the evenings and at weekends, the family members can practise the skills they are learning in treatment. Progress is monitored, and input provided as needed, by the treatment staff.

Hybrid programs are also possible, such as five-day residential treatment. The child may receive active treatment from Monday to Friday and then spend the weekend at home, progress during that time being reviewed when the parents bring the child back to the treatment centre on Monday morning. Some treatment programs have staff on call during the weekend, so that parents, or children, can telephone them to discuss problems that arise during the weekend.

Some residential and day treatment programs use the 'therapeutic community' concept. This may be especially useful for adolescents. The treatment is structured so that the main therapeutic agent is the community and the considerable pressure it can exert on the individuals in it. Related to this concept is the *positive peer culture*, a treatment approach in which group process and the influence of the young person's peers are used as the main change-promoting agents (Vorrath & Brendthro, 1985).

Other environmental changes

These may need to be considered but the influence of the neighbourhood culture is even harder to modify than that of the school, unless the family can move to another neighbourhood. In considering whether to suggest or endorse such a move, it is well to bear in mind that neighbourhood influences are not usually the central problem but just contributory factors. The functioning of the family system is more important in the majority of instances.

Medication

This has only a small role to play in the treatment of conduct disorders, unless there are associated conditions such as epilepsy or attention-deficit hyperactivity disorder. The proper control of epilepsy is important regardless of whether there are associated behaviour problems. Occasionally it may be necessary to use tranquilizers such as phenothiazine drugs or haloperidol to control acutely and violently aggressive young people, but in adequately staffed units this should rarely be necessary. Other drugs that may have a limited role in the treatment of these disorders are discussed in Chapter 21.

As a general rule, medication is not an effective treatment for conduct disorders. Indeed their use has a number of drawbacks. The *artificial* control of symptoms by medication may preclude the possibility of teaching the necessary skills to parents, child and others who may be involved. If symptoms are pharmacologically repressed it is hard to work constructively on them. Yet another problem is that the use of medication may give the young person and other family members the message that there is a magical pharmacological solution to the problems, whereas in reality what is needed is the learning of new social skills, the incorporation of new values and beliefs, the acquisition of improved relationship skills and, usually, changes in the way the family system functions. Ever present also are the danger that drug dependence may develop and the risk of undesired side effects. For example, while it may be possible to achieve some control over aggressive behaviour by the use of tranquillizing drugs, this is often at the cost of some sedation which may impair the child's school performance.

Treating associated conditions

Reading retardation

This and other educational problems, when they are present, should be tackled energetically using appropriate remedial education techniques. Although the academic problems which many of these children have may not cause the behaviour problems, their persistence makes it harder to improve the child's self-esteem as well as making for difficulties in adjustment in school. By the time they present for treatment, many of these children are so retarded in their reading that much of the school work their classmates are doing is beyond them. They may even be unable to read the instructions relating to mathematical and other tasks.

Depression

If present, this should receive appropriate treatment. As mentioned above there have been reports suggesting that behavioural improvement is often seen in depressed children with conduct disorder symptoms when the depression resolves, the symptoms returning with recurrence of the depression.

Severe emotional deprivation

This presents a special therapeutic challenge. It is present in the background, past, present or both, of many children who display antisocial behaviour. Children who have suffered such deprivation from early in life, or through a long period during their childhood, often seem to lack the capacity to form deep and satisfying emotional relationships. When this is so, establishing helpful relationships with the child can be very difficult. In some cases a long period of treatment in a specialized residential treatment setting offers the best hope of effecting improvement, but skilled care and continuity of staffing are required.

Theoretically a good foster home might be better for such children when their own family cannot provide for their emotional needs, but few foster parents have the emotional and personality resources to cope with such children. They may get little response from these children over a long period, while at the same time being subject to constant, and often very distressing *testing out* behaviour. Such behaviour reflects the difficulty these children have in trusting people. Their behaviour seems often to be designed, at an unconscious level if not at a conscious one, to find out whether their present caretakers do really care about them. Those responsible for the care and treatment of these children often face hard choices. While a substitute family setting in which the child's angry, rebellious and generally objectionable behaviour could be contained and worked through would usually be the ideal treatment setting, the risk of failure and rejection from the home, with its damaging consequences for the child, is seldom worth taking. Schemes have however been devised in various centres to train specialized foster parents, and to provide them with the necessary support to provide care for these children in their homes – a challenging task!

Outcome

Many minor and some major conduct disorders clear up with little or no treatment. Some are related to difficulties children and their families experience in surmounting developmental hurdles; when these are overcome the behaviour problems may subside. In other cases psychosocial stress, in the family or outside it, contributes and when the stress lessens or disappears the behaviour problems may resolve. Much depends on the basic stability of the family, parental attitudes, the child's personality and temperament, and whether there are continuing stresses facing child and family.

Despite the above, the outcome for many children with conduct disorders is not good. Those with severe conduct disorders, especially those that have appeared in court, tend in adult life to have a high incidence of psychiatric illness and often engage in antisocial and criminal behaviour (Robins, 1966; Rutter, 1980b). The fact is that severe and persistent antisocial behaviour, particularly when it has its origins in early childhood, is inclined to have a poor outcome. Long term treatment is often necessary and there is a case for regarding such children as suffering from a chronic disorder which requires continuing monitoring and follow-up at least into early adult life (Shamsie, 1992).

The combination of conduct disorder symptoms with reading retardation seems often to lead to a particularly poor outcome, at least in boys with severe reading problems, of average ability and below from mainly working class backgrounds – findings reported by Maughan, *et al.* (1985). These children tended to have high rates of early school leaving, unstable work records and seriously depressed skill levels.

Chapter 7

Hyperkinetic and Attention Deficit Disorders

Definitions, descriptions and prevalence

It has long been recognized that some children are strikingly more active than others. When the degree of activity reaches a certain level children may be deemed *hyperactive*. Often associated with hyperactivity is a short attention span, which is the essential feature of *attention deficit disorders* (ADD). It has also been suggested that ADD may occur without co-existing hyperactivity.

Both the definition and the classification of these disorders have been, and remain, the subject of much debate. As Lucas (1992) points out, the concept of attention deficit disorder, 'although the focus of intensive research in the USA, has not impressed the majority of UK psychiatrists with its validity'.

A 'hyperkinetic syndrome of childhood' has long been recognized and was listed in ICD-9. ICD-10 recognizes *hyperkinetic disorders* and divides them into two main subcategories, *disturbance of activity and attention* and *hyperkinetic conduct disorder*. It also lists *other hyperkinetic disorders* and *hyperkinetic disorder, unspecified* (the use of which is not recommended).

The classifications previously put forward by the American Psychiatric Association (DSM-III and DSM-III-R) have emphasized problems of attention at the expense of hyperactivity. DSM-III had categories for attention-deficit disorders with, and without, hyperactivity. This changed in DSM-III-R which simply listed the category, *attention-deficit hyper-activity disorder*. DSM-III-R also grouped attention-deficit disorders along with conduct disorders and oppositional disorders under the general rubric of *disruptive behaviour disorders*. This was presumably an acknowledgement of the close relationship between ADD and conduct disorders, the symptoms of which often co-exist. This close relationship is also reflected in the ICD-10 category of *hyperkinetic conduct disorder*.

DSM-IV presents the division of the conditions in three subtypes:

(1) Attention-deficit/hyperactivity combined type (ADHD-CT). This is to be diagnosed if six or more symptoms of inattention and six or

more of hyperactivity-impulsivity have persisted for six months or more.

(2)   Attention-deficit/hyperactivity disorder, predominantly inattentive type (ADHD-I) – with six or more inattention symptoms and fewer than six hyperactivity-impulsivity symptoms.

(3)   Attention-deficit/hyperactivity disorder, predominantly hyper-active-impulsive type (ADHD-HI) – with the pattern of symptoms the reverse of (2).

Disruptive behaviour, hyperactivity, conduct disorders, oppositional behaviour and problems of attention often, in various combinations, occur together. It is unclear how far the delineation of specific syndromes within this rather complex spectrum of conditions is a valid exercise, and there seems to be agreement only on the need for a great deal more research.

According to ICD-10, the cardinal features of hyperkinetic disorders (HD) are impaired attention and overactivity. These should be present in more than one situation – such as home, classroom or clinic. Children with HD have short attention spans, breaking off from tasks before these are finished, changing frequently from one activity to another, and appearing to lose interest in one task because they become involved in another.

Overactivity, as described in ICD-10, is manifested in excessive rest-lessness, especially in situations where calm is required. These children fidget more than other children, they may run and jump around, get up when they should remain seated, and behave in unduly noisy and talkative ways. When are these behaviours sufficient to justify a diagnosis of HD? ICD-10 suggests that it is a matter of whether the activity is excessive in light of the context in which it occurs, and of the child's age and intelligence level. DSM-IV has similar criteria for DHD-HI, but emphasises also the impulsivity of these children.

Associated symptoms, which are neither sufficient nor necessary for the diagnosis, include disinhibition in social relationships, reckless behaviour in dangerous situations, and the impulsive flouting of social rules, for example talking out in class when this is not appropriate.

Causes

No single cause for these disorders has been identified. Simple motor overactivity, as distinct from the hyperactivity seen in the disorders we are discussing, may be no more than one extreme of the range of activity levels that exists in any population – just as children may be unusually tall, or short, without having anything wrong with them. Whether the hyperactivity that occurs in children with HD or ADDH can be explained on this basis is not clear. Chess & Thomas' (1984) concept of *goodness of fit* between the temperaments of children and those of their parents may be of help here. It is possible that children at the *very active* end of the spectrum of motor activity may, if they happen to have parents who are temperamentally unsuited to the rearing of very active children, encounter 'problems' which might not be problems for other parents; the less-than-optimal responses of such parents to their children may in turn lead to a worsening of the child's behaviour and have repercussions in the family as a whole. There is some evidence that genetic factors contribute to these disorders. Goodman & Stevenson (1989) studied 128 monozygotic (MZ) and 212 dizygotic (DZ) twin pairs, assessing attention and hyperactivity in each. They found a higher concordance in respect to these behaviours in the MZ same-sex twin pairs than in the DZ same-sex pairs. They concluded that 30 to 50% of the variation in hyperactivity was due to genetic factors. Schachar (1991) has however pointed out that the study had some methodological limitations. He suggests that childhood hyperactivity may be 'one behavioural expression of a heritable temperamental factor that places children at risk for the development of all types of disruptive behaviour' (page 174).

Schachar (1991), in a comprehensive review, points out that we may not be dealing with a single entity but that 'the weight of the evidence points to a generalized neurodevelopmental delay or abnormality underlying hyperactivity'. Evidence for this includes the association of hyperactivity with low IQ, clumsiness, language delay, abnormalities of speech, and perinatal complications. Despite this, it is clear that both hyperactivity and ADD occur in some children who show no evidence of neurodevelopmental delay. Schachar suggests that either developmental delay or attention deficit may have expression in behavioural hyperactivity.

Many other factors have been suggested as possible causes of the conditions we are considering in this chapter. These include diet, the effects of toxins such as lead, and psychosocial disadvantage. There seems to be a valid distinction between *situational hyperactivity* and *pervasive hyperactivity*. The former is limited to certain social situations and seems to be particularly prevalent in school, often affecting children with cognitive impairment and socioeconomic disadvantage. Some believe it is simply a mild form of pervasive hyperactivity, whereas an alternative view is that, unlike the pervasive variety which is more widely generalized, it is predominantly a reactive disorder. (See Schachar (1991) for a discussion of this issue.) It is not difficult to understand how cognitively impaired and socioeconomically disadvantaged children might find school more stressful than other children find it.

The great majority of children with HD and ADD do not have elevated blood lead levels. Evidence that diet plays a substantive role in the causation of these disorders is lacking, though some studies have suggested that diet may have a minor role in some cases (Egger *et al.*, 1985).

How far psychological and psychosocial factors contribute to HD and ADD is not clearly established. Most of us find that our powers of concentration tend to be impaired when we are anxious or tense. The focusing and sustaining of attention are to some extent learned skills, and learning such skills may not occur so well in disorganized and unstable families. Hard data on this are lacking, however. Schachar (1991) points out that recent studies comparing hyperactivity, conduct disturbance and mixed disorders, have found that conduct disorders and mixed disorders, but not hyperactivity, are associated with a rate of parental disturbance greater than that found in control families. Schachar & Waschsmuth (1990) reported a lack of association between both pervasive and situational hyperactivity on the one hand, and parental psychopathology on the other.

Prevalence

Widely differing prevalence figures for these disorders have been obtained in epidemiological studies of child populations. These differences reflect the diagnostic confusion which exists in this area, the differing research protocols used, and the different age groups studied. Schachar (1991) summarized the results of five epidemiological studies reported in the decade from 1981 to 1991. There is agreement among them that ADD alone (that is, without hyperactivity) is relatively uncommon, probably occurring in 1 to 1.5% of the child population. Attention-deficit disorder with hyperactivity (ADDH) is much more common, the prevalence figures that have been found ranging from 6 to 17%. Pervasive hyperactivity defined by parent and teacher questionnaires only – that is, without clinical assessment of the children), ranges from 0.5 to 9.9%, almost a twenty-fold difference. Only one of these five studies estimated the prevalence of the *hyperkinetic syndrome* (as defined by the presence of reports of pervasive hyperactivity, together with the results of clinical interviews with the children); this was a study of 7- and 8-year-old boys and the prevalence rate found was 1.7%.

Epidemiological studies do agree that comorbidity is common. In the five studies summarized by Schachar (1991), comorbidity rates for conduct disorder of 30 to 48%, and for emotional disorder of 14 to 70%, were reported. Using ICD-10, many of these children would presumably meet the criteria for hyperkinetic conduct disorder.

The various epidemiological studies also agree that these disorders are more common in boys than in girls. In the Ontario Health Study, the overall percentages for hyperactivity in the age range 4 to 16 were 8.9 for boys and 3.3 for girls. The disproportion was greater in the 4 to 11 age group (10.1:3.3) than in the 12 to 16 age group (7.3:3.4) (Offord, *et al.*, 1987).

Description

The main features of these disorders were set out in the opening section of this chapter. Regardless of how this group of conditions is classified, it is clear that there is a group of children who present with motor hyperactivity, restlessness, impaired attention and impulsivity. Although readily distractible, they attend only briefly to distracting stimuli.

Onset is usually before the age of three but many of these children do not come to professional attention until they start school. It often seems, in retrospect, that hyperactivity was manifest even in early infancy, and some mothers report that the child was unusually active *in utero*.

Most often the hyperactive behaviour has become apparent when the child started to walk, though some parents, especially those who have had non-hyperactive children previously, realize that the child is different sooner than that. These children are typically on the go all the time, they concentrate on things poorly, and they may interfere with furniture, ornaments, the contents of drawers and other items to an unusual extent. Sleep disturbance is often reported, though some seem to be so tired after a day of frantic activity that they sleep well.

Entry into school may precipitate a crisis. Up until that time the parents may have been able to cope with the child's behaviour, but the additional demands which school makes upon the child, especially the need to attend to what is being taught and the tasks set, may cause problems for child and teacher. The child may fail to respond to the disciplinary measures used by the teacher, and may disrupt the class and display other problem behaviour such as failure to comply to instructions, aggression towards other children, and noisy, over-talkative behaviour.

These children's non-compliance and failure to complete tasks set them are not wilful behaviours. Nevertheless the children may be blamed and even punished for their misdeeds. This may lead to secondary emotional disturbance. In due course they may fall behind in their school work and become disheartened, even depressed. Much however depends on how early their disorder is diagnosed, and how it – and they – are dealt with by those caring for and teaching them.

The early chapters of *Hyperactive Children Grown Up* (Weiss & Hechtman, 1986) are a good source of information about how these conditions affect individuals at different stages of childhood, adolescence and young adult life.

Assessment and treatment

Assessment and treatment should go hand in hand. A rational treatment plan can only be developed on the basis of a comprehensive assessment of child and family, and also of the child's situation at school. It is necessary to establish the type and severity of the child's motor activity and/or attention problems; the situations in which these are more, or less, marked or completely absent; whether there are any associated learning difficulties or perceptual problems; and whether there are such associated psychiatric problems as conduct disorder or emotional disorder. A good understanding of the child's social situations at home, at school and in the local community is also needed. Depending on this assessment, any combination of the following may be required.

Medication

Although it is no panacea and is seldom, if ever, an adequate treatment on its own, medication has an established place in the treatment of these disorders. Methylphenidate, a cerebral stimulant, in appropriate doses, usually improves concentration and classroom behaviour and decreases impulsivity. At the same time, previously purposeless activity becomes more goal directed. The drug has also been found to improve on-task behaviour, test-taking attitudes, the organization and sustained deployment of effort, accurate and efficient information processing, and the correction of errors subjects make (Douglas, *et al.*, 1986). The amphetamine group of drugs, the most commonly used one being dextroamphetamine sulphate, have similar effects and were actually introduced before methylphenidate. Pimozide is another stimulant drug which sometimes proves helpful when the previously mentioned drugs prove ineffective or have serious side effects.

While the short-term benefits of these drugs seem established, their longer-term effects are less clear. Despite their use, some children still fail at school, have problems in their relationships with peers, and develop antisocial behaviour.

The action of these drugs is probably not specific to children with hyperkinetic or attention-deficit disorders, since dextroamphetamine has been shown to reduce the activity levels in normal prepubertal children (Rapoport, *et al.*, 1978).

Drugs with tranquillizing properties, such as chlorpromazine, thioridazine and haloperidol may also reduce activity levels, but often at the cost of undue sedation. The antidepressant imipramine, and related tricyclic drugs, have also been reported to be of benefit in some cases.

Dosage, side effects and other information about these drugs are to be found in Chapter 21.

Behaviour modification

Within limits, conditioning procedures, especially operant conditioning, can improve attention span and decrease impulsive behaviour. Cognitive behavioural approaches can also help children with poor impulse control (Kendall & Braswell, 1985). Teaching behaviours that are more adaptive, such as *stop-and-think* procedures, are generally to be preferred to symptomatic treatment using medication.

Parental counselling

The parents of hyperactive children often need much help and support in managing these children. This may range from advice on the arrangement of the home, so that breakable items and things that might present dangers to the child are out of reach, to instruction in behaviour therapy methods designed to modify specific behaviours.

Intervention in school

Their situation in school is the most difficult one for many children with ADD and HD, since the ability to concentrate is necessary in most learning situations. The short attention span of these children is often a real impediment, both to academic learning and to achieving calm and attentive classroom behaviour. In such cases, counselling and support for teachers and other school staff may be helpful. This may involve instructing school staff in the application of behaviour therapy programs, and in the assessment of the effects of treatment, for example by using the Conners Teachers' Rating Scale (Conners, 1969), a useful means of assessing the response of children to medication and other treatments. Remedial educational help may also be needed by children whose academic progress has been impaired as a result of their attentional problems and hyperactivity.

Outcome

Hyperactivity tends to lessen with increasing age, but other features of these disorders may persist well into adult life. *Hyperactive Children Grown*

Up (Weiss & Hechtman, 1986) is a mine of information about the outcome in these children and reviews other studies as well as presenting the authors' own findings. These authors consider the *core symptoms* to be inappropriate restlessness, attentional difficulties, and impulsivity. Though these may lessen in adolescence, they are often still present, but the presenting symptoms are now usually poor school performance, relationship difficulties, and antisocial behaviour, the latter being present in about 25% of these young people. As a group, hyperactive adolescents have lower self-esteem and poorer social skills, and they are more impulsive than normal controls.

By the time they reach adult life, one-third to one-half of these individuals are indistinguishable from normal adults, but a higher percentage of subjects than of controls engage in antisocial behaviour. Their use of alcohol and cannabis products is greater and they report more malaise, score lower on self-rating scales, and have impaired social skills. Some 20% meet the criteria for *antisocial personality disorder*, but most are gainfully employed and economically self-sufficient. As a group, though, they hold jobs for shorter periods, are laid off or quit more often, and have lower status jobs than control subjects. Their work performance is also rated as inferior by their employers. The children studied by Weiss & Hechtman (1986), on which most of the above outcome data are based, were not treated using the methods currently advocated, and whether modern treatment approaches result in better outcomes is not clear.

An interesting feature of the book by Weiss and Hechtman (1986) is a chapter written by one of the subjects in the authors' follow-up study. This gives a rare published insight, from the perspective of adulthood, into what it is like to grow up as a hyperactive child. A further source of information on these children is *The Overactive Child* (Taylor, 1986a).

Chapter 8

Anxiety and Emotional Disorders

Definition and classification

Since child psychiatry's early days, a distinction has been made between disorders whose primary feature is an excessive level of anxiety, whether this is expressed directly or indirectly, and disorders of social behaviour – the conduct and oppositional defiant or *disruptive* disorders. Many terms have been used for the former group of conditions. These include *neuroses, emotional disorders, anxiety disorders, somatoform disorders* and *stress-related disorders*.

DSM-IV has a category for *other disorders of infancy, childhood or adolescence*. One of these is *separation anxiety disorder*. Otherwise all anxiety or emotional disorders are listed in the general section of DSM-IV, which can be used for both adults and children. Here we find a variety of conditions which may be regarded as expressions of or reactions to anxiety. They are divided into three groups:

(1) Anxiety disorders:

- Panic disorders, with or without agoraphobia.
- Agoraphobia without a history of panic disorder.
- Specific phobia.
- Social phobia.
- Obsessive compulsive disorder.
- Post-traumatic stress disorder.
- Acute stress disorder.
- Generalized anxiety disorder.
- Anxiety disorder due to a (specified) general medical condition.
- Anxiety disorder not otherwise specified.

(2) Somatoform disorders:

- Somatization disorder.
- Undifferentiated somatoform disorder.
- Conversion disorder (associated with psychological factors or with both psychological factors and a general medical condition).

- Body dysmorphic disorder (or dysmorphophobia).
- Hypochondrias (or hypochondriacal neurosis).
- Somatoform disorder not otherwise specified.

(3)   Dissociative disorders:

- Dissociative fugue.
- Dissociative amnesia.
- Dissociative identity disorder.
- Depersonalization disorder.
- Dissociative disorder not otherwise specified.

ICD-10 has a list of six categories of 'emotional disorders with onset specific to childhood':

- Separation anxiety disorder of childhood.
- Phobic anxiety disorder of childhood.
- Social anxiety disorder of childhood.
- Sibling rivalry disorder.
- Other childhood emotional disorders.
- Childhood emotional disorder, unspecified.

Like DSM-IV, ICD-10 also lists anxiety disorders in its general section, though under the general heading *neurotic, stress-related and somatoform disorders*. The main categories (though each is subdivided into up to 14 subcategories) are:

(1)   Phobic anxiety disorders.
(2)   Other anxiety disorders.
(3)   Obsessive-compulsive disorder.
(4)   Reaction to severe stress, and adjustment disorders.
(5)   Dissociative [conversion] disorders.
(6)   Somatoform disorders.
(7)   Other neurotic disorders.

The clinical usefulness, in day to day child psychiatric practice, of making the distinctions between the many subgroups listed in DSM-IV and ICD-10 is open to question. More important than assigning a specific label categorizing each child's condition is achieving an understanding of the symptoms, their meaning and how they have arisen in the context in which they are troublesome, with a view to developing an effective treatment plan.

Prevalence

Emotional disorders were found to be present in 2.5% of the 10- and 11-year-olds in the Isle of Wight study (Rutter, *et al.*, 1970b). In the London borough studied later, the prevalence was found to be about twice that found in the Isle of Wight (Rutter, *et al.*, 1975a). In the Ontario Child Health Study (Offord, *et al.*, 1987) the prevalence rates listed in Table 8.1 were found for emotional disorder and somatization – the latter being defined as the presence of recurrent, multiple and vague physical symptoms without evident cause; many of these symptoms may have been somatic expressions of anxiety.

The differences between the Isle of Wight and Ontario may be due to difference in the age ranges studied and in the research methods and definitions used, as well as to real differences in the populations. A striking feature is the much higher overall prevalence of emotional disorder (11.9%), as compared with conduct disorder (2.7%) in girls. In boys the overall prevalence rates for the two groups (emotional 7.9%; conduct 8.1%) were similar, but these figures conceal the fact that emotional disorders were more common in younger boys and conduct disorders in adolescent boys.

Table 8.1 Prevalence rates for emotional disorder and somatization.

Age	Emotional disorder	Somatization	Age	Emotional disorder	Somatization
Boys 4–11	10.2	—	Girls 4–11	10.7	—
12–16	4.9	4.5	12–16	13.6	10.7
4–16	7.9	—	4–16	11.9	—

Causes

As with all psychiatric disorders, we need to consider genetic, constitutional, physical, temperamental and environmental factors.

The role of genetic factors in the aetiology of anxiety disorders is not well established but is probably significant. For example, it appears that in some family trees there is a genetic relationship between obsesssive-compulsive disorder, Gilles de la Tourette's syndrome and chronic tics (See Chapter 15). Autosomal dominant transmission is apparently involved and the inherited disorder may be expressed either as chronic tics, Tourette's syndrome or obsessive-compulsive disorder (Pauls & Leckman, 1986).

The threshold for the development of neurotic anxiety – that is to say anxiety that is of a degree that appears excessive when related to the subject's life situation – varies from person to person. Precisely how genetic, constitutional, temperamental and environmental factors contribute to this variation is not known. In practice we are limited to making clinical judgements. These are based on the history of the child's past anxiety-proneness, and consideration of how far other factors, such as the way parents handle and respond to the child and the stability of the family system, can explain current anxiety levels and ways of reacting to stress. It is clear, though, that some children are more anxiety-prone than others.

Physical disease and disorders may contribute to the development of anxiety in either of two ways. They may cause the child to become anxious, for example as a result of having severe attacks of asthma which may realistically arouse fears of dying; or they may provoke anxious and overprotective attitudes in parents and others concerned with the child's care. Negative reactions by other children may also be experienced by children with chronic physical disorders.

Sometimes the appearance of anxiety symptoms marks the culmination of a long series of stresses. The adverse or unhelpful attitudes of parents and others over the years may have cumulative effects. Relevant questions are: how much has the child been allowed to mix with other children, and to make his or her own decisions, as opposed to having them made by others? Has too much been done or decided for the child? How secure is the relationship of the child to the parents and the rest of the family? Children's capacities in coping with stress seem to be related to such factors. Those brought up by worrying, anxious parents, perhaps themselves suffering from neurotic conditions, tend to become that way also. It is however impossible in clinical practice to know how far this is due to the operation of genetic factors and how far to the existence of an anxious and perhaps overprotective environment in the home. Nevertheless it does seem that children of parents who see the world as an insecure, unsafe and threatening place tend to view it that way also.

The concept of emotional maturity is helpful in understanding anxiety disorders. As they grow up children normally learn gradually to cope with an increasing range of stressful situations. Their capacity to deal with stress without becoming unduly anxious is a measure of their emotional maturity. Childhood is normally characterized by decreasing dependence on parents, the child becoming progressively able to cope with more and more challenges without support from others. When this process is slowed, halted or even reversed, the likelihood of neurotic symptoms appearing increases. Anna Freud (1966) defined *fixation points* as those at which development may be held up, as a result of excessive frustration, excessive gratification or traumatic experiences. The point at which fixation occurs depends on development to date. Fixation tends to occur when a developmental phase has not been negotiated successfully, and the relevant conflicts have not been resolved.

How do family and other environmental factors work to cause, or contribute to, the disorders we are discussing? According to psychodynamic theory, consciously felt anxiety is usually due in part, and often almost entirely, to causes of which the subject is unaware at the conscious level. The repressed feelings and memories are believed to be concerned with difficulties over the handling of sexual, aggressive and other impulses. Such difficulties are likely to arise in children who have experienced unsatisfactory and insecure relationships with their parents, especially during their early years. The processes of development outlined in Chapter 1 have been distorted. The anxiety and guilt which may arise as a response to the Oedipal conflict, for example, are more easily, quickly and satisfactorily overcome in the context of secure relationships with the parents. If these relationships are tainted by anxiety and unpredictable, gross changes of parental mood, children tend to have difficulty dealing with the stresses associated with the many demands of growing up and accepting increasing responsibility for themselves. Children who do not feel able to depend on and trust their parents may come to see the world generally as threatening and hostile. Yet because of children's different strengths, temperaments and personalities, there is much variation in how they respond to situations of this sort.

Behaviourists, such as Eysenck (1959), view the genesis of neurotic symptoms rather differently. They regard neurotic symptoms as learned behaviour. The symptoms themselves are the neurosis and, behaviourists in their purest culture would say, there is no need to postulate unconscious or other underlying causes. Indeed they believe that behaviours generally, whether considered normal or abnormal, are due to the effects of environmental contingencies.

State-dependent learning

Rossi (1986a; 1986b) draws attention to the concept of *state-dependent learning* and its relevance to the development of psychiatric symptoms. Information learned and experiences undergone can often be recalled only in situations and states similar to those in which they were first learned or experienced – that is, they are *state-bound* or *state-dependent*. Rossi goes on to suggest that:

'So-called "psychological conflict" is a metaphor for competing patterns of state-dependent memory and learning. Reframing therapeutic concepts in terms of state-bound patterns of information and behaviour renders them immediately (1) more amenable to operational definition for experimental study in the laboratory, and (2) more available for active, therapeutic utilization than the traditional process of "analysis" and "understanding" (Rossi, 1986b, page 233).'

The idea that symptoms and behaviours may be understood in terms of state-dependent learning is supported by evidence from epidemiological studies. Both the Isle of Wight (Rutter, *et al.*, 1970b) and the Ontario Child Health studies (Offord, *et al.*, 1987) found that children were rarely identified as disturbed both by their parents and by their teachers. Of the children with neuroses identified in the Ontario study, 50% of the boys and 23.9% of the girls were identified by their parents only; 43% of the boys and 64.6% of the girls either by the teacher or the youth concerned; and only 6.9% of the boys and 11.5% of the girls by both sources. These findings suggest that children's emotional disorders are highly context- or state-dependent.

Family systems theory (see Chapter 2) can also help us understand how environmental factors may lead to the development of undue anxiety in a child (or in other family members). Certain family situations may be particularly stressful for children (Barker, 1984):

- The child may be called upon to be a peacemaker between parents and other family members.
- The child may be called upon to be a mediator.
- The child may attempt to detour conflict in the family.
- The child may play the role of ally, supporting one or other family member – for example, the child who feels the obligation to sit up all night to protect the mother from the alcoholic father when he comes home.

All the above are dysfunctional roles for children who, if they find themselves attempting them, may develop anxiety disorders. Other dysfunctional family scenarios which may be associated with anxiety in children are those that tend to infantilize them, so that emotional development is delayed. In other instances we encounter children upon whom pressure is brought to shoulder responsibilities which are too great for their age and level of development, even though their emotional maturity may be age-appropriate. The relationship between anxiety and various patterns of family dysfunction is discussed further by Barker (1984).

Yet another way of looking at the relationship between anxiety and family functioning is to use the concepts of attachment theory. Heard

(1982) discusses the roles of *care-giving* and *care-seeking* behaviours, which she considers to be built-in, interpersonal and complementary; also that of exploratory behaviour which may be contrasted with attachment behaviour. The caregiver normally assists the child in dealing with anxiety-provoking situations; these stimulate attachment behaviour and lead the child to go to the caregiver for help when this is needed. Heard (1982) describes two forms of ineffective caregiving. In the first, this is experienced as underactive, fear-evoking and unresponsive; in the second it is experienced as overactive, fear-evoking and impinging. Children may react to ineffective caregiving in various ways:

- by continuous unassuaged attachment behaviour;
- with frustrated, inhibited and anxious exploratory behaviour;
- by anxious exploration;
- with frustrated and inhibited exploration.

In all of these situations there is failure of the care-giver to respond in such a way as to terminate the attachment behaviour and relieve the anxiety which led to it. Attachment theory on its own – like the other theories mentioned above – does not provide us with an adequate understanding of anxiety disorders. For one thing, it begs the question of why some parents have difficulty acting as effective caregivers. In many instances such difficulties are related to personal problems of the parents themselves and perhaps to characteristics of the family system.

Finally, we must not overlook the wider social environment, especially the school. Academic and social problems in school may contribute to the development of any of the disorders we are considering in this chapter, especially in anxiety-prone children.

To summarize the various approaches to understanding the anxiety disorders of children, the individual psychotherapist might be most concerned to examine the child's intrapsychic processes for factors there, while the behaviourist would probably be more interested in investigating the child's learning experiences and exploring the environmental contingencies maintaining the symptoms. The family therapist will look primarily at the family system and seek to understand its role in the genesis and maintenance of the symptoms, and the therapist with a particular interest in attachment theory will no doubt look closely for problems of attachment. The geneticist is likely to be interested primarily in the degree to which genetic factors contribute, while others may pay special attention to the *goodness-of-fit* between the temperaments of child and parents, and yet others may consider issues of state-dependent learning. These approaches are not mutually exclusive and the rounded clinician will take them all into consideration when dealing with each anxious child.

Categorization and description

ICD-10 distinguishes anxiety (or emotional) disorders specific to child-hood from the anxiety (or neurotic) disorders of adult life though DSM-IV considers only separation anxiety as specific to childhood. The preamble to DSM-10's description of the 'emotional disorders with onset specific to childhood' states that the validity of this distinction is 'uncertain'. It does however make the point that many emotional disorders occurring in childhood 'seem to constitute exaggerations of normal developmental trends rather than phenomena that are abnormal in themselves'. Such conditions are thought to have a generally better prognosis.

Both DSM-IV and ICD-10 recognise *separation anxiety disorders*. This is anxiety manifest upon separation, or the threat of separation, from attachment figures, usually the parents and more often the mother than the father. In DSM-IV, separation anxiety disorder is defined as a disturbance lasting at least four weeks, characterized by recurrent excessive distress when separation from home or major attachment figure occurs or is anticipated, or by worries about separation from or harm coming to a major attachment figure; reluctance or refusal to be separated from, or to go to sleep without being near to, such a person; and excessive distress, perhaps with physical symptoms such as headaches, abdominal pain or vomiting, on separation, or the threat of separation from an attachment figure. There may be nightmares with separation themes. The symptoms of school refusal, discussed later in this chapter, are often present.

ICD-10's description of this disorder is very similar. It specifies also that there should be no generalized disturbance of personality development.

ICD-10 defines 'phobic anxiety disorder of childhood' as conditions in which there are 'developmentally phase-specific' fears when:

- they appear during the developmentally appropriate age period;
- there is an abnormal degree of anxiety; and
- the anxiety is not part of a more generalized disorder.

ICD-10 defines a 'social anxiety disorder of childhood'. This category is to be used only for conditions arising before the age of six years that are 'both unusual in degree and accompanied by problems in social functioning'. The symptoms must not be part of a more generalized emotional disturbance. There is a persistent or recurrent fear and/or avoidance of strangers, who may be adults, peers or both. There is normal attachment to parents or other familiar people. The social avoidance is beyond the range of normal for the child's age and there must be 'clinically significant problems in social functioning'. This category takes in the 'avoidant disorder of childhood' described in DSM-III-R.

Yet another category described in ICD-10 is that of *sibling rivalry disorder*. It is defined as occurring following the birth of a sibling (usually the immediately younger one). There is evidence of sibling rivalry or jealousy of an abnormal degree with associated psychosocial problems.

As we have seen, in addition to disorders which are defined as having their onset during childhood or adolescence, both ICD-10 and DSM-IV identify other emotional disorders which may have their onset at any time in life. ICD-10 lists the following:

- Phobic anxiety disorder.
- Other anxiety disorders.
- Obsessive-compulsive disorder.
- Reaction to severe stress, and adjustment disorder.
- Dissociative [conversion] disorders.
- Somatoform disorders.
- Other neurotic disorders.

Each of the above disorders is further subdivided.
The DSM-IV categories were listed above.

Anxiety in children

Anxiety disorders are rarely diagnosed in infancy. Infants can certainly appear upset, as evidenced by crying, sleeplessness and irritability, but whether such reactions are of the same nature as the anxiety states of older children is unclear. Many things that may cause such behaviour – hunger, cold, physical diseases, tension in the family and disruption of routine, and how far anxiety, or its infantile equivalent, is responsible is hard to determine.

According to DSM-III-R, 'avoidant disorder of childhood' may develop as early as two-and-a-half, and 'separation anxiety disorder' at pre-school age. In practice it is difficult to distinguish these disorders with confidence before about four or five years of age, that is before the use of mental defence mechanisms develops. Moreover, during this age period – four to five – many children whose emotional development is proceeding quite normally display irrational fears of such objects as flies, birds, dogs, earthworms, wind, the dark and other things they have not yet become familiar with and do not understand. In older children such fears are not normal and might be found in children with neurotic/anxiety disorders. The patient's age, and the normal stress tolerance for that age, must always be taken into account.

Anxiety disorders in children tend to be less fixed and chronic than such disorders in adults, so that the response to treatment and the prognosis are generally better. They often disturb the family and people in the child's environment as much as, or more than, they do the child. In this respect neurotic children differ from neurotic adults, who often live their lives without causing distress to others.

As is implied by the variety of diagnostic categories listed above, the clinical manifestations of emotional/anxiety disorders are quite varied. In many cases the anxiety is directly expressed. These children may be shy, timid and clinging, emotionally immature, overdependent on their parents and poor at mixing with other children. They may fear loss of family, or death or other disaster. They may have difficulty getting to sleep and their sleep may be disturbed by dreams, nightmares or frequent waking. There may be *free-floating anxiety* – that is anxiety that comes to be associated with any situation the child experiences. Such anxiety is often perceived as arising from within, rather than from the environment. Distractibility and impaired concentration may accompany feelings of general apprehension.

Common somatic manifestations of anxiety are loss of appetite, feelings of nausea, abdominal pain, diarrhoea, vomiting, headaches, dry mouth, rapid heart beat, cold and clammy hands, dizziness, sweating, increased frequency of micturition and palpitations. Restlessness and feelings of tension may be present. Symptoms of this type characterize the generalized anxiety disorders listed above.

Panic attacks may occur in the course of an anxiety state. They are characterized by the sudden onset of extreme fear, sometimes with a sense of impending doom and often with such physical symptoms as shortness of breath, palpitations, sweating, faintness and trembling or shaking. Subjects who suffer panic attacks may or may not also have agoraphobia (see below).

The features of separation anxiety have been outlined above. It is distinguished more by the context in which it occurs – separation from an attachment figure – than by the symptomatology.

Exactly how the anxiety disorders of children should be subdivided is unclear. A good formulation specifying the various factors considered to be associated with or responsible for the anxiety (or other symptoms) the person is experiencing may be more useful. Basing one's understanding and treatment of the clinical problem on such a formulation is better than using a diagnostic label.

Phobic states or disorders

In phobic states there is persistent and irrational fear of specific objects, activities or situations. This leads to avoidance of the objects or situations. The fear sometimes appears to be due to the defence mechanism of displacement, that is, it is transferred from its true, but unconscious, source to the phobic object. Thus the agoraphobic person who is afraid of going out of the house (agoraphobia being the fear of open spaces) is effectively prevented from having to deal with many situations which might be met with away from the security of home.

The phobic object or objects may change during the course of the illness. While they may dominate the clinical picture, phobias are sometimes but one feature, even a minor and transient one, of a neurotic disorder which may have as its main feature anxiety symptoms such as those described above. There is an almost infinite variety of phobic objects, for example, buses, dogs, cats, doctors, insects, heights, enclosed spaces, shops, crowds, snaked, dentists and so on.

Monosymptomatic phobias, or *simple phobias*, are sometimes encountered in children. The child has a severe and perhaps handicapping fear of a particular object or situation. Such isolated phobias may differ in their aetiology from other neurotic disorders, in that they are not usually accompanied by general emotional immaturity and their development is more easily understood on the basis of learning theory. They may often be examples of state-dependent learning, fear and avoidance of a particular situation being learned in the course of experiencing a single frightening situation. The subject then re-experiencies these emotions when again placed in that situation or a similar one. These phobias respond better to behaviour therapy (see Chapter 21) than the more complex phobic disorders.

Agoraphobia is uncommon in childhood and early adolescence, though it sometimes starts in late adolescence. Its main feature is severe and handicapping fear of being alone or in public places from which escape is difficult.

The essential feature of social phobia, which may occur in late childhood or adolescence, is a persistent, irrational fear of situations in which the subject is exposed to possible scrutiny by others. It may be manifest when the subject is asked to speak or perform in public, or when using public lavatories, eating in public, or writing in the presence of others. As in the other phobic conditions we have discussed, the subject recognizes that the fear is excessive or unreasonable, and is consequently distressed by it.

The term *school phobia* has been used to describe a certain form of reluctance to go to school. It is a complex condition better described as *school refusal*. It is discussed in a later section.

Helpful discussion of the fears and phobias of childhood are those of Berecz (1968) and Ferrari (1986).

Obsessive-compulsive disorders

These disorders are characterized by obsessional thoughts, that is, thoughts and ideas which intrude and persist despite conscious awareness of their unreasonableness and resistance to them; and by compulsive actions related to such thoughts.

The *prevalence* of obsesssive-compulsive disorders (OCD) in children and adolescents may be about 1.9% though only a minority of those with the condition come to psychiatric attention (Whitaker, *et al.*, 1990).

The essential *clinical feature* of obsessive-compulsive disorder is the repetitive intrusion into the subject's life of thoughts which are unwelcome and which the subject would like to banish. Such thoughts are often acted out in compulsive rituals. The thoughts and resulting actions are not *ego-systonic* – that is, they are not in harmony with the subjects's view of the world. This distinguishes them from delusional beliefs. A common symptom of OCD is the urge to clean and wash things. The obsessive man will know that he does not need to wash his hands repeatedly many times daily, or perhaps even hourly, but is unable to resist the urge to do so. The deluded man, on the other hand, is firmly convinced that his hands (or whatever he is washing) are dirty and must be washed. No rational argument will convince him otherwise.

In clinical practice it is necessary to distinguish between the minor obsessions and compulsions of childhood and the more serious ones that cause distress to the subjects and/or their families. Behaviours such as avoiding the cracks in concrete paths, touching lamp standards as they are passed, and feeding and bedtime rituals, are quite common, especially in younger children. The symptoms of OCD are more severe and persistent, there is conscious resistance to them, and they interfere with the child's life. They can be quite complex. One boy had to shut the dining room door three times and then touch each corner of the table before he could start eating a meal. Even more complex dressing, eating and other rituals occur.

Whether children who have rituals and 'superstitious' ideas when young are more likely to develop OCD later is unclear, though it has been suggested that this may be so (Leonard, *et al.*, 1990).

The symptoms of OCD in children most often appear around age six, though psychiatric help may not be sought until later.

OCD often co-exists with other psychiatric disorders. Its relationship with tic disorders has been mentioned earlier. Others that may co-exist include major depression and other depressive disorders, and any of the *anxiety* disorders mentioned above. It is not unusual to see children in whom a variety of anxiety/neurotic symptoms appear either in succession or simultaneously.

Impulsions, originally described by Bender & Shilder (1940), should be distinguished from compulsions. Examples of impulsions are behaviours such as constantly looking at an object, drawing the object, being pre-occupied with an object in fantasy or thought, hoarding things, counting repeatedly and being repeatedly preoccupied with numbers. The behaviour resembles compulsive behaviour but there is a lack of conscious resistance to it. Impulsions are more common in younger children – aged about four to ten – while obsessive-compulsive phenomena tend to be seen more in older children and adolescents. Sometimes impulsions give way to obsessive-compulsive behaviours and both types of behaviour may be present around puberty.

Hysteria, conversion disorders and dissociative states

These disorders fall into two broad groups:

(1) Those characterized by physical symptoms which may suggest organic disease, although there is no other evidence of such disease. Both DSM-IV and ICD-10 call these *somatoform disorders*.
(2) Dissociative disorders, in which there are psychogenic changes in the subject's consciousness, identity or motor behaviour.

In both of the above groups of conditions the subject is consciously unaware of the underlying problem and is not malingering – that is, consciously fabricating or elaborating symptoms. The symptoms are real to the patient who is imperfectly aware, or quite unaware, of their psychogenic cause.

(1) Somatoform disorders – disorders with physical symptoms

(a) Somatization disorders
The terms which have been used for these conditions in the past include hysteria and Briquet's syndrome. Their main feature is summarized in ICD-10 as 'repeated presentation of physical symptoms, together with persistent requests for medical investigations, in spite of repeated negative findings and reassurances by doctors that the symptoms have no physical basis'. In children the requests for investigations may come as much, or more, from the parents as from the young person. There may be multiple physical complaints, often described in dramatic, vague or exaggerated terms. The complaints may include visual problems, paralyses, seizures, pain in any part or parts of the body but especially the

back and abdomen, dizziness, shortness of breath, headache and abnormal skin sensations, such as itching, burning, tingling and numb feelings. In older female patients there may be complaints of menstrual pain and excessive menstrual bleeding. Depression and anxiety often accompany the physical symptoms.

The DSM-IV manual states that diagnostic criteria are usually met before age 25, and disorders of this type occur quite frequently in children who have not yet reached puberty. They may not meet all the DSM-IV diagnostic criteria, either because there are as yet too few symptoms or because they have not yet been present for several years.

(b) Conversion disorders (or conversion hysteria)

Many of those who meet the DSM-IV criteria for somatization disorder would in the past have been regarded as having conversion disorders. In these conditions the symptoms are understood as representing the *conversion* of anxiety into some physical form. ICD-10 defines various 'dissociative disorders of movement and sensation'. The possible clinical manifestations are legion. They include complete or partial paralysis of any part of the body, lack of motor coordination, inability to stand or walk, trembling or shaking of any part of the body, speech problems, convulsions and loss of sensation in any part of the body, usually distributed in a way which is not compatible with a neurological lesion. Along with loss of normal sensation, or on their own, there may be tingling or other abnormal sensations. Partial, but very seldom total, loss of vision may be reported.

(c) Hypochondriacal disorder

The essential feature of these disorders is what ICD-10 describes as 'a persistent preoccupation with the possibility of having one or more serious and progressive physical disorders'. Those with these disorders are inclined to interpret normal or everyday sensations as evidence of disease. They often have persistent somatic complaints and may also be unduly preoccupied by their physical appearance. The patient's beliefs about being ill persist despite reassurance by physicians that they do not have the illness(es) they fear they have. There may be associated depression and overt anxiety. This condition is uncommon before puberty but is sometimes seen in adolescents.

(d) Somatoform autonomic dysfunction

This is a new category appearing in ICD-10. The symptoms are those of dysfunction of one of the bodily systems which are under the control of the autonomic nervous system – which is responsible for bodily functions that are outside conscious control. Symptoms include palpitations, sweating, flushing, tremor, feelings of tightness or of being bloated or distended. There are subjective symptoms referred to a specific organ or bodily system, but no evidence of organic disease.

(e) Persistent somatoform pain disorder (Pain disorder associated with psychological factors in DSM-IV)
This is a term used for conditions in which there is complaint of persistent, severe and distressing pain, with associated emotional conflict or psychosocial problems which appear to be the main causative influences.

Primary gain is a term used when the symptom serves to keep an internal conflict or need out of conscious awareness. Thus aphonia (the inability to speak except, usually, in a whisper), or paralysis of an arm, may be a reaction to an argument in a person who has an inner conflict about the expression of rage; the symptom thus has symbolic significance in relation to the conflict.

Secondary gain is the term used when the symptom enables the subject to avoid situations that are unpleasant or anxiety-provoking to the person.

(2) Dissociative Disorders

Children have the capacity to dissociate, that is to leave the real world to exist for a while in another one of their own construction. Not infrequently they do this when experiencing severe abuse, especially sexual abuse. Fully developed dissociative disorders are however relatively rarely met with in childhood. The following dissociative disorders are described.

(a) Psychogenic (or dissociative) amnesia
In this condition there is loss of memory for some past period of time, or for particular events or persons.

(b) Hysterical or dissociative fugue
Patients with this disorder suddenly leave their current lives, often to travel elsewhere to start again with a new identity. Typically they have no memory of their previous lives or indentities.

(c) Depersonalization disorder
In this disorder there are feelings of altered perception or experience of the self, with the loss of a sense of one's own reality, sometimes accompanied by a similar alteration in the perception of one's surroundings ('derealization').

(d) Multiple personality disorder (or dissociative identity disorder in DSM-IV)
In this condition the person displays two or more distinct personalities
and identities at different times, usually with sudden transitions from one
to another.

   None of these dissociative disorders is common in children, but a history of severe abuse, especially sexual abuse, during childhood is said to
be regularly found in the histories of adults with multiple personality
disorder. It seems that many of those who have suffered such abuse have
learned how to avoid pain by dissociation and that this sometimes
becomes a pattern of behaviour which persists into adult life.

The relative frequency of the anxiety disorders of children

Reliable data on the frequency with which the various anxiety disorders
occur are few. Cultural factors undoubtedly play a part in determining
how anxiety is expressed and handled. Turgay (1980) reviewed research
on conversion disorders in childhood. He pointed out that the incidence
of such disorders varies greatly in different cultures. In Turkey, where
Turgay has studied conversion disorders, they seem to be more common
than in western countries. An example of a culture-specific neurotic
syndrome is the so-called *brain fag syndrome*, probably better called *school
anxiety*, which has been described in children living in various parts of
Africa (Prince, 1960; German, 1972). The strikingly florid presentation of
some of these children is unlike anything commonly seen in western
psychiatric practice. This condition occurs in African children who are
subject to intense and often unrealistic pressures to perform in school at a
level they feel to be beyond them. Guiness (1986) describes it as not
'associated so much with personality or intelligence factors as with
sociocultural stresses and ... the historical development of education in
Africa'. The extended family system with its attendant obligations, the
high regard for education, the perceived economic advantages of a good
education and the immense difficulty which achieving success presents in
an educational system based upon European practices of times gone by,
combine to put the child in an intensely anxiety-provoking situation.
Prevalent beliefs about bewitchment add to the anxiety of all concerned.
The result can be severe, incapacitating headaches, abdominal pains, loss
of vision, difficulty in hearing and florid conversion symptoms. These are
often closely associated with the times when school attendance is
required. It is easy for such children and their families to believe that
someone who wishes the family ill has cast a spell over the child and
anxiety about this can further exacerbate the symptoms. In extreme cases

the emotional disturbance becomes so great that the child may appear out of touch with reality – a *psychogenic psychosis*.

A word of warning

Caution is in order in attributing physical symptoms to psychogenic causes. There is a real danger of misdiagnosing organic disease. Moreover the two may co-exist. A common combination is *pseudoseizures* and true epileptic seizures; indeed the former most often occur in subjects who also have, or have in the past suffered from, epilepsy. As well as trying to establish that organic disease is *not* present, it is desirable to establish also that there are adequate psychological causes for the symptoms. If the symptoms can be understood on neither basis, it is better to leave the diagnosis open until further information is available and the progress of the condition has been observed for a longer period.

School refusal (school phobia)

The main feature of school refusal is reluctance to attend school associated with anxiety and, often, depressed mood. It is sometimes called school phobia because these children appear frightened to go to school. It is usually associated with separation anxiety.

Prevalence

School refusal probably has a prevalence of 1 to 2% of the school population (Weiner, 1982). It seems to be more common in early adolescence than at other ages, but may occur at first entry to school and on changing to a new school. When the onset is in the teen years there are often associated depression and difficulties in school.

Clinical picture

While fear of school, implied by the term *school phobia*, can be a feature of this condition, it is not usually the primary one, though at first sight it sometimes appears to be. Separation anxiety, and the fear of leaving home are generally more important. Berney, *et al.*, (1981) found that separation anxiety was 'moderate or marked' in 87% of 51 children aged 9 to 15 with school refusal.

School refusal should be distinguished from truancy, the wilful avoidance of school (see Chapter 6). Truancy is often associated with other oppositional or conduct problems and there is not the high level of anxiety seen in children with school refusal. It is this anxiety, sometimes accompanied by depression, that makes it difficult for children with school refusal to go to school. If attempts are made to force the child to go to school, increased distress usually results, though in some cases this is the best way to manage the problem. Physical symptoms such as poor appetite, nausea, vomiting, pains and diarrhoea are common, especially at breakfast time. They may disappear once the time for going to school has passed. This may lead parents and school staff to think that the child is malingering. In more severe cases symptoms persist and may be present throughout the day; there may also be sleep disturbance. There is usually exacerbation of the symptoms when the child is faced with pressure to attend school.

These children are often emotionally immature and so have difficulty coping with the everyday stresses of life at school. They may find relationships with other children difficult and they become acutely anxious away from what they feel is the safety and protection of home and family. School attendance may finally cease in response to a minor additional stress like a change of teacher, bullying by other children or transfer from one school to another. The emotional immaturity of these children is often manifest also in their, often covert, aggressiveness. Having been raised in anxious and often indulgent environments, they have not learned to accept frustration and to channel their aggressive drives into socially useful and constructive activities. Their anger may seldom have been aroused, since they have always been given their way. When this situation changes they may become both panic-stricken and very angry. Their anger is often expressed verbally but some become physically violent with their parents, for example if the latter try to force them, by physical means, to go to school. Anger may also be expressed silently through refusal to speak or cooperate, both with parents and with therapists and others trying to help.

Either anxiety or depression may dominate the clinical picture in these children. They may also feel resentful because they are aware, unconsciously if not at a conscious level, of their inability to fulfil age-appropriate roles. Depression is seen more often in adolescent school refusers than in those in younger age groups. Bernstein & Garfinkel (1986) reported that 69% of 26 early adolescent, chronic school refusers met DSM-III criteria for either major depression or adjustment disorder with depression.

A word is in order about the family constellations seen in these patients. Skynner (1975) commented on the frequent combination of an anxious and overprotective mother and a weak, passive, ineffectual or absent father.

The treatment of anxiety disorders

(a) Psychotherapy

Psychotherapy, in one form or another, plays a major role in the treatment of the disorders discussed in this chapter. It usually needs to involve child and parents and is often best focused on the family system as a whole. The diagnostic assessment and resulting formulation should indicate where the main therapeutic efforts are required.

Individual therapy

This may or may not involve the working through, with the child, of unconscious conflicts. Whether it need do so will depend on the severity and chronicity of the disorder, and on the child's response to changes in the environment, especially the family environment.

Work with the parents

This is needed when there is evidence of overanxious, overprotective or otherwise unhelpful attitudes to or handling of the child. In many such cases one or both parents have their own psychiatric problems and these may require treatment.

Family therapy

This is often needed. When the child's disorder appears to be related to the way the family system as a whole functions, treatment designed to promote change in the functioning of the family system often proves to be the best approach. In school refusal, especially in adolescence when the family psychopathology is often complex and chronic, family therapy can be particularly valuable.

When family systems problems are prominent features – and they often are – I prefer to address these problems first. This may lead to amelioration or resolution of the child's symptoms. If it does not, individual work with the child may be needed, perhaps combined with further therapy for the parents.

(b) Behaviour therapy

Behavioural approaches are often effective in the treatment of phobias, especially monosymptomatic ones. The procedure of *systematic desensitization* (see Chapter 21) is an established treatment for monosymptomatic phobias. The essence of this approach is the gradual introduction of the phobic object or situation while the subject is in a state of relaxation.

Behaviour therapy can also contribute to the treatment of obsessive-compulsive disorders. The procedure of *response prevention* (Stanley, 1980), which consists essentially of consistently preventing the compulsive behaviour, can be effective when ritualistic behaviours are prominent. One often finds that by the time a child comes for treatment the other family members, and others who have contact with the child, have fallen into the habit of giving in to the rituals; that is, they modify the environment so that the child is allowed extra time to dress, eat meals, prepare to go to bed and so on. This usually leads to a worsening of the symptoms.

Behavioural analysis may reveal that various environmental contingencies are reinforcing or promoting any anxiety symptoms. The response of family, teachers and others to the symptoms of children with any of the disorders mentioned in this chapter may serve to reinforce those symptoms. When this is so, an appropriate behaviour modification program is often indicated.

Behaviour therapy is discussed further in Chapter 21.

(c) Daypatient and inpatient treatment

Children living in particularly insecure and anxiety-provoking home environments can often benefit from a period of daypatient or inpatient treatment, while therapy is conducted with the family and/or the parents. This can be an effective, if drastic, way of countering the effects of anxious parental overprotection, such as is often present in severe school refusal.

(d) Pharmacotherapy

Drugs have but a small part to play in the treatment of childhood anxiety disorders, unless there is associated depression – and even in those cases, their value is open to question. Sometimes, however, antidepressant medication is helpful, and imipramine has been reported to be of value in school refusal (Klein, *et al.*, 1980).

Small doses of anxiolytics such as diazepam or chlordiazepoxide may occasionally be helpful in bringing about a temporary reduction in the anxiety level of an acutely anxious child, particularly when this is a reaction to severe, current environmental stress which cannot be immediately alleviated. These drugs should not be prescribed for more than a few days; a week is a reasonable maximum.

The disadvantages of the use of anxiety-relieving drugs generally outweigh any merits their use may have. At best they are a symptomatic treatment, and much more important than simply removing the symptoms is dealing with the causes and associated factors. Prescribing medication for the child tends to give the message that the problem is simply the child's, whereas it is usually as much that of the family or wider social environment. It may also be taken to mean, by the child and those concerned with the child's care, that there is an easy pharmacological cure for the problems, which in reality are usually related to such issues as relationships, emotional maturity and family functioning. The model of a 'magical' chemical cure for human problems, though often implied in present-day advertising is not one we should offer our young people.

The cautionary note above about the use of drugs requires some modification in the case of obsessive-compulsive disorders (OCD). Clomipramine (also known as chlorimipramine), has been shown to be effective in the treatment of OCD in adults, and there is evidence that it is of value in children also. Summarizing this evidence, Green (1991) suggests that 'clomipramine is the drug of choice for children and adolescents with severe obsessive-compulsive disorder...'

(e) Special points about the treatment of school refusal

When there are family systems problems associated with school refusal, for example the combination mentioned above of an over-involved mother and child and an uninvolved father, these need to be addressed in family therapy. But whatever treatment is employed with family and/or child, it is necessary to consider when the child should return to school. With children who are still attending, even with difficulty and with symptoms, efforts to make the school environment temporarily less stressful and to provide emotional support to the child at school are well worthwhile. When school attendance has only recently broken down, an early return to school is usually advisable. With more severe and chronic cases some delay, while a sound treatment plan is developed and work is done with the family, may be justifiable.

Whether it is done early in treatment or later, the return to school needs to be well planned and carefully orchestrated. All concerned should first be agreed on the plan. These will include the parents, school staff including the child's teacher(s), the family doctor and any other medical or paramedical professionals who are involved, and any others who are active in the treatment of child or family. The child should be aware of the plan and, if possible, agree to it, though this is not essential. A meeting of the above people to work out and agree upon the plan is desirable. Planning done over the telephone or by letter is not usually very effective. By the end of the meeting everyone should know exactly what is to happen on the day appointed for the child's return to school. It must also be agreed what is to be done if the child refuses to get up, leave the house, or enter the school or classroom, or resists resuming attendance in any other way.

Firm, calm handling of the return to school is desirable. It may sometimes be necessary to take the child to school physically, even if not properly dressed, in order to break the cycle of events that has seemed to make attendance impossible. Usually, though, once these children realize that all concerned with their care are agreed about the timing and other details of their return, they resume attendance with little difficulty. The plan should provide for what is to happen if the child becomes acutely anxious at any point. Whatever this is, it should scarcely ever be that the child returns to or remains at home.

In a minority of very severe cases a period of psychotherapy with the family or some combination of members of the family may be required before plans are made for the child's return to school. Attempts to force severely anxious and depressed children and those who have had repeated severe panic attacks to attend school too early can aggravate the problems. In some such cases a period of treatment in a daypatient or inpatient unit, combined with psychotherapy for the family or for child and parents, proves a more effective and expeditious approach (Barker, 1968; Hersov, 1980).

Blagg & Yule (1984) described a 'flexible, behavioural approach' involving:

- a detailed clarification of the child's problems;
- a realistic discussion of child, parental and teacher worries;
- contingency plans to ensure maintenance once the child has returned to school;
- *in vivo* flooding, that is enforced return to school, under escort if necessary;
- follow-up, consisting of frequent contacts until the child has been attending full-time for at least six weeks, then careful steps to ensure return after genuine illness, holidays and long weekends, at the start of a new academic year, and after any reorganization of the child's timetable.

These authors reported the rapid return to school of 28 out of 30 treated using the above approach. A comparison group treated in a hospital unit did less well and another one treated by home teaching and outpatient psychotherapy did very poorly.

The role of drug therapy in these disorders is not clear, though there is some evidence, as mentioned above, that imipramine may be helpful. It should not however be considered as anything more than an adjunct to the other measures I have outlined. It may be more likely to be helpful when there is evidence of a depressive disorder in addition to the school refusal.

Sometimes the parents and/or the child request a change of school, class or teacher. Such changes can be helpful, especially if there are real-life stresses at school or the child has gained the reputation of being a 'cry baby' or 'crazy' in the class or school. In itself, however, it is seldom an adequate treatment. It may represent an attempt by child or parents to deal with anxiety or guilt by projection on to outside sources, such as the school or a member of the school staff.

All the treatment approaches mentioned in this chapter are discussed more fully in Chapter 21.

Outcome

The outlook is usually good for neurotic and anxiety disorders developing in childhood. Many anxiety symptoms clear up completely, with or without treatment, and are not followed by any observable psychiatric abnormality. This applies particularly to the milder cases, and to disorders occurring in children whose emotional development has been satisfactory. It is also more likely when the symptoms develop in response to severe, but short-lived, environmental stress.

In some, especially the more severe, cases the symptoms are more persistent, especially in the absence of suitable treatment. Emotionally immature children, overdependent on their parents, tend to do less well unless their overdependence is resolved. Constitutional predisposition, suggested by a positive family history and the appearance of symptoms with little apparent environmental cause, may be associated with a poorer outlook. This seems to apply at least in some cases of OCD. A review by Zeitlin (1990) suggests that there is often recurrence of this condition in adult life.

Further reading

A useful source of further information is the edited book *Anxiety Disorders of Childhood* (Gittelman, 1986).

Chapter 9

Mixed Disorders of Conduct and Emotions

Many children present with combinations of symptoms which do not fit easily into the established diagnostic categories.

In child psychiatric practice we often meet children who display both antisocial behaviours and emotional symptoms. The symptoms of conduct disorder and of oppositional defiant disorder may co-exist with emotional symptoms such as anxiety and depression. There has been uncertainty how to classify the conditions of such children. The alternatives have been to opt for one diagnosis, choosing it on the basis of which symptoms are the more prominent, or are reported to have appeared first; to make dual diagnoses; or to have categories for *mixed disorders*.

In acknowledgement of the existence of a large group of children who display a mixture of antisocial behaviour and emotional symptoms, ICD-10 has proposed a category of 'mixed disorder of conduct and emotions'. In the ICD-10 manual, these disorders are described as 'characterized by the combination of persistently aggressive, dissocial, or defiant behaviour with overt and marked symptoms of depression, anxiety or other emotional upsets'. This new diagnostic category is offered tentatively, with the statement that 'insufficient research has been carried out to be confident that this category should indeed be separate from conduct disorders of childhood'. It does not appear in DSM-IV.

Despite its tentative presentation in ICD-10, this category of disorder merits a short chapter of its own for three reasons. The first is that these mixed conditions are common. Defining them as a specific type of disorder is likely to draw the attention of both clinicians and researchers to a group of disturbed children who may otherwise fail to get the attention they merit.

The second reason is that these disorders, however they are dealt with in a diagnostic scheme, illustrate the important point that in child psychiatry we do not, for the most part, deal with discrete, easily defined clinical entities. We deal, rather, with complex, continuously variable reactions to equally complex combinations of aetiological factors in immature, incompletely developed personalities. Creating child psychiatric diagnostic categories is in large measure an artificial process, designed to create order where order does not truly exist. It is justified in that it can facilitate communication between professionals and because it is necessary to describe clinical groups for research, epidemiological and related purposes. But it is much easier to define physical diseases. Thus tuberuclosis is any condition due to infection with the tuberculosis bacillus, a peptic ulcer is a certain type of ulceration of the lining of the stomach or duodenum, and so forth.

A third reason for having a category for these mixed disorders is the therapeutic challenge they present. Once a disorder is defined, more attention may be directed to the development of approaches to treatment and prevention.

Definition

For a diagnosis of *depressive conduct disorder*, one of the two main sub-categories of mixed disorders appearing in ICD-10, there should be:

- the symptoms of conduct disorder of childhood, as they are defined in the ICD-10 manual; and
- 'persistent and marked depression of mood, as evidenced by symptoms such as excessive misery, loss of interest and pleasure in usual activities, self-blame, and hopelessness.' There may also be disturbances of sleep or appetite.

ICD-10 also lists a subcategory of 'other mixed disorders of conduct and emotions'. In these disorders, there is the combination of conduct disorder of childhood with 'persistent and marked emotional symptoms such as anxiety, fearfulness, obsessions or compulsions, depersonalization or derealization, phobias, or hypochondriasis'. Anger and resentment neither contradict nor support the diagnosis.

Finally, ICD-10 has a 'residual' category for 'mixed disorders of conduct and emotions, unspecified'.

Clinical features

Children whose disorders fall into these *mixed* categories may have quite a wide variety of symptoms – almost any combination of the symptoms described in Chapters 6 and 8, provided that they meet criteria for conduct disorder set out in ICD-10. In practice these are often insecurely attached children from chaotic, poorly organized families. They have lacked not only appropriate social training but also an adequate degree of emotional stability and security. In older children, and especially in adolescents, there may be a serious degree of depression along with the antisocial behaviour. These children's self-esteem is usually low and they feel, unconsciously if not consciously, that they are failures and they have little sense of personal accomplishment or self-worth.

Treatment approaches

Despite the unquestionable fact that there are many children with mixed disorders, the literature on their treatment is limited. These disorders do not appear as separate categories in standard textbooks such as those of Lewis (1991) and Rutter, Taylor & Hersov (1994). The approach of most writers has been to regard these children as suffering from whichever condition seems most prominent and to regard the other symptoms as associated problems, with the implication that the main therapeutic effort should be addressed to the principal disorder. Data are lacking on whether this is the best approach. What does seem clear is that these are complex cases requiring comprehensive assessment and, usually, multifaceted treatment plans.

In view of their complexity, and the lack of systematic research about how to treat them, these are clinical situations in which a comprehensive, in-depth case formulation is invaluable.

It is clear that much further research is needed on how best to tackle the problems of these children. They are essentially multiply handicapped. Almost any combination of the treatment methods discussed in Chapter 21 may be needed. Addressing problems in the family system, once these have been defined, is usually as important as work with the presenting child.

Outcome

There are as little systematic outcome data concerning these mixed disorders as there is empirically based information on how best to treat them. Clinical experience suggests however that, without effective treatment, these children tend to do rather badly. By contrast, children with *pure* anxiety or depressive symptoms who have previously received and responded to appropriate social training within a stable and secure family setting, are likely both to cooperate with treatment for their anxiety or depressive disorder and to function well once such treatment is successful.

Similarly the child displaying antisocial behaviour, if emotionally stable and securely attached to parents, will often respond well to therapeutic interventions. In either of these two types of case, the stability and proper functioning of the family system are important. They provide a background of security which children with these mixed disorders often seem to lack.

When a child has neither secure attachment in a reasonably stable family setting, nor a background of proper social training – including good parental models – the therapeutic challenge is considerable and the outcome often disappointing.

Chapter 10

Major Affective Disorders and Suicide

The essential feature of major affective disorders is an abnormality of mood. This may be in the direction of depression or of mania, that is elated mood. Mania, and its lesser form, hypomania, are uncommon before puberty but are encountered more frequently in adolescence.

Classification

Apart from disorders characterized by anxiety, neither DSM-IV nor ICD-10 recognizes any category of affective disorder occurring specifically in childhood. The only possible exception is the *depressive conduct disorder* of ICD-10, discussed in the previous chapter. Otherwise mood, or affective, disorders appear in the general sections of both classifications. These categories may be used for patients of any age. The main ICD-10 categories are:

● Manic episode, subdivided into hypomania, manic episode without psychotic symptoms, and manic episode with psychotic symptoms, and also 'other' and 'unspecified' manic episodes.

● Bipolar affective disorder, which has ten subcategories, with also some further subdivisions. The subcategories specify whether the current state is one of depression or mania, or is mixed, and how severe it is.

● Depressive episode, which may be mild, moderate or severe, with the severe category being divided into episodes without or with psychotic symptoms. There are also 'other' and 'unspecified' depressive episodes.

● Recurrent depressive disorder, a category for use when there are repeated episodes of depression without intervening episodes of mood elevation or overactivity. This category is subdivided according to whether the condition is in remission or, if it is not, how severe the current episode is.

● Persistent mood [affective] disorders. These comprise cyclothymia, in which there is persisting instability of mood, with periods of mild depression and mild elation; dysthymia, a long-standing depression of mood of insufficient severity to meet the criteria for a depressive disorder; and 'other persistent mood [affective] disorders'.

- Other and unspecified mood [affective] disorders.

DSM-IV has broadly similar categories and both the classification schemes also have categories for adjustment disorders with depressed mood. ICD-10 lists adjustment disorders with brief and with prolonged depression and with mixed anxiety and depressive symptoms. Adjustment disorders are discussed in Chapter 15.

DSM-IV, like its predecessor, has a category of *dysthymic disorder*, its main feature being a chronically depressed mood lasting most of the day, and of at least two years' duration. Low self-esteem, lack of energy, poor concentration and difficulty making decisions are common features, but the criteria for a depressive disorder are not met. In children, irritability, rather than depressed mood, may predominate.

Depression in children and adolescents

It has long been clear that children can suffer from moods of depression, but whether, and how frequently, they also have conditions analogous to the major depressive disorders of adulthood has been the subject of dispute. In recent years it has been increasingly accepted that they can suffer *adult-type* depression; how often this happens is uncertain. The existence of adult-type depression in adolescents is generally accepted and there is also evidence of a continuity of depressive symptomatology from before puberty, through adolescence into adult life, though there are important differences, including response to medication, in the different age ranges (Jensen & Saunders, 1991). It is not surprising that children appear to be more reactive to their family environments than older subjects tend to be. It also appears that co-morbidity – the simultaneous presence of symptoms of other disorders such as conduct disorders, oppositional behaviour or anxiety-related syndromes – is common in depressed children, probably more so than in adults.

Despite difference in presentation and associated symptoms, Puig-Antich (1986, page 345) has stated that the phenomenology of major depression is 'quite similar from age 6 to senescence'. He states also that the developmental variations that do occur are 'minor compared to the steadiness of the symptomatology'.

Depression, like other problems affecting children, must be considered in the light of the developmental processes that occur during childhood. Developmental, as well as other, aspects of childhood depression are examined in *Depression in Young People: Clinical and Developmental Perspectives* (Rutter, *et al.*, 1986).

Prevalence

A study by Whitaker, *et al.*, (1990) suggested that about 4% of 14- to 17-year olds may have major depression, the rate being higher in girls (4.5%) than in boys (2.9%). The rate of major depression is almost certainly lower in pre-pubertal children. Kashani, *et al.*, (1983), in a study in New Zealand, found 1.9% of 9-year-olds to be suffering from 'major depression' while 3.6% had 'minor depression'. Rutter (1986) points out that the sex ratio changes over the time of puberty, there being more pre-pubertal boys than girls with depression, whereas after puberty the number of girls increases. Moreover depression before puberty is often associated with – and possibly at least partially caused by – other disorders such as serious academic problems. Pre-pubertal depression also tends to be associated with a family history of alcoholism and/or antisocial behaviour. Onset after puberty occurs more often in girls and is usually *primary*, that is, not associated with another disorder, and there is more often a family history of major affective disorder, usually depression.

The changes in the prevalence patterns over the adolescent age range have been explored, and the literature has been reviewed, by Cohen, *et al.* (1993a and b).

Manic conditions are considerably less common than depressive ones in adolescents, and are even more uncommon before puberty. They may however be confused with other disorders, such as attention-deficit (Chapter 7) or conduct (Chapter 6) disorders (Carlson, 1990a).

Causes

Affective disorders may present as either primary or secondary conditions, as indicated in Figure 10.1.

Genetic factors probably play a significant role in predisposing to primary depressive disorders in children. In clinical practice, it is usually hard to separate the effects of growing up in a family in which a parent suffers from an affective disorder or alcoholism from predisposing genetic factors. According to Akiskal & Weller (1989), the concordance for depression in monozygotic twins reared together is 76%, whereas for dizygotic twins it is only 19%, and for monozygotic twins reared apart it is

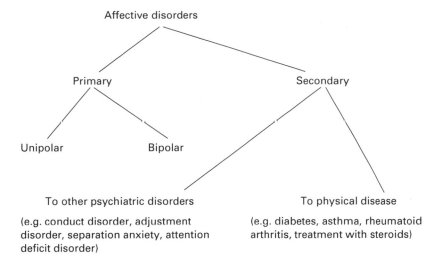

Fig. 10.1   The types of affective disorder.

67%, suggesting a role also for environmental factors even when there is genetic loading. Children of parents with affective disorders show a high rate of psychiatric problems and Cytryn, *et al.*, (1986, page 179) state that:

'Already at the age of 12 months the infants of manic-depressive parents [that is, those suffering from bipolar disorders] show disturbances in attachment behaviour and dysregulation of affect ... similar to the central characteristics of adults with affective illness.'

Regardless of the relative roles of genetic and family environmental factors in causing affective disorders in children, we need to be aware that the children of parents with affective disorders are more at risk of developing psychiatric disorders generally and depressive ones in particular.

Environmental stress often seems to contribute to depression, though there are few data on which stresses are most likely to do so. Separation from an attachment figure has been blamed and Bowlby (1980) has claimed that separation experiences contribute to the later development of depression. While it appears that bereavement, especially the loss of a parent, can lead to depression, grief reactions tend to be briefer in young children than in adolescents and adults. But this is a complex issue because the bereavement may involve many things in addition to the loss of a loved one – for example, the break-up of the home, geographical moves, the arrival in the family of a step-parent, financial problems, and emotional problems in other family members, especially the surviving parent.

Children may lose parents other than by death. The separation and/or divorce of parents are common stresses, and parents may also be lost, at least for a while, because they are imprisoned or admitted to hospital. As with bereavement, it can be difficult to separate out the effects of parental separation, divorce or imprisonment from those of the marital strife or otherwise disturbed family environmental situations which often precede these events.

'Learned helplessness' (Seligman & Peterson, 1986) is a term that was originally used to describe the state of dogs that had been subjected to a series of electric shocks over which they had no control. The dogs showed motivational, cognitive and emotional deficits and their state bore some resemblance to human depression. It has been suggested that children's sense of security and their self-esteem may become impaired by being over time in painful and unpleasant situations over which they have no control. An important aspect of self-esteem is the possession of a sense of mastery over the environment. It is reasonable to suppose that such a sense might be lacking in some measure in children brought up in families in which events occur in random fashion and cannot be predicted or anticipated. This is very much the situation in the *chaotic* family (Barker, 1993b).

There are a number of biological correlates of depression in children, some of which are similar to those observed in adults while some are different (Jensen & Saunders,1991). There are also several biochemical theories of depression and no doubt there are biochemical changes in the brain which correspond to, and indeed are part of, the depressive process. There has however been little research on the biochemical correlates of childhood depression.

As indicated in Figure 10.1, depression sometimes appears as a secondary phenomenon accompanying such other conditions as conduct disorders, adjustment disorders, separation anxiety and attention-deficit disorders. It may be difficult to determine which is the primary condition, particularly when conduct disorder and depressive symptoms co-exist. This has no doubt been a factor in the proposal that mixed disorders of conduct and emotions, specifically *depressive conduct disorder* be recognized as distinct disorders, as discussed in Chapter 9.

Depression may also complicate physical illnesses such as those listed in Figure 10.1. Some drugs used in the treatment of physical illnesses, for example cortisone, prednisone and related compounds, may lead to depression. So also may the chronic abuse of barbiturates, cocaine and other 'street' drugs.

Description

The essential feature of all depressive disorders is depressed mood, that is a mood of sadness and gloom, which may be accompanied by tearfulness.

Typically the subject looks unhappy and may express feelings of misery and hopelessness. There is loss of energy and of interest in things which usually interest the person. Self-blame and feelings of unworthiness and guilt, such as are not justified by the circumstances, are other common features. Of course, feelings of depression are familiar to all of us, but in depressive illnesses these are of greater severity and duration.

A variety of other symptoms usually accompany the feelings of depression and some combination of these is required to make the diagnosis. These include:

- Change in sleep pattern, usually insomnia though sometimes excessive sleepiness.
- Change in appetite, usually diminished appetite but sometimes an increase in appetite.
- Weight changes associated with the appetite changes.
- Slowing of thought processes and of bodily movements.
- School problems. These may be academic or social, with either withdrawal or episodes of aggressive behaviour.
- Suicidal thoughts or behaviour.

Eliciting these symptoms in young children can be difficult, and normal children tend to exhibit quite rapid changes of mood. They may be crying one minute and laughing the next. To make a diagnosis of a depressive disorder, however, it is necessary to have evidence of a sustained period of depressed mood, together with at least some of the other symptoms listed above, rather than a series of brief periods of unhappiness. The limited vocabulary and capacity to conceptualize of younger children may make it hard for them to explain what they are experiencing. Sometimes depression is conveyed better in their play or their drawings or paintings than in their conversation.

Self-blame and feelings of guilt are common in depression. One depressed 12-year-old said that her 'nervous state' was responsible for her father's difficulties at the office, her mother's anaemia and general ill-health and the bad behaviour of her brother and sister. She also had difficulty getting to school and entertained suicidal thoughts.

In adolescence, depression of psychotic intensity, that is with delusions and hallucinations, is encountered more often than in younger children. Well developed delusional systems are uncommon but hallucinations with depressive content are reported more frequently; they may take the form of voices telling the young person that he or she is a worthless, bad person, responsible for various evil things.

While the onset of depression in adolescents may be acute, it is more often insidious and the depression may not be immediately obvious.

Rather than presenting with depressed mood, the adolescent may present with anxiety – perhaps about going to school – panic attacks or somatic symptoms such as headaches or abdominal pain. The presence of depression may only be revealed by appropriate questioning, in response to which the young person may talk about how she or he has felt like weeping, can get little or no pleasure out of life and may even have been considering suicide, or perhaps running away. Fatigue, irritability, poor concentration, difficulty in coping with school work which previously did not present difficulty, and sleep and appetite disturbances may also be revealed on questioning. There may or may not be a history of stress in the family, school or wider environments.

The term *anaclitic depression* was coined by Spitz (1946) to describe a condition of misery, crying, withdrawal and failure to thrive in babies and young children suffering from severe deprivation of parental care. This was apparently an environmentally determined reaction to a gross lack of care, such as may be found in large, poorly run institutions which, fortunately, are rare in developed countries. It is probably unrelated to the depressive conditions seen in later childhood.

In assessing children it is important to bear in mind that the parents are not always aware of depression in their children. The children tend to be better sources of information than their parents. Brent, *et al.* (1986), in a study of childhood suicidal behaviour, found poor correlation between the reports of the children and those of their parents. They recommended that the more serious report should be given the greater weight.

Several self-report and parent-report scales and some semi-structured interview schedules have been devised to assist in the diagnosis of childhood depression. Their greatest use is probably in research, but they can be of help in the assessment process and in monitoring the response to treatment. They have been reviewed by Costello (1986).

Associated conditions

As discussed in the previous chapter, depression is often associated with conduct disorder symptoms. Another important association is with eating disorders, about one-third of patients with such disorders also having affective disorders, most often depression. As we have seen above, anxiety symptoms of various sorts also accompany depression in many subjects.

Suicide and suicidal behaviour

Suicidal behaviour in children and especially in adolescents has become a subject of increasing concern as its incidence has been climbing in many

Major Affective Disorders and Suicide   125

jurisdictions and it seems to be occurring more frequently at younger ages. The existing state of our knowledge in this area was reviewed by Carlson (1990b). Suicide rates increase with age with males predominating. According to the studies reviewed by Carlson (1990b), shooting, hanging and carbon monoxide poisoning are the leading methods used by males. The predominance of shooting probably reflects the fact that the studies reviewed were from the United States, where guns are more readily available than in many other countries. Girls used overdoses, carbon monoxide and firearms with about equal frequency.

Incidence of suicide

This varies substantially according to the population and age range studied. Thompson (1987) studied the rates of suicide in subjects younger than 20 in the Canadian province of Manitoba during the years 1971 to 1982. He found rates to be much higher in Native American boys than in other groups.

In the USA in 1986, the age-specific mortality from suicide in 5- to 14-year old children was 0.8 per 100 000 with most of these occurring near the top of this age range. In the age range 15 to 24 the rate was 12.8 per 100 000, this accounting for about 16% of all deaths in this age bracket. These rates have been increasing steadily since the early 1960s. The rates for males are consistently higher than those for females (Pfeffer, 1991).

The rates of attempted suicide

These are more difficult to estimate for several reasons, though it is generally accepted that they are higher for girls than for boys, and also higher than completed suicides, especially in girls. Exactly what constitutes a suicide attempt is not always clear. Many people take minor overdoses of sedative or other drugs, cut their wrists or indulge in other minor acts of self-harm, without having a wish to die. Such behaviour is sometimes referred to as *parasuicide* and it is commonly seen in teenage girls who are under stress of one sort or another. Rather than being an attempt at suicide, the act is rather a cry for help or attention, or an attempt to draw attention to some need or problem. Sometimes, though, the subject miscalculates and the outcome is fatal. In practice, it is hard to draw the line between parasuicide and true suicide attempts, though to whichever category an 'attempt' belongs there is usually a need for psychiatric assessment and, often, treatment.

Frequency of suicidal behaviour

In clinical populations, especially inpatients in psychiatric units the frequency is naturally much greater than that in the general population. For example, Myers *et al.* (1985) reported that 61 (17.5% – 40 boys and 21 girls) of 348 children aged 5–13 admitted to a psychiatric unit had engaged in suicidal behaviour, defined as 'any self-destructive statement or action expressed with explicit desire to kill oneself, and offered whether spontaneously or upon interview'. A wish to be dead did not qualify. Seven were aged 5–7, and 25 were in the age range 8–10, the remainder being 11 or older. This is a rather lower percentage than others that have been reported. Most of the suicidal children were diagnosed as having either depressive or conduct disorders. Depression was diagnosed in 30% of the suicidal children but in only 3% of the non-suicidal admissions. A conduct disorder diagnosis was made about equally frequently in the two groups.

When the family histories of the suicidal children were compared with those of the non-suicidal admissions, they were found to contain significantly more abused mothers, abusive fathers and reports of suicidal behaviours by other family members. The children had also experienced recent stressful life events more often than their non-suicidal fellow inpatients. The results of this study are similar to those of other studies.

Seriousness

Suicidal behaviour should not be taken lightly. Although in many cases, especially in the pre-pubertal age group, it does not presage actual suicide, it is often an indication that there are serious problems in the family, the child, or both. Some children threaten suicide in imitation of the behaviour of other family members. Such children may have no intention of killing themselves but living in a household in which members make such threats can promote feelings of insecurity and be stressful in other ways. In some families threatening, or talking about, suicide is a family-sanctioned way of expressing distress. Suicidal behaviour in any family member is often an indication that there is serious psychopathology in the family.

In adolescence the risk of suicide is generally greater than it is in younger children. The assessment of suicidal risk is an important part of the psychiatric examination and is discussed in Chapter 18. The presence of suicidal ideation or intent, or a history of past attempts, should alert the clinician that there may be serious family problems or that the suicidal individual may be in emotional difficulty – or both. It may be that the young person or the family are having difficulty negotiating a stage in the life cycle. On the other hand, the subject may be suffering from a major psychiatric disorder, perhaps especially a depressive one. Many adolescent suicides are impulsive rather than planned acts. The ready availability of a means of suicide, such as a gun or drugs which are lethal in overdose, results in the fatal act. Some adolescents kill themselves in the context of the abuse of alcohol or other drugs which adversely affect their judgement.

Attempted suicide always justifies careful psychiatric assessment of the suicidal individual and the family. The depression which is often present may clear up, though perhaps only temporarily, after the attempt. This often happens when the young person is in hospital and is being treated solicitously by the family and others. The underlying problems may continue, however, and if they are not addressed in treatment, there may be repeated attempts at suicide.

Mania and manic disorders

In mania, and its lesser form, hypomania, the mood disturbance is in the direction of elation. Manic subjects typically feel excessively happy, though irritability may predominate. They are hyperactive, constantly on the go and lacking in judgement. They may spend their money as if they are millionaires. They sleep less than usual, their self-esteem is inflated and they may engage in many reckless and often ill-judged activities. Their speech is rapid and pressured and may contain many jokes and puns. There may be *flight of ideas*, the rapid flitting from one subject to another associated one, though the process may be so fast that others miss the association. The manic subject is readily distracted and often starts things but does not finish them. Delusions of grandeur, such as thinking one is the king, or God, or enormously wealthy, or possessed of special powers, are common. Hallucinations, which may reinforce the delusional ideas, sometimes occur.

The term *hypomania* is used for milder forms of this condition. There is elation and excess activity, often combined with some of the other features mentioned, but the full picture is not present and there are no delusions, hallucinations or psychotic behaviour.

Manic disorders are rare before puberty, though some well documented cases are on record. Mania is often one part of the mood cycle in bipolar disorders. It has been suggested that manic conditions in pre-pubertal children are liable to be confused with attention-deficit hyperactivity disorder. In adolescence it can be hard to differentiate manic disorders from schizophrenia.

The diagnosis of child and adolescent mania is discussed and the literature reviewed by Carlson (1990a). She makes the important point that attention-deficit and conduct disorders are usually chronic, with onset before the age of six or seven, whereas mania is episodic. Hyperactive conduct disordered children may boast and appear grandiose though they are not usually truly elated.

Bipolar affective disorders (manic-depressive psychosis)

Manic or hypomanic states are often episodes in the course of bipolar affective disorders. The subject has periods of depression alternating with periods of mania or hypomania, often with periods of normal mood in between. A manic or depressive episode may last from a few days to many months and the periods of normal mood in between these episodes may be similarly varied. Children in whom bipolar disorder appears before puberty have a particularly virulent form of the disorder (Carlson, 1990a). Onset is much more common in adolescence and indeed the usual age of onset is in adolescence or early adulthood.

According to Hassanyeh & Davidson (1980), who reported five boys and five girls with onset of bipolar disorder before age 16, mania is easier to diagnose in this age period than depression which, they report, was sometimes diagnosed retrospectively. They warn, however, that mild cases of mania and hypomania can easily be mistaken for manifestations of conduct disorder. This is especially so when restlessness, hostility, irritability and verbal abuse predominate. In addition to displaying euphoria, hyperactivity, pressure of speech, flight of ideas, grandiosity, sleep disturbance and distractibility, manic adolescents often hurled verbal abuse at their parents and denied that anything was amiss, even in the face of wildly disturbed behaviour. In the girls, sexually provocative behaviour, including wandering about the house naked, was common. The manic patients' rooms were in a state of total disorder, the 'bomb-in-the-room' syndrome. In their depressed phases these patients showed depressed mood, self-depreciation, agitation, sleep disturbance, diminished socialization, changed attitudes towards school, somatic complaints, lack of energy, loss of appetite and/or weight, suicidal ideation and psychomotor retardation. Two of the depressed patients presented in stupor (a state of depressed consciousness, short of unconsciousness, in which the subject appears dazed and unresponsive). Others showed severe psychomotor retardation – that is, a slowing of both thoughts and actions.

Treatment of affective disorders

Children's moods are very sensitive to the environment and depressive feelings are often reactive to environmental factors. They may meet the criteria for an adjustment disorder (see Chapter 15) and, if so, the main need may be either to lessen the stress to which the child is reacting or to provide support until the stress has lessened or no longer exists.

When the stress is chronic and/or severe the therapeutic task is more difficult. Apart from general family instability, there may be parental alcoholism or drug abuse; physical violence towards the children or between the parents; sexual abuse; emotional rejection; physical neglect; or some combination of these factors. The family system may be such that the child plays the role of family scapegoat, which can be quite stressful.

A prime focus of treatment should be the alleviation of any stresses the child is facing. There may be a need for family therapy; counselling of the parents; temporary removal of the child to a treatment centre or other placement while steps are taken to change the stressful circumstances; intervention in the school to alleviate stress there; or treatment of depression, alcoholism or other psychiatric problems in a parent or parents. A supportive relationship with a therapist may be helpful, especially when the stress is likely to be short-lived and when active steps are being taken to deal with the source of stress.

The role of antidepressant drugs in the treatment of childhood depression is unclear. Although Puig-Antich (1980) reported encouraging results, subsequent studies have not been so encouraging. The evidence for the efficacy of these drugs in depressed children and adolescents has been reviewed by Jensen & Saunders (1991). They conclude that the results of treatment with tricyclic antidepressants such as imipramine or nortriptyline are generally disappointing, though they suggest that one reason for the poor results of many clinical trials of these drugs may be due to the mixing of patients with *reactive* depressions with those who suffer from *biologic* depression. Indeed there is some evidence that children with *pure* depression or depression associated with an anxiety-related disorder, show a higher drug response rate and a lower placebo response than those in whom the depression was associated with a conduct or oppositional disorder.

My own clinical experience suggests that in quite a small majority of pre-pubertal children in whom there is a strong family history of depression, and in whom the depression is a recurrent phenomenon in the absence of substantial environmental stress, the response to tricyclic antidepressants tends to be good. All this suggests that a particularly careful clinical assessment is in order before the use of medication is considered. It has also been suggested that immaturity of the nervous and endocrine systems of children may affect the response to antidepressants.

In the management of subjects with depression, the possibility of suicide must always be borne in mind. If the risk appears high, admission to a hospital unit for children or adolescents may be advisable, though in some well functioning families sufficiently close observation may be possible in the home. Admission to hospital, or temporary placement in some other situation out of the home, may also serve to relieve stress while work is done to lessen the stress. Periodic assessments of suicidal risk are advisable as long as the depression persists.

Lithium carbonate is effective in preventing the recurrence of attacks of mania and depression in many subjects with bipolar disorders. Its use, and that of other drugs, together with other treatment methods that may be of value in children and adolescents with affective disorders, are discussed further in Chapter 21.

Outcome

Major affective disorders tend to resolve in time, even without treatment, provided suicide does not intervene. This applies in childhood and adolescence as much as it does in adult life. Unfortunately the risk of recurrence is quite high and it seems that it is even higher in children with primary affective disorders – that is, those that do not appear to be secondary to severe stress or other psychiatric problems. With onset in adolescence the risk is less than with pre-pubertal onset, but greater than with onset in adult life.

When the affective condition, usually depression, is secondary to continuing stress or is associated with conduct, oppositional or attention-deficit disorder, the outlook often seems to depend on the progress of the associated disorder. As a general rule, the more the condition is a response to environmental circumstances, the better the outlook is, providing the adverse circumstances are temporary or can be alleviated, or the child removed from them. If the cause appears to be more *endogenous* – that is, in so-called *primary* cases – the outlook is generally less good. Heavy genetic loading for affective disorders, alcoholism or anti-social behaviour may be poor prognostic signs.

Chapter 11

Pervasive Developmental Disorders

Originally introduced to diagnostic schemes in DSM-III, the term *pervasive developmental disorder* has now been embraced also by ICD-10. It takes in, but is not confined to, autistic disorders, a long-recognized group of disorders with early onset. As summarized in the ICD-10 manual, the main features of these disorders are 'qualitative abnormalities in reciprocal social interactions and in patterns of communication [and a] restricted, stereotyped, repetitive repertoire of interests and activities'. While in the great majority of cases there is some degree of impairment of cognitive functioning, some of these children are of average or higher intelligence. Mental retardation is thus not a necessary feature. DSM-IV defines autistic disorders in similar terms.

Autism

Many terms have been used for the disorder first described by Leo Kanner (1943; 1944) as *early infantile autism*. DSM-IV used the term *autistic disorder*, while ICD-10's term is *childhood autism*.

For many years children presenting with the syndrome that Kanner described were regarded as suffering from a psychotic disorder (see Chapter 13) coming on very early in life. Some considered it a form of schizophrenia and argued that one could not expect schizophrenia starting before the subject had learned to talk, and while cognitive development was still at an early stage, to present in the same way as in older persons. For example, auditory hallucinations would be unlikely in a child who had not started talking.

Subsequent research has demonstrated so many differences between autism and schizophrenia that it is now generally agreed that these conditions are distinct disorders (Rutter & Garmezy, 1983). Autistic children exhibit delays and abnormalities in the development of a range of psychological functions, with onset early in life. Psychoses, on the other hand, are characterized by the loss of reality contact in people who previously have maintained a conventional relationship to and understanding of their environment. In as far as autistic children appear to be out of touch with reality, this is secondary to a gross failure of the developmental process to take its usual course.

Prevalence

On the basis of reported studies, Zahner & Pauls (1987) concluded that the prevalence of autism is about four to five cases per 10 000. Much depends, however, upon the strictness of the criteria used for making the diagnosis. In addition to autistic disorders, DSM-III-R also had a category of 'pervasive developmental disorders not otherwise specified'. This was not precisely defined and was often used for disorders which have many of the features of autism but do not completely meet the criteria for autistic disorders. ICD-10 has categories for *atypical autism* and for 'other pervasive developmental disorders' and 'pervasive developmental disorder, unspecified'. If some or all of the cases which can be classified in these *residual* groups are included, this is reflected in higher prevalence rates. On the other hand, if very strict criteria are used, prevalence rates as low as 2 per 10 000 are found.

Autistic disorders are about three times more common in boys than girls but there is some evidence that girls tend to be more seriously affected (Lord, *et al.*, 1982).

Causes and associated conditions

Genetic, organic cerebral, environmental, biochemical and immunological causes have all been suggested for autism. Good evidence that genetic factors are involved was provided by a study of 21 pairs of same-sexed twins, one or both of whom had autism (Folstein & Rutter, 1977). Eleven were monozygotic (MZ), that is, *identical* and ten dizygotic (DZ), or *fraternal*. Four of the MZ, but none of the DZ pairs were concordant for autism. In addition, six of the non-autistic co-twins (five MZ and one DZ) showed some serious cognitive disability, either speech delay, IQ below 70 or scholastic difficulties. Thus there was 36% concordance for autism in MZ twins as compared with none in DZ twins; and 82% concordance for cognitive disorder in MZ pairs, as against 10% in DZ pairs. These findings could not be explained on the basis of brain damage at birth. It seemed that in some cases the disorder resulted from an inherited cognitive defect plus brain damage.

There are other reasons to believe that genetic factors are involved. The rate of autism in the siblings of autistic children is about 50 times that in the general population, and there is a family history of delayed speech in about 25% (Bartak, *et al.*, 1975). Also 15% of the siblings of autistic children show evidence of language disorders, learning difficulties or mental retardation, whereas this applies only to 3% of the siblings of children with Down's syndrome (August, *et al.*, 1981).

The relationship between autism and the 'fragile X' chromosome abnormality has been the subject of much discussion and controversy. While there is agreement that this abnormality is associated with mental retardation, reports of whether and, if so, how often it is associated with autism have been conflicting. Summarizing the results of studies that have screened autistic males, Hagerman (1992) reports an 'overall yield of fragile X-positive individuals' of about 7% which, he points out, makes fragile X the most common known medical cause of autism. Although autism has been reported in females, Hagerman (1992) concludes that it is rare but that it 'appears to be on the continuum of shyness and social anxiety that are very common in fragile X girls'. To quote Hagerman (1992, page 1133) again:

'The significant finding is that a spectrum of autistic features is seen throughout all individuals affected by fragile X, which reflects an impairment in brain function caused by fragile X.'

The *autistic features* of the fragile X syndrome include such behaviours as gaze avoidance, hand-flapping, stereotypies, attentional problems and impulsivity. These can all interfere with the individual's social relationship capacity. How often a diagnosis of autistic disorder is made in these children may depend largely on how many autistic features are considered to be needed to make the diagnosis.

It does seem clear that autism is not simply a reaction to the environment. Some of the early reports of this condition favoured explanations based on psychodynamic theories and even proposed that the condition was due to certain parenting styles. Such theories, as least as explanations for the development of autism, are not now generally accepted, though the stability and other characteristics of the autistic child's family are important influences on how such children develop.

It seems clear that abnormalities of brain functioning are at the basis of autism but precisely what these abnormalities are is unclear. Bishop (1993) points out that because the majority of autistic children are mentally retarded, it is 'not surprising to find widespread neuropathology associated with autism'. The abnormalities reported vary greatly however and which of them are responsible for the specifically autistic features, as opposed to the associated mental retardation, remains to be elucidated. On the basis of his review of research, however, Bishop (1993) suggests that abnormalities in the frontal lobes of the brain, and in an area of the frontal and temporal cortex known as the *mesolimbic cortex*, are strong contenders for the sites of the trouble.

Autistic syndromes have been reported in children with congenital rubella (Chess, 1977) and following infantile spasms (see Chapter 13).

Another theory is that some cases of autism may have an immunological basis. Stubbs, *et al.* (1985) studied human leucocyte (white blood cell) antigens (HLA) in the parents of autistic children. They found that the parents shared HLAs very much more often than parents of normal children are believed to do, and offer an ingenious explanation of how this might be related to autism in the children.

While Kanner (1943; 1944) stated that the parents of autistic children lack emotional warmth and are detached and of obsessional personality, subsequent research has produced no firm evidence of this. Moreover it has been suggested that the reported parental attitudes, when they are observed, could be reactions to the behaviour of these children, especially their lack of emotional responsiveness. It seems unlikely that adverse parental attitudes or handling could be solely or even mainly responsible for so severe a condition coming on so early in life. Moreover, autism has not been shown to be associated with child abuse or neglect. On the other hand the way autistic children are reared, and the type of care they are given, certainly can affect their development. Given that their autistic child tends to withdraw into his or her own world and shun contact with reality, the parents may either accept this, or they may take active measures to counter such behaviour. The same applies to the responses of teachers and others with whom the child comes into contact.

Description

Kanner (1943; 1944) described four main features of 'early infantile autism':

- autistic aloneness;
- delayed or abnormal speech;
- an obsessive desire for sameness;
- onset in the first two years of life.

These have remained the basis of the diagnosis but the criteria have been refined and clear evidence of onset before age two is not required by all definitions. As the ICD-10 manual puts it:

'Usually there is no prior period of unequivocally normal development but, if there is, abnormalities become apparent before the age of 3 years'. (Page 253.)

DSM-IV also stipulates that the symptoms should start before age three. The four main areas of functioning which are affected in autism are:

(a) social interaction
(b) communication
(c) behaviour, the range of which is restrictive and repetitive
(d) cognitive function.

(a) Social interaction

There is a qualitative impairment of reciprocal social interaction. This is the *autistic aloneness* described by Kanner. Autistic children seem unable to appreciate the feelings of others and to respond to social cues as normal children do. They do not intuitively modify their behaviour in response to the signals others give and to the context as non-autistic children do. There is a lack of empathy, of understanding of the feelings and emotional reactions of others. They tend to 'do their own thing' regardless of who is around or what is happening in their environment. They seem unable to 'read' their environment as other children do. The able and committed parents of one 14-year-old boy described how they made a practice of teaching their son everything he would have to do when he went to a party or other social event; but woe betide them if they missed a step or something unexpected happened at the party, because the boy could never figure out, from the context, what he should do.

The parents often report that their autistic children were unresponsive infants who did not seem to want to be kissed or cuddled. They may have failed to assume the posture appropriate for being picked up or nursed. The social smile has often developed late and these children are typically slow to distinguish between parents and strangers, approaching either without discriminating between them. A related behaviour is gaze avoidance, the failure to make eye to eye contact with people. While autistic children may look at people, they fail to do so when it is appropriate, for example during a conversation or when requesting something. These children often appear more interested in a person's spectacles or facial contours, than with the individual as a person. *Indicating behaviours,* such as drawing people's attention to things by showing them or alternately looking at them and making eye contact with the other person, have been found to occur less often than in retarded children or normal children at similar developmental levels (Mundy, *et al.,* 1986).

(b) Communication

Both verbal and non-verbal language are affected. Not only do these children fail to develop normal or, sometimes, any speech, but they also fail to communicate effectively by gesture, body movements or facial expression. They differ from children with developmental language disorders (see Chapter 12) who point to what they want, pull people towards things and generally make their wishes known in non-verbal ways. Also when autistic children do develop speech, they fail to use it for social communication in the normal way. They may exhibit *echolalia*, the repeating of words or phrases spoken by others. They usually use these out of context and inappropriately. The echolalia may be immediate or delayed. If delayed, the words or phrases may come out of the blue much later, resulting in the production of what seems to be nonsense. Many autistic children acquire a few stock phrases which they repeat in parrot fashion, with little or no relation to what is going on around them. Their speech is often stilted and monotonous, without the usual intonations and inflexions.

It seems that these children's failure to speak normally is but one manifestation of a profound defect of language function, often present from the early months, though in some cases speech starts to develop normally and is then lost, partially or completely.

(c) Behavioural abnormalities

The behaviour of these children is characterized by rigidity, stereotypies and inflexibility. The range of their behaviour is usually quite limited. As the ICD-10 manual puts it, they tend 'to impose rigidity and routine on a wide range of aspects of day to day functioning'. Some autistic children get very upset by minor changes in routine, or the moving of furniture in their house, wearing different clothes, or even a change in the order in which books are placed in a bookcase. While they can be taught new skills, they have difficulty generalizing these to new situations or tasks. Their play is stereotyped and repetitive. Typically it is neither symbolic nor imaginative and toys are rarely used as the objects they represent. Thus an autistic child may use a toy telephone to bang on the floor or to swing to and fro on the end of its cord, but will probably not imitate adults' use of a telephone by speaking into the mouthpiece as other children do. A word of caution is in order here, however, because lack of symbolic play is common, though less so, in retarded non-autistic children, so that its discriminative value is limited. In some ways the rigidity and repetitiveness of these children's activities is a behavioural equivalent to their stereotyped and repetitive language.

Ritualistic behaviour is common in these children, for example checking and touching rituals and dressing in particular ways. When their
rituals are interrupted, these children may become anxious or angry.
Rocking, twirling, head-banging and similar repetitive behaviours are
often seen, especially in mentally retarded autistic children. They are not
confined to autistic children, however, and may be seen in non-autistic
retarded children, especially the more severely retarded, and in those
with seriously impaired hearing or vision.

Other non-specific behavioural abnormalities often encountered in
autistic children include overactivity, disruptive behaviour and temper
tantrums, which may occur for little or no obvious reason. Overactivity
may alternate with underactivity. Such self-destructive behaviours as
violent head-banging or biting the arms, wrists or other parts of the body
may occur. Other common symptoms are sleep disturbances, fears and
phobias, wetting and soiling, and impulsive acts. All these, while not
confined to autistic children, are particularly hard to deal with in such
children because it is difficult to communicate effectively with them.

(d) Cognitive abnormalities

These are complex and extensive (Rutter, 1983) and they extend well
beyond the problems with the use of language mentioned above.

As we have seen, a majority of autistic children are mentally retarded
but in all of them, whether retarded or not, there is an abnormal pattern of
cognitive functioning. Memory may be excellent, and indeed in some
areas it may be phenomenal, and visuospatial tasks may be well
performed, but these children are poor at symbolization, understanding
abstract ideas and grasping theoretical concepts. They may be preoccupied with things like train or bus timetables or the different models of
cars or aeroplanes. One 11-year-old boy knew the numbers of all the main
highway routes in the UK. He had spent many hours poring over maps
and one had only to ask him how to get from one city or town to another,
and the route and road numbers would pour forth immediately and
accurately. Abstract or creative thought, however, were beyond him.

Atypical autism

Atypical autism is a term that appears for the first time in ICD-10, though
DSM-IV's 'pervasive developmental disorder not otherwise specified'
seems to cover similar conditions. These categories reflect the reality that
there are children who display many *autistic* features but who do not
exhibit the full picture. Atypical autism, according to ICD-10, is to be used

for pervasive developmental disorders which differ from autism either in their age of onset, or because of failure to fulfil all three of the sets of diagnostic criteria – that is, impaired social interaction, communication problems, and restricted, stereotyped, repetitive behaviour. According to ICD-10, this condition arises most often in children with a very low level of functioning which results in their having little scope for exhibiting the specific behaviours required for a diagnosis of autism. The ICD-10 manual also states that atypical autism can also occur in individuals with a severe specific developmental disorder of receptive language (see Chapter 12).

Rett's syndrome (ICD-10) or disorder (DSM-IV)

First described by Rett in 1966, this syndrome is now included as a category of pervasive developmental disorder by both ICD-10 and DSM-IV. Occurring in girls, it is characterized by apparently normal early development and then, usually with onset between the ages of 7 and 24 months, the gradual loss of manual dexterity and speech. Many of these children display *autistic* features such as impairment in social interaction and language, and stereotypies, particularly those involving hand-wringing. This condition is clearly a degenerative neurological one and by middle childhood these children have developed a variety of other neurological problems, affecting especially motor function. Eventually they develop severe mental handicap and gross motor disabilities. The syndrome is well reviewed by Tsai (1992) who also discusses the pros and cons of classifying Rett's syndrome as a pervasive developmental disorder.

Other childhood disintegrative disorder

ICD-10 suggests the use of the above term for pervasive developmental disorders, other than Rett's syndrome, in which there is normal or near-normal development for the first two years of life followed by the loss, over a period of a few months, of various previously acquired social and communicative skills, together with behavioural deterioration. DSM-IV uses the term *childhood disintegrative disorder*.

These children may become irritable, restive, anxious and overactive. The loss of skills and behavioural disturbance may be progressive but in many cases it stabilizes after a period of some months of deterioration. By that time there is usually a profound loss of language, regressed functioning in the areas of play, social skills and adaptive behaviour generally, together with loss of bowel and/or bladder control. There is usually a loss of interest in the environment, together with stereotyped, repetitive movements and autistic-like impairment of social interactions. According to ICD-10 they are not correctly identified as cases of dementia because they differ in three key aspects. There is no evidence of an identifiable organic disease or damage; the loss of skills is sometimes followed by a degree of recovery and the impaired socialization and communication has 'deviant qualities typical of autism rather than of intellectual decline'.

These disorders are an ill-defined group, probably of varied aetiology, requiring more research before we can be confident about how they should be classified.

Asperger's syndrome

This is another disorder that appears for the first time in both ICD-10 and DSM-IV. In the previous edition of this book it was discussed as a category of personality disorder, partly because children fitting Asperger's description of the syndrome are sometimes referred to as suffering from 'schizoid personality disorder of childhood'. The new classifications, however, list it in their sections on pervasive developmental disorders, possibly because it has by some been considered to be a variant, or milder form, of autism.

In 1944 Asperger described what he called 'autistic psychopathy of childhood'. Wolff & Barlow (1979) described 17 such children and compared them with intelligent autistic children and with normal children. Since then there has been increasing interest in this group of children, with many published reports and much discussion of what may be the true nature of the disorder.

Children with Asperger's syndrome are distant, aloof and lacking in empathy and in these respects resemble autistic children. Gillberg & Gillberg (1989) list the following diagnostic criteria:

- Severe impairment in reciprocal social interaction. These children do not play or interact with others in a reciprocal way; they lack interest in being in the company of other children; they fail to understand and react appropriately to social cues and consequently display odd social behaviours.
- 'An all-absorbing, circumscribed interest in a subject'. This is invariably taken to extremes and tends to exclude interest in other subjects.
- The attempt to introduce and impose stereotyped routines, or the subject's special interest, in all or almost all aspects of life.
- Speech and language problems. Language development is delayed, it

tends to be 'formal and pedantic' and often flat and staccato, though 'superficially [perfectly] expressive'.

- Non-verbal communication problems. These included limited or clumsy gestures and inappropriate facial expressions.
- Motor clumsiness. (This is one of the features that distinguishes these children from those with autism who are typically agile.)
- They find group activities, especially rough games, stressful. Other features are obstinacy and aggressive outbursts when they are under pressure to conform; preoccupation with their own systems of idea and beliefs, for example electronics, dinosaurs or space travel; emotional detachment; rigidity, which may be of obsessional proportions; sensitivity, sometimes with accompanying paranoid ideas; learning problems which may be present despite above-average or average assessed intelligence; and, in a minority of cases, bizarre antisocial behaviour.

Asperger's syndrome is commoner in boys than in girls, the male:female ratio being 9 or 10 to 1. Referral is often the result of school-related problems such as school refusal, running away, temper outbursts, suicidal threats, stealing and mutism.

This seems to be a distinct group of children whose presentation, in some respects, falls somewhere between that of autistic children and that of normal children. This does not necessarily mean that children with Asperger's Syndrome simply have mild degrees of autism, though the ICD-10 manual suggests that this may sometimes be the case. Like autistic children, they show stereotypies and tend to impose patterns on their environment, and they have linguistic handicaps and lack perceptiveness for meaning. On the other hand, they do not show the repetitiveness and the motivation for tasks of cognition and memory of autistic children, and they do not show the general delay or retardation in language or in cognitive development that are so common in autistic children. Their motor clumsiness also presents a contrast with the agility so common in autistic children.

'Residual' categories

Both ICD-10 and DSM-IV have residual categories for 'other' and 'not otherwise specified' pervasive development disorders. This acknowledges that there are a number of children who present clinical pictures which resemble those of the conditions described above, but who do not meet all the listed diagnostic criteria. DSM-III included 'infantile autism, residual state', a term which described children who had met the criteria for autism in the past, but who had experienced a degree of recovery and no longer met the full criteria. This term was dropped in DSM-III-R and did not reappear in DSM-IV.

Differentiating PDDs from other conditions

Pervasive developmental disorders require to be distinguished from the results of deafness, various forms of mental retardation, developmental language disorders and the psychotic disorders discussed in Chapter 13.

The history and clinical presentation usually provide good evidence that the problem is failure to respond to people, rather than inability to hear. Nevertheless it is usually wise to arrange audiometry to confirm this. These children can be hard to test and in difficult or doubtful cases the measurement by electroencephalogram (EEG) of the responses evoked in the cerebral hemispheres by auditory stimuli may be helpful in determining whether there is any hearing loss.

While mental retardation and PDD often co-exist, retarded children who do not suffer from PDD usually relate freely with people, are not preoccupied with sameness and are more generally retarded. By contrast, the retardation seen in children with PDD is more patchy and tends to be confined to particular functions while others, such as memory or mathematical skills, may even be possessed at an advanced level.

Children with developmental language disorders (see Chapter 12) are not usually withdrawn and respond to people normally and communicate freely by non-verbal means. Echolalia and pronoun reversal are much less common than in autistic children. Bizarre behaviours, rigidity, stereotypies and lack of symbolic and imaginative play are not features of developmental language disorders.

Treatment of PDDs

No treatments are available which remedy the ill-understood basic causes of the PDDs. Treatment is therefore symptomatic. Nevertheless there is much that can be done to help these children and their families.

Lord & Rutter (1994) provide an excellent summary of how treatment may be approached. The essence of the task is to foster social and communicative development; enhance learning and problem-solving; decrease behaviours which impede learning; and assist families in coping with their autistic members. Educational and behavioural methods remain the mainstays of treatment. A basic principle is that children – like adults also – generally learn more from doing things than from having things done for them.

Like all children, autistic children have a need for active meaningful experiences. Particular experiences are needed to counter the various problems autistic children have in the area of cognitive development. Thus for self-isolation planned periods of interaction are needed; for impaired understanding, simplified communication and individual teaching; for specific cognitive defects, learning tasks which capitalize on the skills the child does possess while helping develop those that are weak; and for lack of initiative, a more structured and direct teaching approach than is used with normal children. Language skills, social skills and the capacity to learn, can all be promoted using similar principles. Their essence is the careful assessment of the child's strengths and weaknesses, and the systematic building up of skills where these are weak, while capitalizing on the areas of strength.

Some of the implications of this approach are that the treatment should aim to counter social isolation by ensuring that the child experiences periods of interaction. It should break learning down into small steps specifically suited to the child's progress to date. Teaching should take place in structured, individualized situations. It is also important that personalized caretaking is enhanced by the avoidance of residential care in early childhood. The treatment task, the essence of which is teaching things which autistic children find it much harder to learn than normal children do, is both complex and challenging. A sound knowledge of behaviour therapy principles, as outlined in Chapter 21, and by Murdoch & Barker (1991) is necessary for effective treatment.

An important part of the treatment of these children is the teaching of communication skills. This is often a long and difficult task. It has been suggested that the use of both non-vocal methods of communication, namely sign language and symbols, as well as verbal methods may be helpful. This has been called *total communication*. Although these children often have as much difficulty with non-verbal as with verbal communication, a combination of the two may promote faster development than either alone. While it is clear that many children can learn to use signs to communicate their needs, the part that sign language should play in treatment is at present a matter of dispute among those treating these children.

Treatment should be a joint venture of the planners of the programme, the professional behaviour therapists, the speech therapists and teachers concerned, and the parents. Treatment is usually best carried out in the home and a neighbourhood school, preferably in a small class or group, with increasing opportunities for the autistic children to mix with their non-autistic peers as their communication and social skills improve. Residential treatment is to be avoided if this is at all possible. These children are liable to become institutionalized because of their tendency to withdraw from social contacts and their communication difficulties. Some parents become highly skilled behaviour therapists and can provide almost constant therapeutic experiences for their children. These children are at a great advantage, since the amount of therapeutic work done with them may be much greater than would otherwise be possible if it were carried out only by mental health professionals who are rarely available to the extent that parents are. Another advantage they have is that the treatment by the parents is carried out in their natural home and family environment.

Medication is sometimes helpful in the management of autistic children. There is some evidence that the use of haloperidol can lead to decreased level of social withdrawal, hyperactivity, stereotypies, fidgetiness, and emotional lability (Gadow, 1992). Other drugs which have been reported to be of value in treating some of the symptoms of autistic disorders include fenfluramine, a drug which has some similar actions to amphetamine; the opiate antagonist naltrexone; propanolol; and the anxiolytic buspirone. None of these is an established treatment but there is some evidence that each of them may be of value in lessening certain of the symptoms. The relevant literature is summarized by Gadow (1992). There is less information on the value of drugs in the treatment of pervasive developmental disorders other than autism, but both haloperidol and fenfluramine may be of value (Gadow, 1992).

An important aspect of the management of these cases is providing appropriate help for the families. The presence in a family of a severely disturbed child places a great strain on the other family members. Emotional support and, sometimes, relief care can lighten the burden experienced by parents and other family members. Generally speaking, children who can remain at home with their families do better than those who are removed. Some parents experience feelings of guilt about having a severely disturbed child. It is important to make it clear they are in no way responsible for their children's problems. On the contrary, many of these parents are much to be admired for the devoted way they respond to the challenge of rearing their developmentally disordered children. The experience of being 'co-therapists' can itself help guilt-ridden and despairing parents gain new hope and more positive attitudes towards their children's problems. In many parts of the world there are organizations of parents and others interested in the problems of, and services for, autistic and other similarly handicapped children. Many parents find it helpful to become active in such societies.

The literature on the treatment of children with PDDs other than autism is scant compared with that on autism, but approaches similar to those that have been outlined for autistic children are usually needed. In all cases a careful assessment of the child to determine which are the areas in which development is going awry is a necessary prerequisite to the development of a treatment plan. Some of these children are less severely handicapped than many autistic children. They may be able to attend either regular school classes or classes for children with learning disorders, while being given special help in the areas in which their development is abnormal.

Outcome

Some autistic children show a measure of improvement, often starting at about four to six years of age. The better the level of functioning early on, the better the outlook. Those with intelligence quotients below about 50 (assuming that they have cooperated in the testing and the results are valid), and those who have acquired no speech by the age of five years, mostly remain severely handicapped and often eventually require long-term residential care. An average or higher non-verbal IQ and some speech at age five are hopeful signs.

About two-thirds of all autistic children remain severely handicapped in adult life. Some remain in the care of their families for a period of years but many are eventually admitted to institutions, often when their parents can no longer care for them. Lotter (1978) found that fewer than one-fifth of adult autistic subjects were working and surviving in the community. Some of these are to be found living and working in sheltered situations. Well-planned long-term active treatment, combined with constructive care in a concerned family and avoidance of residential care (except for short-term admission which may give the family a break or tide them over a crisis) all probably improve the outlook. Some useful speech is acquired by about 50% of autistic children but few acquire normal language skills. Epilepsy develops in about one fifth of autistic subjects, often during adolescence (Deykin & MacMahon, 1979).

The residual signs of their disorder seen in adult autistic individuals include emotional coldness and the appearance of being aloof, lack of empathy for others, a limited social life and great difficulty in making friends. There is continuing evidence of their language disorder, with poor comprehension of abstract concepts and the use of repetitive, stilted, mechanical or echolalic phrases.

Rumsey, *et al.*, (1985) reported a detailed study of 14 men, with a mean age of 28, who had well-documented histories of autism. Half had had the diagnosis made by Leo Kanner. They were a predominantly high functioning group, 12 having performance IQs in the average range. Social relationship difficulties, concrete thinking and stereotyped, repetitive behaviours were particularly common. Language skills 'ranged from normal to complete mutism'.

Lord & Rutter (1994) summarize the literature on the course and outcome in autism. Wolff (1991) has reported on the adult outcome in 32 children diagnosed as suffering from *schizoid personality disorder* of childhood – a group having much in common with Asperger's syndrome. She found that, in adult life, three-quarters of the children met the DSM-III criteria for schizotypal personality disorder (see Chapter 15) and two developed schizophrenia. As a group they were 'more solitary, lacking in empathy, oversensitive, with odd styles of communicating, and often with circumscribed interests'.

Chapter 12

Specific Disorders of Development

In addition to the pervasive developmental disorders discussed in the preceding chapter, both ICD-10 and DSM-IV list other categories of disorders of psychological development. In DSM-III-R these were grouped together in Axis II of the diagnostic system, but in DSM-IV they are promoted to Axis I. These are disorders in which there is delayed development in a specific area or areas, other aspects of development being largely or entirely unaffected.

ICD-10 offers us four subgroups of specific developmental disorders. These are:

(a) Specific disorders of speech and language.
  • specific speech articulation disorder
  • expressive language disorder.
  • receptive language disorder.
  • acquired aphasia with epilepsy.
  • other developmental disorders of speech and language.
  • developmental disorder of speech and language, unspecified.

(b) Specific developmental disorders of scholastic skills.
  • specific reading disorder
  • specific spelling disorder
  • specific disorder of arithmetical skills
  • mixed disorder of scholastic skills
  • other developmental disorder of scholastic skills
  • developmental disorder of scholastic skills, unspecified.

(c) Specific developmental disorder of motor function.

(d) Mixed specific developmental disorders.

The DSM-III-R categories are broadly similar:

• Developmental arithmetic disorder.
• Developmental expressive writing disorder.

- Developmental reading disorder.
- Developmental articulation disorder.
- Developmental expressive language disorder.
- Developmental receptive language disorder.
- Developmental coordination disorder.
- Specific developmental disorder, not otherwise specified.

DSM-IV, as we saw in Chapter 3, has a somewhat simpler approach, listing four categories of *learning disorder* affecting, respectively, reading, mathematics and written expression, plus a 'not otherwise specified category'; *motor skills disorder* – that is developmental co-ordination disorder; and *communication disorder* – including expressive language, and receptive language disorder, phonological disorder (formerly developmental articulation disorder); stuttering; and a 'not otherwise specified' group.

These disorders have their onset during infancy or childhood; there is impairment or delay in the development of functions that are strongly related to biological maturation of the central nervous system; and they have a steady course without the remissions and relapses that are characteristic of many mental disorders.

Any of these disorders may affect a child without there being a general psychiatric disorder. All occur more frequently in boys than girls.

Speech and language problems (ICD-10) and Communication disorders (DSM-IV)

The rate at which language is acquired varies widely in normal children. At least in borderline cases, deciding when language development is sufficiently delayed to justify a diagnosis of specific developmental language disorder is difficult. There is a continuum between rapid language development and very slow development. Cases at either end of the continuum present no difficulty but the decision as to where on the continuum to draw the line between 'normal variation' and 'delay' is essentially an arbitrary one. DSM-IV states that in the case of expressive language disorder the child's scores on standardized measures of expressive language development should be 'substantially below those obtained from standardized measures of both non-verbal intelligence and receptive language development'. ICD-10 suggests that a delay that falls 'outside the limits of 2 standard deviations may be considered abnormal'.

From a practical clinical point of view it is important to be aware that there is a continuum ranging from very rapid to very slow language development. Severe delay is often accompanied by other difficulties such as emotional and behavioural problems and, later, difficulties in learning reading and spelling. ICD-10 suggests that four main criteria should be considered when children with language delay are assessed: severity, course, pattern and associated problems.

On the matter of *severity* ICD-10 suggests the 'two standard deviations' measure as a useful guideline, while pointing out that this is less useful in older children, since there is a natural tendency to improvement as children get older. If, despite a currently mild degree of impairment, there is a history of severe delay at earlier ages, one is likely to be dealing with the sequelae of a significant disorder as opposed to a normal variation.

The *course* of the child's language development also helps distinguish normal variations from serious developmental problems. In the former, language development pursues its normal course, or something close to it, but occurs later than in the average child. In the latter the development is not just somewhat slower than normal but in addition speech and/or language skills are qualitatively impaired, so that there is also an abnormal language *pattern*. Finally if language delay, or a history of late speech and language development, is accompanied by such *associated problems* as scholastic difficulties, relationship problems and/or emotional or behavioural difficulties, the delay may well be more than just a normal variation.

The importance of language disorders to the child psychiatrist lies primarily in their association with other problems. The child whose language development is delayed but who is otherwise developing normally – and there are many such children – does not present a psychiatric concern. Most such children will develop normal language skills in due course, with or without some help, which may be provided by a speech therapist. On the other hand, the psychiatrist encounters many children in whom language problems are part of a complex pattern of difficulties affecting school progress, relationships, self-esteem, behaviour and the emotions. Being aware of the possibility that a developmental language disorder may be a major contributing factor, and being able to recognize, or at least suspect it, is therefore important.

Reading and spelling problems

Problems with learning to read are commonly found among boys referred for psychiatric attention. Difficulty learning to spell is often an associated problem. These problems are considerably less common in girls. In technologically advanced societies, in which success usually depends on having a high level of formal education, inability to read well constitutes a serious handicap.

The prevalence of reading disorders, when allowance is made for the general intelligence of the children studied has been variously found to be between 4% (Rutter, *et al.*, 1970b), and 10% (Berger, *et al.*, 1975), the latter figure being derived from a study in inner London, the former from the Isle of Wight study. A study in New Zealand yielded a prevalence rate of 7% (Silva, *et al.*, 1985). The boy:girl ratio found in these studies has ranged from 3.3:1 to 7:1. If the level of general intelligence is not taken into account, the prevalence of reading delay is higher, since children with below average intelligence naturally tend to progress more slowly. Taking into account general intelligence seems logical in evaluating reading delay, but there is only a moderate correlation between measured IQ and reading – the correlation being about .5 to .6 (Rutter & Rutter, 1993, Chapter 6).

Causes

The *causes* of specific developmental reading disorders are not fully understood. The predominance of boys suggests biological susceptibility, perhaps genetically determined. Boys with a 27,XXY chromosome complement have deficiencies in reading and/or spelling skills as well as impaired development of language, especially (Walzer, 1985). The vast majority of children with reading and language problems have normal chromosomes, however. It does seem that the causes of these problems are complex. The association of reading problems, delayed development of language, and speech problems suggests an underlying biological deficit but this is ill-understood. A study of 13-year-old twins suggested that genetic factors may be more important in the aetiology of spelling difficulties than of reading difficulties, at least at this age (Stevenson, *et al.*, 1987).

Goswami (1992) suggests that the key factor in learning to spell is the child's phonological skills – that is, the ability to associate particular sounds with particular letters. Phonological skills are also important in learning to read and many children with severe reading difficulties lack adequate phonological skills. On the other hand, there is also an established association between specific developmental language disorders and reading difficulties, although in the general population most children with phonological problems develop language normally (see Rutter & Rutter, 1993, pages 204–210).

Clinical picture

The *clinical picture* is that of a child, more often a boy, with a history of a serious delay in learning to read. This may have been preceded by delay in the acquisition of speech and language skills, while development in other areas has been relatively normal. There are also often writing and spelling difficulties.

Associated emotional, social and behavioural problems may be reported, but the most common association is with antisocial behaviour. Whether the reading problems cause the antisocial behaviour, or *vice versa*, or whether there are common factors underlying both sets of problems, has not been clearly established, though it is not difficult to see how inability to read, or difficulties in school as a result of a reading problem, might affect adversely a child's self-esteem and ability to function in various areas.

McGee, *et al.* (1986), in a longitudinal study of over 900 children, found significant associations between both specific reading retardation and reading backwardness (that is, retardation in reading that is part of a pattern of generally delayed development) on the one hand, and problem behaviour on the other. The teachers of the children with reading problems reported behaviour problems from the time of entry into school, principally hyperactive and aggressive behaviours. It may be that when these children enter school they already have poor pre-reading skills and poor social adjustment. On entering school they are liable to experience failure both in reading and in making the necessary social and behavioural adjustments, exacerbating their overall difficulties.

The terms *dyslexia* and *developmental dyslexia* have been used for the problems of children with specific reading difficulties. They are probably best avoided, however, because they suggest that dyslexia is a *disease*, whereas in reality we are dealing here with a complex delay in development with varying and usually multiple causes. There is no objection to describing a child as dyslexic, provided one realizes that this is only a way of using a Latin word to say that the child has a reading problem. Better than bestowing a label is the making of a comprehensive functional diagnosis, taking into account all contributory and associated factors.

Assessment and treatment

The *assessment* and *treatment* of children with reading, spelling, and other academic difficulties are the province of the educational psychologist and remedial teacher. Appropriate tests of cognitive function and academic attainment should be performed. If behavioural or other problems are also present, child and family should be assessed, as set out in Chapter 5. In addition to the necessary educational measures, the family may need advice, support or family therapy, especially when there are associated behavioural or family problems. In these sometimes complex cases, a team approach often proves fruitful.

Outcome

The *outcome* in cases of reading and spelling disorders depends on the severity of the disorder and the help available to the child in school and at home. Many children overcome their reading problems, often with extra help from teachers and/or parents. Some seem eventually to reach a state of reading readiness, but if reading problems are not detected, assessed and treated in good time either behavioural or emotional problems, or both, may develop, along with progressive failure at school. The ability to read is necessary for success in other school subjects. Inability to read may lead to general, chronic school failure. This is damaging to the child's self-esteem, with all the unfortunate consequences that follow.

Spelling problems may be less handicapping in this age of word processors and computers, and even electronic typewriters now have built-in spell-checks which can greatly assist the poor speller.

Arithmetic problems

ICD-10 and DSM-IV have categories for *specific disorder of arithmetical skills* (ICD-10) or *mathematics* (DSM-IV). These disorders are characterized by specific impairment of mathematical skills such as cannot be explained by the child's level of general intelligence or what ICD-10 calls 'grossly inadequate schooling'. The skills referred to are the basic ones of addition, subtraction, multiplication and division, not the more complex ones such as algebra, trigonometry and geometry. The difficulties should not be due to the direct effects of impaired vision, hearing or neurological function.

Assessment and treatment

This requires the use of standardized tests, preferably individually administered. The level of attainment in arithmetic and the child's general intelligence level must be measured.

As with reading problems, *treatment* is the sphere of the teacher, assisted as necessary by the educational psychologist. Mathematical difficulties are on the whole less handicapping than reading problems, though they too may lead to emotional difficulties. The advent of computers and especially of small, low-priced electronic calculators has, I believe, lightened the burden of children who have difficulty learning mathematics.

Developmental disorders of motor function

Variously known as *specific disorders of motor function* (ICD-10), *developmental coordination disorder* (DSM-IV), *the clumsy child syndrome* and *devel-*

opmental dyspraxia, this condition is characterized by serious impairment of the development of motor coordination which cannot be explained as an aspect of generally retarded development. Also, the condition is not part of any other specific congenital or acquired neurological disorder. There is often some associated impairment of the performance of visuospatial tasks.

Children with this disorder are characteristically late developing motor skills such as dressing, feeding and walking. They experience difficulty in writing, drawing and copying. They perform badly at ball games, tend to break crockery and are poor at handicrafts. In severe cases the clumsiness may be so great that it interferes with the child's school work, games and physical education. Intelligence is normal when assessed using verbal tests, though the child tests at a lower level on non-verbal tests. In verbal tasks these children usually function well but because of their inability to write, or because they can only write legibly if they go extremely slowly, they may be thought to be intellectually dull or even retarded. In other instances they are regarded as lazy and the view is taken by others that they could to better if they tried harder.

Clumsy children, as these are often called, do not usually show evidence of an abnormality in their ability to carry out voluntary movements; their problem is that they are unable properly to coordinate these movements to perform particular tasks. In a sense, the condition is analogous to developmental reading disorders, in which the subject can see the writing but cannot organize it into the meaning it represents.

Children with this disorder may present at psychiatric clinics or offices, sometimes with secondary disorders and sometimes because the nature of their problems has not been recognized and they are thought to have an emotional/behavioural problem rather than a developmental/neurological one. Careful history-taking usually reveals the true state of affairs. This is confirmed by asking the child to write and draw. Comparing the results with the child's verbal productions, which typically are at a much higher level, can confirm the diagnosis. Psychological testing of verbal and non-verbal skills can provide further confirmation and can refine the diagnosis, pinpointing the child's disabilities more precisely.

Treatment involves explaining the nature of the disability to child, family and teachers. Special teaching and training aimed at developing the child's motor skills is indicated and consultation with, and treatment by, an occupational therapist often proves valuable. Modification of the child's school environment may be needed. These children should be relieved of motor tasks that are beyond them, for instance in games and physical education activities that require much motor coordination. The demands made on them in areas such as writing and drawing should reflect the level of their coordination skills. At the same time the areas in which they function well – generally non-verbal ones – should be capitalized on. Their motor disability should not be allowed to prevent them from expressing their knowledge. Some clumsy children learn to use typewriters or computers better than pens and pencils.

The possibility of secondary emotional disorders developing is ever present in these children. Persistent, especially unrecognized, coordination problems can cause school failure as well as inability to compete successfully with other children in games. These can lead to a lowering of self-esteem, peer group relationship problems and emotional problems such as anxiety or even depression.

A good description of this condition was provided by Walton, *et al.* (1962) who called it developmental dyspraxia. *The Clumsy Child* (Gubbay, 1975) is a useful source of further information.

Mixed specific developmental disorders

Various combination of the specific developmental disorders occur and it is important to be aware that the presence of one does not exclude the possibility that there may be others. The combination of language and reading and spelling disorders is one of the more common.

Chapter 13

Schizophrenia and Other Psychoses of Childhood

The essential feature of psychotic disorders is altered contact with reality. The psychotic person is attempting to adjust to a subjectively distorted view of his or her world. By contrast, individuals with neurotic/anxiety disorders are adapting in morbid ways to their real-life situations.

It can be difficult to discover whether young children are psychotic because their limited verbal skills make it hard for them to explain their subjective experiences. Moreover children who are developing normally usually have a rich and vivid fantasy life. While theoretically the distinction is clear – fantasy is recognized as such by the subject – for the observer, distinguishing between fantasy and delusion in young children can be a challenge.

Another difficulty we face when confronted with a child who may be psychotic, stems from the distortion of personality development and learning that result from psychotic processes arising in childhood. Intelligence, at least as measured by many tests, is manifested largely through such learned behaviours as verbal and motor performance skills. Children who have failed to learn such skills because they have been involved in their psychotic world, rather than the real world, cannot give evidence of their intelligence, or their intellectual potential, in the usual ways. As time passes, and the psychotic process continues, the child's level of intellectual functioning may gradually fall. The end result may be a child presenting with both symptoms of a psychotic disorder and of mental retardation, and it may not be clear which is the primary condition.

Childhood schizophrenia

Nowadays a clear distinction between autistic disorders and childhood schizophrenia is generally accepted, though this has not always been so. Autism is regarded as a severe disorder of the development of a range of psychological functions, rather than as a condition in which the subject has lost contact with the real world.

Neither DSM-IV nor ICD-10 have separate categories for childhood schizophrenia, as distinct from schizophrenia occurring in adulthood. The same diagnostic criteria apply regardless of the age of the patient. Nevertheless, making a firm diagnosis of schizophrenia is often difficult in children, both because of the difficulty in distinguishing between fantasy and delusion, and because children's limited verbal skills make it difficult for them to describe their subjective experiences. Nevertheless the condition has been reported in children as young as five years of age, though it seems to be very rare before the age of seven (Tanguay & Cantor, 1986). Whether the disorder occurs before the age of five is a matter of dispute.

Prevalence

The *prevalence* of schizophrenia in pre-pubertal children is lower than that of autistic disorders, occurring at perhaps seven-tenths the prevalence of the latter condition (Tanguay & Cantor, 1986). There may be a predominance of boys but it seems that this is less marked than in autism. In each of three series of cases of childhood schizophrenia reviewed by Russell, *et al.* (1989) the boys outnumbered the girls. When the figures for the studies are added together, the boys outnumber the girls 63 to 29, but these studies were not based on samples from epidemiological surveys. After puberty schizophrenia occurs more frequently and late adolescence is a common time for its symptoms to appear.

Causes

The *causes* of schizophrenia are not fully understood. Genetic predisposition plays a role in both adults and children. Research in adults has provided evidence that environmental factors play a part, certainly in predisposing to relapse in schizophrenic patients discharged from hospital, and perhaps in precipitating the disorder. There is evidence that a high level of expressed emotion in families is associated with a higher relapse rate (Leff & Vaughn, 1985), but whether similar processes operate in childhood is not known. It has been suggested that another combination of behaviours, known as *communication deviance* (CD), may contribute to the development of schizophrenia (Singer, *et al.*, 1978; Wynne, 1981). CD consists of various forms of vague, ambiguous, wandering, illogical and idiosyncratic language, in some ways similar to, though less severe than, the disordered thinking of schizophrenic subjects. It may be present in the parents' language patterns for years before the onset of schizophrenia in their offspring, and does not invariably lead to schizophrenia.

Despite the various family and environmental factors that have been implicated or inferred, the consensus of opinion nowadays is that the causes of schizophrenia are basically biological. There is evidence of genetic predisposition. Various biochemical abnormalities have been reported and many theories have been proposed regarding the biological causation and correlates of schizophrenia. Most research has, however, been carried out in adult, rather than child, populations.

Clinical picture

The main features of the *clinical picture* are as follows:

(1) Delusional beliefs

Delusions are false beliefs held despite evidence to the contrary such as would be accepted by others. The delusions of schizophrenic patients may include delusions of persecution by others (paranoid delusions); delusions of reference (for example that items in newspapers or advertisements, or on television, refer to oneself); belief that thoughts are being put into, withdrawn from or broadcast from one's head (thought insertion, withdrawal or broadcasting); and the belief that one's thoughts are controlled by some external force. *Delusional perceptions* arise fully fledged on the basis of a genuine perception which would be regarded as commonplace by others.

(2) Thought disorder

Associations become loosened, so that the subject's thoughts move from one subject to another apparently unrelated or distantly related one. Sometimes the process resembles the 'knight's move' in chess. Although these patients may talk a lot, it is hard to grasp what they are saying. Poverty of thought, that is to say the existence of little content, may be observed despite the copious production of speech. In extreme cases talk may become completely incoherent.

(3) Hallucinations

These typically occur in clear consciousness and are most often auditory. They may consist of voices repeating the subject's thoughts out loud or anticipating them; or two or more hallucinatory voices may be discussing or arguing about the patient who is referred to in the third person; or voices may comment on the subject's thoughts or behaviour.

(4) Disorders of affect

The subject's emotional reactions are often blunted, flattened or inap-

propriate. Thus painful experiences may be described with a smile and
there may be sudden, apparently inexplicable changes of mood.

(5) Volitional disorders

These patients may feel that their impulses, acts and emotions are
under external control. They may say they feel like robots or as if
they have been hypnotized. Lack of interest and drive, with failure to
initiate activities or follow them through, often lead to a falling off in
school or work performance. In extreme cases catatonia – the assumption
of a rigid, unmoving posture – may be observed though it is rare in
children.

(6) Other features

These include social isolation, often combined with preoccupation with
fantasy or with delusional or illogical ideas; and loss of a sense of identity.
These patients may be puzzled about who they are, the meaning of their
existence, and the nature of the world around them.

A detailed description of the symptoms of a series of 35 schizophrenic
children is provided by Russell, *et al.* (1989). Although the age of onset,
based on information available later, was thought to have been between
3 and 11 years, with a mean of 6.9 years, only five of the subjects were
under the age of 8 at the time of diagnosis. This is a reflection of the often
insidious onset of the disorder and the difficulty of deciding when criteria for making the diagnosis are met. There is also a natural reluctance,
on the part of many mental health professionals, to make a diagnosis
with such serious implications in a child until there is ample evidence to
support it.

Of the 35 children reported by Russell, *et al.* (1989), 28 (80%) presented
with auditory hallucinations, 22 (63%) with delusions, and 14 (40 %) with
thought disorder. Visual, tactile and somatic hallucinations were less
common and were reported only by children who also had auditory
hallucinations. The above symptoms occurred in various combinations.
Nineteen (54%) of the children presented with both hallucinations and
delusions, 10 (29%) with delusions and thought disorder, and 8 (23%)
with hallucinations, delusions and thought disorder.

In this series of 35 children, 24 also met the diagnostic criteria for other
conditions. These were: conduct disorder (10), atypical depression (9),
dysthymia (4), enuresis/encopresis (5), elective mutism (1), separation
anxiety disorder (1), and oppositional disorder (1). In two cases there was
evidence of 'physical/sexual abuse'. The report by Russell *et al.* (1989)
contains much other useful information about the clinical features of
childhood schizophrenia.

Precursors of schizophrenia

A number of *precursors of schizophrenia* have been reported and it seems clear that individuals who develop schizophrenia, whether before or after puberty, may exhibit various abnormal behaviours long before a diagnosis of schizophrenia is warranted (Kolvin, *et al.*, 1971; Green, *et al.*, 1984), though this may be no more than another way of saying that the onset is often insidious. Barbara Fish has long believed that schizophrenia may occur in infancy and early childhood. She has described a patient who developed an acute schizophrenic illness at age 19 (Fish, 1986). He was the son of a woman with chronic schizophrenia and had been studied from birth as part of a research project. Fish states that 'on the research observations he had deviate development from his first day'. He was late smiling and rocked 'endlessly' on his rocking horse when young. By six years of age there was 'much more severe psychopathology', with difficulty in social relationships. When 9 years 7 months he was diagnosed as having 'a severe personality disorder with schizoid and paranoid traits'. While single case studies must be regarded with caution, the onset of this young man's schizophrenic illness seems to have been the culmination of a long, perhaps lifelong, period of abnormal development. This may apply to other cases. It is apparent also that the diagnostic criteria set out in both DSM-IV and ICD-10 are not easily applicable to infants.

Nuechterlein (1986) reviewed the literature on childhood precursors of adult schizophrenia. These may include attentional and information processing abnormalities; neurological *soft signs* (minor neurological abnormalities not indicative of structural lesions of the nervous system which would be within normal limits if the child were younger); abnormalities of the autonomic nervous system (that which supplies the heart, blood vessels and various glands and the function of which is largely outside conscious control); and defects of social functioning and communication.

Treatments

There are few satisfactory data on what *treatments* are helpful for prepubertal children with schizophrenia. According to Cantor & Kestenbaum (1986) those that have been used include 'parentectomy', psychoanalysis for both child and parents, behaviour therapy, milieu therapy, family therapy, educational therapy and a variety of psychotherapeutic techniques such as movement and paraverbal therapy. These have been offered 'with or without psychopharmacological intervention and alone or in combination with other approaches'.

In 1983 Beitchman pointed out that systematic studies of the treatment of childhood, as opposed to adult, schizophrenia have largely been lacking, and this remains true ten years later. In practice, pre-pubertal children seem usually to be treated using regimens similar to those used with adolescents and adults. In adolescence, approaches similar to those used with adults are often productive. The main features are:

- family intervention;
- the use of antipsychotic drugs;
- long-term support of the patient by a therapist who also coordinates the work of a multidisciplinary team.

Family intervention is distinct from family therapy. The idea that schizophrenia was a consequence of certain patterns of family functioning has been virtually abandoned. But intervention designed to help other family members provide an environment that is as helpful as possible to their schizophrenic member – for example by reducing the expressed emotion or communication deviance mentioned above – seems to be of value (McFarlane, 1983). While there is a lack of hard data on how this might help children, as opposed to adults, theoretical considerations might suggest that family work would be even more important with children.

The value of antipsychotic drugs is well established in adults with schizophrenia. The widely used phenothiazine drugs and haloperidol have recently been joined by several new compounds, though their use in children and younger adolescents has not been much investigated to date. Because the long-term use of these drugs carries the risk of producing serious side-effects, caution is advisable in their use and doses should be kept as low as possible. Treatment is a long-term endeavour. Therefore the younger the patient when treatment commences, the greater the caution that is needed.

Long-term support by a therapist for both the child and the family is a must. It is doubtful whether any specific form of psychotherapy affects the schizophrenic process itself, but over the years these children and their families usually encounter a wide range of difficulties. These may be educational, social or vocational, or they may concern the child's individual development and relationship with his or her world and the people in it. Cantor & Kestenbaum (1986) discuss various ways in which therapists may help these children with such problems. They suggest that the therapist should be prepared to function as 'auxiliary ego, as facilitator of sensory perceptions, and as coordinator of a multi-disciplinary team'.

Outcome

Schizophrenia is a serious disorder at any stage of life but in childhood its implications are particularly grave. Occurring in a personality which is incompletely developed, it may stunt or block completely the normal processes of psychological growth, in addition to causing symptoms as outlined above. The outlook is therefore generally better the later the onset, and it is generally best when the onset of the condition is sudden and it occurs in a child or adolescent whose personality development and relationships have previously been normal. In such cases there is sometimes complete remission.

The short-term response to medication may be gratifying, but it is not always maintained and lifelong medication has serious drawbacks. A major need is to help the young person handicapped by schizophrenic symptoms make the best possible adjustment in society. Many of these children and adolescents become chronic schizophrenics in adult life. At some point, often when their families are no longer able or willing to care for them, they may require admission to an institution or group home for long-term care.

Reactive psychoses

Psychotic reactions to severe stress may occur in children as they do in adults. DSM-III-R lists *brief reactive psychoses,* in which psychotic symptoms appear in response to psychosocial stress such as would be 'markedly stressful to almost anyone in similar circumstances'. The clinical picture is one of emotional turmoil presenting in a person who was previously functioning well, together with at least one of the following:

- incoherence or loosening of associations;
- delusions;
- hallucinations;
- behaviour that is grossly disorganized.

DSM-IV describes *brief psychotic disorders* which, it states, may occur with or without marked stressors.

In ICD-10 such disorders are similarly listed in a section entitled *acute and transient psychotic disorders* – which may or may not be associated with acute stress.

The symptoms last for a few hours or days but clear up quickly – according to DSM-IV the duration may be up to one month 'with full remission of all symptoms in that time'. This can present a problem to clinicians who cannot know whether the diagnostic criteria are met until after recovery. ICD-10 is less rigid in its diagnostic criteria.

The condition may occur in middle childhood or adolescence. It does not seem to be as common in western cultures as in some others. In Africa it may occur as a complication of school anxiety (the *brain fag* syndrome – see Chapter 8), and its presentation may be quite dramatic. It may be exacerbated by the subject's belief that he or she has been bewitched.

Short-term administration of major tranquillizers such as the phenothiazine drugs or haloperidol, together with reassurance and nursing in calm and quiet surroundings, usually lead to rapid improvement and resolution of the psychotic symptoms within a few days. The nature of any causative stress should be determined and if it is continuing, steps should be taken to remove or alleviate it. Therapy with child or family, and sometimes liaison with the school, may be needed to guard against recurrence. The longer-term outlook is usually favourable.

Toxic confusional and delirious states

In these conditions there is diffuse, general impairment of brain function, with a state of delirium or confusion. In delirium, consciousness is clouded and the subject's awareness of the environment is altered. Orientation for time, place and person is impaired. Attention is ill-sustained and the stream of thought is disordered. Illusions, the misinterpretation of sensory stimuli (as, for example, when an inanimate object is perceived as a monster about to attack one); bizarre or frightening fantasies; and hallucinations, often visual, may occur. In severe cases the subject appears completely out of touch with reality.

Confusional states are characterized by milder degrees of disorientation and confusion, without the full picture of delirium.

These conditions may be acute, coming on quite suddenly, or subacute, starting gradually over the course of a few hours. Any of the following may be responsible for these states:

- systemic infections, especially when there is a high fever;
- metabolic disturbances, for example hypoglycaemic reactions in diabetics;
- acute brain injury;
- acute infections of the brain;
- some rare forms of epilepsy;
- chemical intoxication by drugs.

Children, especially in their first few years, are particularly prone to develop delirious reactions during acute febrile illnesses such as measles, pneumonia and other childhood infections. The advent of antibiotics, in those parts of the world where they are freely available, has greatly reduced the frequency of these reactions.

Chemical intoxication is a frequent and important cause of these conditions. It occasionally results from the proper use of medically prescribed drugs but, principally in adolescents, a more important cause is the abuse of prescription drugs and the use of 'street' drugs.

Prescription drugs which, if abused, may be responsible for confusional states include, but are not limited to, sleeping compounds of various sorts, codeine-containing analgesics, and benzodiazepine tranquilizers such as diazepam and triazolam. Among the 'street' drugs used by young people are marijuana, lysergic acid diethylamide (LSD or 'acid'), mescaline, phencyclidine (PCP or 'angel dust'), 'magic mushrooms', amphetamine drugs, cocaine (which can cause a severe psychosis with paranoid delusions), and heroin. A serious problem in some demographic groups is solvent, petrol (gasoline) and glue sniffing (Sudbury & Ghodse, 1990). This is sometimes encountered in quite young children, often well short of puberty. These substances can cause both short-term confusion and long-term brain damage.

Treatment

The *treatment* of delirious and confusional states is primarily the treatment, or removal of their causes. Medical conditions should receive the appropriate therapy, the use of any causative drugs should immediately be stopped and any necessary treatment given to deal with drug overdoses.

Educational and other measures are usually required for young people who are abusing drugs. Drug abuse and its treatment are discussed further in Chapter 18.

Chapter 14

Enuresis and Encopresis

Both ICD-10 and DSM-IV include enuresis and encopresis in their listings of the psychiatric disorders of childhood and adolescence. In ICD-10, 'nonorganic' enuresis and encopresis appear in the section covering 'other behavioural and emotional disorders with onset usually occurring in childhood and adolescence'. DSM-IV lists *encopresis* and *enuresis* under the heading *elimination disorders*. While these conditions have traditionally been listed among the psychiatric disorders of children they are really in that borderline territory where psychiatry and paediatrics overlap. Enuresis and encopresis may exist on their own, together, or as part of another psychiatric disorder.

Enuresis

Nonorganic enuresis, as ICD-10 calls it, is characterized by 'involuntary voiding of urine, by day and/or by night.' It must be abnormal in relation to the subject's mental age and is not due to poor bladder control resulting from a neurological disorder, nor to epilepsy or to a structural abnormality of the urinary tract. DSM-IV defines *enuresis* (*not due to a general medical condition*) a little differently, in that it may be involuntary or intentional, though it is usually involuntary.

The essence of this disorder is the inappropriate voiding of urine, often while asleep at night (nocturnal enuresis), or during the day (diurnal enuresis), resulting in wetting of the bed or the child's clothes. The DSM-IV definition of enuresis requires that the wetting occur at least twice a week over a period of three months. The child must have a chronological age of at least five, or if developmentally delayed, a mental age of at least five. In reality, the age at which children become continent of urine varies quite widely and to set a specific age as separating normal from abnormal development in this area is arbitrary.

Prevalence

The reported *prevalence* of enuresis varies according to the population studied and the criteria used to make the diagnosis. According to DSM-IV, at age five, 7% of boys and 3% of girls are enuretic. At age ten prevalence rates are down to 3% and 2%; and at 18 years old 1% of males are enuretic and fewer than 1% of females. In reality there are wide variations from country to country. Thus in Australia and North America rates three times higher than those in Sweden have been reported. The British rate is nearer the Swedish one, rather than that of what the *British Medical Journal* (1977) once called the 'bed-sodden states of America'.

Verhulst, *et al.* (1985) reported the prevalence of nocturnal enuresis in boys and girls between the ages of 4 and 16, based on a study of 2600 Dutch children. At age 5, 17.9% of boys and 10% of girls wet the bed at least once a month, while 14.1% of boys and 6.7% of girls were wet at least twice a month. At nearly all ages the prevalence in boys was greater than that in girls. Prevalence declined more rapidly between the ages of four and six in girls than it did in boys. Bedwetting was rare in girls from the eleventh year onwards, and in boys from the thirteenth year. These findings are in general agreement with those of other studies.

Daytime wetting is considerably less common than nocturnal wetting and occurs more frequently in boys than in girls. A large scale study of 7-year-olds in Scandinavia yielded an overall prevalence of enuresis of 9.8%, 6.4% being wet only at night and 1.8% only by day, while 1.6% wet both at night and by day (Jarvelin, *et al.*, 1988).

Causes

While enuresis may be due to organic neurological conditions or to various disorders of the urinary tract, in most cases there is no demonstrable physical cause. When there is a demonstrable physical cause, the condition is not considered a psychiatric one and does not meet either the ICD-10 or the DSM-IV criteria. In girls with diurnal enuresis, however, urinary tract infections are quite common. Of a group of enuretic girls reported by Halliday, *et al.* (1987), 212 had had previous infections and 12 had one or more episodes while being treated. It seems that diurnal enuresis predisposes to infection, which in turn may exacerbate the enuresis.

The bladders of enuretic children tend to be functionally, though not anatomically, smaller than those of non-enuretics. As a group, enuretic children pass urine more frequently than non-enuretic children but this does not seem to be related to their functional bladder capacities (Shaffer, *et al.*, 1984).

Enuresis tends to run in families and genetic factors may be involved. Jarvelin, *et al.* (1988) found that, in the population of 3206 children they studied, the risk of a child being enuretic was 7.1 times greater if the father had been enuretic after the age of four, and 5.2 times greater if the mother had been enuretic.

Although unusually deep sleep has been suggested as a cause of nocturnal enuresis, evidence that enuretic children sleep more deeply than other children is lacking. There is an association between enuresis and emotional disorder but most enuretic children are not emotionally disturbed. Enuresis may however be a feature of the regressive behaviour which appears in some children when they are under stress. It may also be present in children with conduct disorders, neurotic disorders or psychoses. Diurnal wetting is probably more often associated with psychiatric disorder than is bedwetting (Berg, 1979).

In most cases, no specific cause can be found for the enuresis. It is often ascribed to delayed neurological maturation, to which genetic factors may contribute. If family disorganization is combined with such delayed maturation and the child receives inconsistent toilet training, delayed achievement of bladder control may be even more probable. Other anxiety-producing stresses may also contribute.

Description

In most cases enuresis is *primary*, that is to say the child has never become dry. In uncomplicated enuresis, the most common variety, the only symptom is the passing of urine while asleep. The child has not learned to control micturition while asleep. About one bedwetter in five also has increased frequency of micturition by day, but without daytime wetting. In another, smaller, number of children there are both increased frequency and wetting by day.

Various emotional symptoms may complicate enuresis. If the child is blamed or punished for wetting the bed or the clothes, this may lead to anxiety or feelings of guilt. Much depends on the family's attitudes towards the problem. Enuresis causes great unhappiness and distress to some children, though if it is sensibly handled this need not be the case.

Secondary enuresis is enuresis starting after the child has achieved continence for a certain, variously defined, period of time – this being set at 3 months in the study of Shaffer, *et al.* (1984) and at 1 year in that of Starfield (1967). It has been suggested that children with secondary enuresis are more likely to have psychiatric disorders than primary nocturnal enuretics, but the findings of a study by Shaffer, *et al.* (1984) did not support this.

In summary, functional enuresis – that is enuresis in the absence of any demonstrable organic cause – may be nocturnal, diurnal or both; it may have been lifelong or it may have started after a period of continence; and it may or may not be associated with evidence of psychiatric disorder. Although it is included in classifications of child psychiatric disorders, this is more, in the words of the ICD-10 manual, 'because of [its] frequency and association with other psychosocial problems'.

Investigation and treatment

In cases of primary enuresis, carefully taken histories from child and parents will establish that lifelong wetting is the main problem. If anxiety or other psychiatric symptoms have arisen, perhaps in response to family members' attitudes towards it, this should also become clear as the history is taken and the current family situation is assessed.

It is important to adopt an optimistic outlook while taking the history. You should let the family know that the problem is a common one and not too serious, despite the inconvenience it may cause. Many parents and children are unaware of the frequency of the complaint and any self-blame should be dispelled as far as possible.

The history should be reviewed for evidence of infection or diabetes. It is important to ascertain that the child has conscious control over micturition, that is to say that the muscles responsible for preventing the voiding of urine are functioning, even though control may lapse from time to time. With some anatomical abnormalities urine is constantly leaking and control is never complete. Urinary infections are often accompanied by painful micturition and increased frequency, though they may be 'silent'.

A physical examination should be carried out and the urine examined for evidence of infection or diabetes. How far further investigation of the urinary tract is necessary when there is nothing in the history to suggest an organic cause is open to question. X-ray studies are helpful when abnormalities are suspected but their routine use may not be justified. When an associated physical problem is suspected, consultation with a paediatrician is advisable.

Three main approaches to treatment are available. Whatever the treatment approach, support and reassurance for child and family are important. The symptom is usually best referred to as 'a delay in learning to control the bladder while asleep' (or 'when excited'), rather than as a serious disease.

(a) Conditioning

This is often used as the treatment of first choice. It involves the use of an *enuresis alarm.* These are devices which wake the child when urine starts to be passed. Many models, marketed by different companies, are available. Early models had two wire gauze sheets, or a pair of metal foil covered sheets one of which is perforated, which were placed in the bed. They were separated by a bed sheet and another bed sheet was placed on top. They were connected by wires to a battery-operated buzzer or bell so that as soon as the bedsheet separating the two metal sheet became wet the buzzer or bell sounded, waking the child up.

Modern technology has considerably refined this apparatus. Rather than have metal sheets, which moved if the child was a restless sleeper, sometimes causing false alarms, the wires are usually connected to terminals which are the two halves of a press fastener. The child wears thin underpants or pyjamas and the terminals are pressed together with the material separating them. Modern electronic circuitry ensures that as soon as the child passes even a few drops of urine the material between the terminals becomes wet enough to complete the circuit and cause the alarm to sound. This wakes up the child who gets up and empties his or her bladder.

Enuresis alarms are available from a variety of munufacturers. In addition to those described above there are 'silent' alarms which use a low frequency vibrator placed under the pillow instead of a buzzer (useful when the child shares a bedroom); 'remote' alarms which can sound in the parents' bedroom; and extra-loud (for the deep sleeper), two-tone and intermittent alarms. Models are also available for daytime use. A flat wetting sensor can be attached to the underpants, connected by a wire to the alarm which can be worn on a belt, in a pocket or strapped on the back (Halliday, *et al.*, 1987).

Some practical points about the use of these alarms are worth mentioning. It is important to get the child's active cooperation in the use of the apparatus. It is easy to sabotage its use, by disconnecting the terminals or switching the alarm off after it has been set. The best plan is for the child to accept responsibility for setting the alarm up, and for changing pyjamas and, if necessary, bed sheets, and re-setting it after each episode of wetting. The need for the child's active cooperation means that it is not usually possible to use the alarm below the age of five or six. It is sometimes necessary to spend time, even several interviews, preparing the child for its use.

When the alarm is first employed, the child may be woken several times each night. This often portends a good result, presumably because the conditioning process is repeated frequently. The amount the child drinks before going to bed should not be restricted and the child should not be 'lifted' to pass urine during the night. Doing either of these things tends to delay the conditioning process.

The alarm is principally of value when there is no evidence of other psychiatric problems. If it is associated with emotional disorder or oppositional behaviour it is often impossible to obtain the child's cooperation. In such cases it is usually best to postpone its use until the associated disorder has been effectively dealt with. Some children are frightened of the apparatus and reassurance may be ineffective until the underlying emotional problems are resolved.

Over 80% of nocturnal enuretics who use the alarm properly become dry. Some of these relapse and not all relapses respond to further treatment, though most do. (Dische, *et al.*, 1983) reported initial arrest of wetting (42 successive dry nights in 95 (84%) of 113 children but 40 relapsed. Of these only 31 were retreated and of these 31, 16 became and remained dry, a long-term success rate of 63%.

(b) Medication

By using various members of the tricyclic group of antidepressants, medication can be effective in controlling enuresis. The drug that has been most widely studied is imipramine but there is evidence that both desipramine and clompramine are effective too (Green, 1991). Unfortunately the relapse rate is quite high. If there is no response, the blood level should be estimated since this may not be dose-related in children. Doses of 25 mg, or if that is not effective, 50 mg at bedtime are usually required. The medication should be continued until the child has been continuously dry for at least one month, and then only gradually reduced, preferably over a period of two to three months. The value of medication is limited by the high relapse rate. I have found, however, that sometimes refractory cases respond when administration of a tricyclic drug, usually imipramine, is combined with the use of an enuresis alarm.

(c) Hypnotherapy

This may be of value and one report has suggested that it may achieve results comparable to those of the enuresis alarm (Edwards & van der Spuy, 1985). Formal trance induction is apparently not necessary.

Outcome

As the figures for prevalence rates at different ages indicate, most enuretic children will grow out of the symptom in time but the spontaneous rate does not justify therapeutic inaction. Tretment is successful in well over half the cases but sometimes secondary emotional disorders or family disorganization stand in the way of the use of the alarm.

Encopresis

Encopresis, or faecal soiling, is the passage of faeces in innapproprate places. It usually involves the soiling of the subject's clothes.

Prevalence

A study in Sweden (Bellman, 1966) revealed a prevalence of soiling at age seven of 2.3% in boys and 0.7% in girls, a male:female ratio of 3.4:1. In the Isle of Wight study of 10- and 11–year-olds prevalence rates of 1.3% in boys and 0.3% in girls were found (Rutter, *et al.*, 1970b). By the age of 16 the prevalence had fallen almost to zero.

Causes

Figure 14.1 summarizes the various ways in which soiling can arise.

Encopresis may be retentive or non-retentive, the difference being a matter of whether or not faeces have accumulated in the colon and rectum

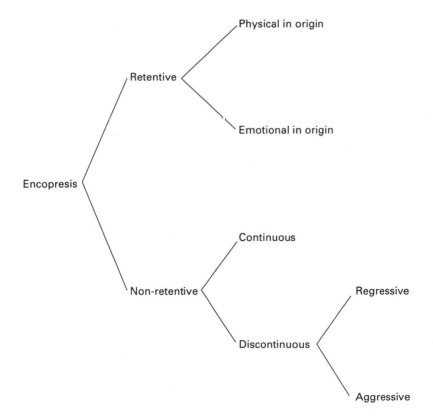

Fig. 14.1 Types of encopresis.

in abnormal quantities. In severe cases the large intestine may be grossly dilated.

Retentive encopresis

Retention of faeces may have physical or emotional causes. Physical ones include anal fissure (a longitudinal fissure in the wall of the anus, which can make defecation very painful), and Hirschprung's disease, a rare condition in which the nerve ganglia are congenitally absent from a section of the colon; as a result, the smooth muscle of this section does not contract properly, so that faeces are not moved on as they should be.

The emotional factors contributing to encopresis are often less clear-cut than the physical ones. It has long been believed that anger arising, usually, in the context of the relationship between the mother (or whoever undertakes bowel training) and the child can be an important factor (Anthony, 1957; Pinkerton, 1958). In these cases a disturbed parent-child relationship is postulated and the soiling is seen arising as a reaction to coercive toilet training.

Attempts at toilet training may have started early, even within the first few weeks of life, and success surprisingly early, though short-lived, may be reported. The subsequent negativistic refusal to defecate may be a reaction to coercive, rigid toilet training by parents who have a high regard for order and cleanliness and over-value early bowel and bladder control. They may also have obsessive personalities. Their encopretic children have been thought to be expressing anger, of which they may be consciously largely unaware, by soiling or by retaining faeces rather than passing them. They may choose this method of expression because issues of bowel control are matters of special concern in their families. The mothers have been said to have an inordinate fear of constipation and a tendency to use laxatives to excess. Their preoccupation with bowel function may date back, and be related, to their own childhood experiences.

As children continue to resist defecating, faeces accumulate in the large intestine. This becomes distended and the faeces in it eventually become hard and impacted. Liquid faeces may pass around the impacted masses and leak out of the anus, the child having no control over this. The end result may be indistinguishable, except perhaps from the history, from encopresis of physical, as opposed to emotional origin.

Emotionally determined retentive soiling as described above seems to be less common now than it was in the 1950s when the papers by Anthony and Pinkerton were written. This may be because of changed attitudes towards toilet training. This nowadays tends to be more relaxed and permissive, and rigid and coercive methods are widely recognized as inappropriate.

Non-retentive encopressis

Non-retentive soiling may be *continuous*, that is present from birth, the child never having been successfully trained.; or *discontinuous*, the child having been trained at some point in time, the soiling returning later.

Continuous soiling is encountered in some children who are poorly cared for in other ways than having lacked proper toilet training. They may present as dirty and badly dressed and show other evidence of ineffective social training. They may have a history of playing truant from school and their academic progress is often below average. The family may be faced with such other problems as debt, unemployment, unsatisfactory housing, or drug and/or alcohol abuse.

Moderate and severely mentally retarded children are late achieving bowel control, amd some of the severely retarded never do so, but they are readily distinguished by their generally retarded development. They do not meet the ICD-10 criteria for *non-organic encopresis*, or DSM-IV's *encopresis*.

Discontinuous non-retentive soiling may be either *regressive* or *aggressive*. Regressive soiling is usually a reaction to some form of stress in the family, such as the birth of a sibling. It may be one feature of a more general emotional regression and is more likely to occur when bowel continence has only recently been achieved. Short-lived episodes of regressive soiling occurring in response to acute stress may be more appropriately classified as adjustment reactions (see Chapter 15). Regressive soiling is akin to the diarrhoea some people experience before potentially stressful experiences such as examinations or important interviews.

Aggressive non-retentive soiling tends to have a psychopathology similar to that of psychogenic retentive soiling, but instead of refusing to defecate at all, the child refuses to do so at the place and time desired. In these cases, too, there is an ongoing battle for control of the child's bowels between child and parent(s). This is graphically described in Anthony's (1957) paper.

Clinical features

The essential clinical feature of encopresis is the passing of faeces in the clothes. It may have been lifelong or it may have commenced after a period of continence. In severe cases of retentive soiling the rectum is found, on digital examination, to be greatly dilated and packed with faeces. Around these, liquid or semi-liquid faecal material is passing and leaking from the anus, the child having no control over this.

The soiling itself may vary from the regular passage of all faeces in the clothes, to staining of underwear or nightclothes. It may occur daily or less frequently – the DSM-IV criteria for the diagnosis of encopresis stipulate a minimum of once a month for at least three months. The child must be over four years old and have a mental age of at least four. In some cases it does not occur at school, yet is reported to happen frequently at home. (This, however, is unlikely to be the case when there is a serious degree of retention of faeces.) When the soiling is thus restricted it suggests a relationship to difficulties in the family.

In asessing these cases it is essential to take a careful history from both parents and child. Details of the bowel training methods used should be sought. Was this coercive or lackadaisical, or even absent? Relaxed, laid back training may be effective in stable families in which the children feel secure and are naturally inclined to want to meet their parents' wishes. It is in the chaotic, disorganized families that inconsistency and the lack of proper training is more likely to lead to encopresis.

Aggressive soilers, whether retentive or non-retentive, often present as clean, well-dressed but inhibited children. They are often doing well at school. They may seem ashamed of their soiling and may try to conceal it, for example by hiding or destroying underclothes – though this may infuriate their parents and may be but another means whereby their aggressive feelings are expressed. They are often reluctant to discuss anything related to bowel function, but may allude to it in play or drawings. In about half of this group associated food refusal is reported by the parents, though these children are usually adequately nourished. They may not engage in rough play and may be less self-assertive than is usual in their age group, their aggressive feelings being expressed instead though refusal to conform in the spheres of bowel and, often, eating behaviour. Typically, the aggressive soiler is a bright, successful pupil at school, in contrast to the 'never properly trained' continuous soiler, who usually is not. A clear history of a period of faecal continence is not always obtained in these cases.

Regressive soiling can usually be distinguished by the presence of other regressive behaviours such as clinging to mother, 'baby talk', infantile feeding behaviour, reluctance to sleep or go to bed alone, or a return to immature patterns of play. There is usually a history of a recent or continuing stressful experience.

The clinical picture is not always as clear cut as the above might imply. Mixed forms of encopresis occur. Some *aggressive* soilers, whether retentive or not, have never achieved faecal continence; and aggressive soiling can occur in socially disorganized, poorly functioning families as well as in rigid, obsessional, materially successful ones. Sometimes there are both aggressive and regressive features as, for example, when the child feels both anxiety about the family or some other situation, as well as hostility towards the parents.

Soiling may be a feature of other child psychiatric disorders. These include pervasive developmental disorders, conduct disorders, adjustment disorders and mental retardation. In such cases the other disorder is usually the primary focus of clinical attention, the soiling being but one feature of a disorder having a number of other clinical features. For purposes of diagnostic classification, the other disorder should usually take precedence.

Investigation and treatment

In investigating and treating encopretic children it is necessary first to establish whether there is retention of faeces and, if so, whether the soiling is due to overflow incontinence. If there has been longstanding faecal retention it can be difficult to discover how the problem first arose. If the original cause was physical, emotional difficulties may have developed as secondary phenomena. If it was emotional, the child's negativistic refusal to defecate may have been complicated by long-standing constipation and dilatation of the large intestine.

Abdominal and rectal examinations, if necessary supplemented by X-ray investigations, usually establish whether there are accumulations of faeces in the large intestine. In Hirschprung's disease, there is a segment of narrow, undilated colon, with a great increase in the size of the colon proximal to it. In psychogenic cases the whole length of the colon is dilated.

Whatever the original cause, when there is a severe degree of faecal retention, this must be treated by appropriate physical means. The long-term administration of a laxative such as Senokot may be sufficient. An alternative is mineral oil. If such measures prove inadequate, rectal suppositories (such as Dulcolax) may be used or, if they prove insufficient, enemas. In severe cases it may be best to initiate treatment in hospital. Even then, enemas and suppositories should only be administered after a good relationship has been established with the child by the nurses looking after the child, and after due explanation of the treatment to the child. Otherwise the child may feel that the treatment is another aggressive attack. Physical measures should always be part of a wider plan of treatment dealing also with the emotional and family problems.

In many cases, treatment in hospital is not needed. When it is, most children become clean within two or three weeks of admission if they are treated appropriately and any faecal retention is relieved. If the encopresis continues it may be because it is being dealt with in a punitive or hostile way, or because dysfunctional interactions between child and parent(s) are continuing. For example, one boy for several weeks handed his mother soiled clothes to take home to wash, unbeknown to the hospital staff.

If there is no retention of faeces, physical treatment is not required. If toilet training has not been provided, the child usually responds to a period of consistent, firm and kind training, using behaviour modification principles (see Chapter 21). This is best carried out at home by the parents who usually need support and guidance in implementing the treatment plan. If the parents are unable to provide the necessary structure and stability, the child may need to be placed temporarily in a hospital, foster home or treatment centre. The administration of a laxative along with the behaviour modification program does not seem to help in cases in which there is no constipation (Berg, et al., 1983).

Treatment specifically for the soiling may not be necessary in regressive soiling. Attention should be directed to removing or alleviating the stress that is responsible for the child's anxiety. If the stress cannot be fairly quickly removed, psychotherapy for the child may be required.

Family therapy or counselling for the parents may be needed. When the encopresis is but one of many family problems, therapy to improve family functioning may be needed before the parents can effectively apply behavioural or other treatments.

Sometimes the attitudes of the parents towards bowel function generally and soiling in particular need attention, especially when there is aggressive soiling in over-controlled children. The mother is often the parent most involved in the battle with the child. Once a trusting relationship with the parents is established, bowel function and related matters, including any misconceptions about the dangers of constipation, may be discussed. Some who have been brought up to be very bowel conscious overrate the importance of bowel regularity. Their fears and anxieties need to be put to rest before the child's symptoms, and how they should be managed, are discussed. The parents should be helped to understand the soiling as a means of self-expression or protest in a child who may feel unable to express angry feelings in other ways. In addition the parents need to come to an understanding that the open expression of aggression is a sign of improvement. Simple explanation of these points is seldom sufficient. Discussion of them over a period of time, in the context of a trusting relationship with the therapist, is usually required. Family therapy interviews can help in this process. They can assist all the members of the family in understanding the issues in the family that have been maintaining the symptoms.

Outcome

Progress and response to treatment depend on the type of encopresis and the openness of the family to change. Regressive soiling generally disappears quite quickly, once the stress to which it is a response is resolved. Aggressive soiling, especially when it is long-standing and accompanied by faecal retention, is harder to treat. When soiling is a feature of a seriously disorganized family system, the outlook depends on the skill of the therapist in engaging these sometimes very difficult families and the responsiveness of the family.

In the great majority of cases encopresis resolves by the mid-teen years but some angry children subsequently display their unresolved aggressive feelings in other ways.

Chapter 15

Other Clinical Syndromes

Adjustment disorders

Adjustment disorders differ from most other diagnostic categories in that their definition rests on their apparent cause, rather than their clinical features. The latter vary considerably. While adjustment disorders may occur at any time of life, children may be particularly prone to suffering from them because of their immaturity and heavy dependence on those caring for them.

According to ICD-10, diagnosis depends on a careful evaluation of the symptoms, and of the subject's previous history and personality, together with an assessment of any stressful event or situation, or life crisis, that may have led to the symptoms. There has to be 'strong, but not presumptive' evidence that the disorder would not have arisen if the person had not experienced the stressful circumstances. Both ICD-10 and DSM-IV require that a period of no more than three months elapses between the onset of the stress and that of the disorder.

DSM-IV defines *adjustment disorder* as the development of 'clinically significant emotional or behavioural symptoms in response to an identifiable psychosocial stressor or stressors', occurring within the prescribed three months. Both ICD-10 and DSM-IV list subtypes of adjustment disorder, according to the predominant symptoms. The ICD-10 subtypes are:

- brief depressive reaction,
- prolonged depressive reaction,
- mixed anxiety and depressive reaction,
- with predominant disturbance of other emotions. (This category is to be used when several types of emotional reactions are reported, for example anxiety, depression, worry, tension or anger, but no one emotion predominates; it is also to be used for childhood regressive reactions such as may be characterized by bed-wetting or thumb-sucking.)
- With predominant disturbance of conduct.

- With mixed disturbance of emotions and conduct.
- With other specified predominant symptoms.

DSM-IV has six subtypes, these being characterized by, respectively, 'depressed mood', 'anxiety', 'mixed anxiety and depressed mood', 'disturbance of conduct', 'mixed disturbance of emotions and conduct', and an 'unspecified category'.

The disorder can be 'acute' (lasting less than six months) or 'chronic', with symptoms persisting longer than six months – though they cannot persist for more than six months after the termination of the stressor or its consequences.

Clinical picture

It will be clear from the above that there is no one *clinical picture* that characterizes adjustment disorders. In practice, the line between, for example, a conduct disorder and an 'adjustment disorder with predominant disturbance of conduct' is a fine one. Drawing it, in borderline cases, may be a matter of weighing the evidence that the disorder is primarily a response to stress in a child who was previously functioning well or at least, if 'conduct' symptoms predominate, did not display significant behaviour problems. It is important also to realize that the line is essentially an arbitrarily drawn one, designed to fit an artificially created framework. More important – much more – than determining which diagnostic category is appropriate to the making of a comprehensive assessment and, when treatment is planned, taking into account all relevant factors, whether these are recent stresses or longer-term circumstances.

The stressful circumstances that may lead to an adjustment disorder are legion. They range from family disasters such as the illness, death or imprisonment of family members or the separation of the parents, to acts of family violence, to problems in school, migration from one city or culture to another, peer group problems, the effects of disasters such as the loss of the family home by fire or one's property as a result of a burglary, and the consequences of war.

Just as there is no one clinical picture, there is also no one treatment approach. When the stress is likely to be short-lived (it may even have ceased although its consequences persist), little treatment may be needed beyond support and reassurance for all concerned. If the stressful circumstances are continuing, efforts should be made to remove or ameliorate them. If this is impossible, continuing psychotherapeutic help may be needed by child and/or family. Occasionally it may be helpful, even necessary, to remove the child to a different situation for a short time, while the various problems are tackled.

Other reactions to stress

ICD-10 and DSM-IV both list *acute stress reactions* (*disorders* in DSM-IV) and *post-traumatic stress disorder* (PTSD). Either may occur in children. The former is defined as occurring in individuals who do not have 'any other apparent mental disorder' and react immediately, or at most within a few minutes, according to ICD-10, to an exceptional stress, for example a natural catastrophe such as an earthquake, a serious accident, a battle or a criminal assault or rape. DSM-IV allows for onset up to one month. Anxiety, dissociative and other symptoms may occur.

Post-traumatic stress disorder, which was listed though not described in Chapter 8, is a delayed and/or protracted response to a stressful situation or event. The symptoms include the reliving of the trauma in 'flashbacks' or dreams, together with feelings of detachment or emotional numbness or blunting. There may also be avoidance of people or particular situations, especially those that are associated with the trauma. Thus if the trauma was the result of a severe automobile accident, the child may be reluctant to travel by car, or perhaps in any sort of motor vehicle. Other symptoms that may be present include lack of energy, attacks of panic or apparently irrational fear, or ongoing anxiety or depression.

Children may display any combination of the symptoms of adjustment disorders, acute stress reactions and PTSD when faced with major stressful events or situations. The May 1986 issue of *The Journal of the American Academy of Child Psychiatry* (Vol. 25, No. 3) contains a series of papers describing children's reactions to a variety of stressful events. These include witnessing the murder of a parent; the Three Mile Island nuclear power station accident; a devastating earthquake; and the events of the Pol Pot regime in Cambodia. The book *No Place to be a Child: Growing Up in a War Zone* (Garbarino, *et al.*, 1991) also contains much information about children's reactions to severe stress. While these are often devastating, it is also apparent children's reactions vary a great deal and some children are extraordinarily resilient.

Treatment

The *treatment* of reactions to severe stress depends on the causes, whether these are continuing and whether the stress can be relieved or the child removed from it. The same principles as outlined for adjustment disorders apply, though special measures are usually needed for children with PTSD. They may require intensive individual therapy. This may be at least partly verbal, but it often needs to include exploration of the child's memories of, and feelings about, the traumatic event(s) using play, drawing, puppetry, storytelling or dramatic re-enactment. Sometimes hypnotherapeutic methods are helpful in exploring the past traumatic events and helping the young person let go of the memories and fears and coming to a new understanding of the present situation. The objectives of the therapy should be the 'ventilation of feelings, exposure and discussion of symptoms, and clarification and interpretation of the child's defences and coping strategies' (Terr, 1991, page 760). Family therapy and group therapy may sometimes be useful and there may be a case for the use of medication, though only as an adjunct, and usually a temporary one.

Very short-term administration of anxiolytic drugs such as diazepam or lorazepam may tide children over acute stress for a few days, but prolonged use of such drugs is not indicated. Terr (1991) suggests that the drugs clonidine or propranolol may help alleviate some of the symptoms of PTSD, but hard data on their value are lacking.

Personality disorders

Many psychiatrists and other mental health professionals are reluctant to use the term *personality disorder* when the subject is a young person whose personality development is incomplete. Nevertheless, a small minority of children show such seriously maladaptive personality characteristics that the diagnosis is justified.

For a diagnosis of a personality disorder to be appropriate there must be severe, well-established problems of personality functioning affecting the subject's life in major ways. The diagnosis implies that the individual has developed inappropriate and seriously abnormal ways of dealing with the daily tasks of living, interpersonal relationships or the handling of stressful situations – or some combination of these.

Causes

Serious distortions of the normal processes of personality development in childhood have been attributed to constitutional, including genetic factors, and also to various environmental circumstances. Organic brain damage appears to play a part in some cases. The aetiology no doubt varies from case to case, with more than one cause operating in many instances.

Extremely unfavourable experiences during early life have long been blamed for personality disorders. Dockar-Drysdale (1968; 1973) and

Balbernie (1974), influenced by the work of Winnicott (1960), suggested that children with certain types of personality disorders have lacked *primary experience*. According to Balbernie (1974), 'The mother in nurturing and care, provides regular, ordered, complete experiences of well-being through which a child learns that it does survive separation'. Lacking this experience, children act out their anxiety, do not feel guilt, lack regard for others' feelings and fail to value themselves. To quote Balbernie again, 'The basis of well-being is the experience of a basic sense of natural order that is internalized'. This has not been provided for children who lack primary experience. They are described as *unintegrated*. These theories led to the concept of *frozen children*, whose primary experience has been interrupted when they and their mothers should be starting to separate out. They survive 'without boundaries to personality, merged with their environment and unable to make any real relationships or feel the need for them'.

Winnicott (1960) described *false selves* and *caretaker-selves*. He wrote:

'The false-self sets up as real and it is this that observers tend to think is the real person. In living relationships, work relationships, and friendships, however, the false-self begins to fail. In situations in which what is expected is a whole person the false-self has some essential lacking.'

Research since the above views on the development of personality disorders were formulated suggests that things are not as simple as Winnicott and his colleagues assumed. Summarizing more recent research, Rutter & Rutter (1993) point out that the belief that personalities are largely determined by experiences in early life is probably incorrect. It often appears to be the case, because very adverse early experiences are so often followed by problems in later life. Rutter & Rutter (1993, page 33) point out, however, that, 'provided later experiences are really good, the ill-effects of early deprivation or adversity are surprisingly evanescent in many respects'. The impression that this is not so has arisen because of the high probability that an adverse early upbringing will be followed by a similarly adverse later childhood. Thus 'early experiences do not have an over-riding importance that is independent of later experiences' (Rutter & Rutter, page 33). Personality development is thus an ongoing process that continues throughout childhood and adolescence and even in adult life, though it is no doubt true that as we get older our personalities do get more fixed and radical change becomes less likely.

It is likely that genetic factors play a part in personality development. It seems also that children's vulnerability to adverse circumstances varies. This may be related to genetic make-up and temperament.

Table 15.1 Categories of personality disorder.

ICD-10	DSM-IV	Main features
Paranoid	Paranoid	Suspicious, jealous, sensitive to slight or imagined insults, affective responses restricted.
Schizoid	Schizoid	Distant, cold, aloof, detached, introspective, unresponsive, few or no close friends.
Dissocial	Antisocial	Lacking feeling for others, disregarding social norms and obligations, failing to plan ahead or learn from failure, poor work and parenting record.
Emotionally unstable	Borderline	Impulsive, unpredictable, with unstable but intense interpersonal relationships. Identity uncertain, mood unstable, fearful of being alone, self-damaging.
Histrionic	Histrionic	Over-dramatic, flamboyant, labile mood, suggestible, drawing attention to self, egocentric, dependent.
Anankastic	Obsessive-compulsive	Rigid, inflexible, obsessive, ritualistic, perfectionistic.
Anxious (avoidant)	Avoidant	Hypersensitive to rejection, avoiding relationships, socially withdrawn, desiring affection and acceptance. Feelings of tension and apprehension.
Dependent	Dependent	Helpless, clinging, passively compliant, lacking vigour.
—	Schizotypal	Social isolation, ideas of reference, 'magical' thinking, recurrent illusions, odd speech, suspiciousness, hypersensitivity.
—	Narcissistic	Grandiosely self-important, with fantasies of success, power, brilliance or ideal love. Require attention and admiration, resent criticism, lack empathy and take advantage of others.
'Other' and 'Unspecified'	Not otherwise specified	—

Personality disorders are quite diverse, as can be seen in Table 15.1. In some categories, such as *schizoid personality disorder* (also known as Asperger's Syndrome and discussed in Chapter 11), the genetic factors may be more important than the environmental ones. In a study of 17 cases by Wolff & Barlow (1979) the children's histories revealed no adequate cause for the disorder. This suggested that, at the least, these children had a strong biological predisposition to the condition. This may or may not apply to other categories of personality disorder.

Both ICD-10 and DSM-IV list a variety of categories of personality disorder but these are derived mainly from studies on adults. Indeed ICD-10's list of personality disorders is entitled *disorders of adult personality*. Table 15.1 lists the disorders as they appear in the two classifications. The respective descriptions of the corresponding categories differ slightly but the categories from each of the diagnostic systems appearing on the same line are broadly similar.

Caution should be exercised in applying these labels to conditions encountered in childhood, and the younger the child, the greater the caution that is advisable. As we have seen above, personality development and maturation are possible, indeed the rule, throughout childhood and adolescence. Only serious, long-standing disorders, especially those that persist in all environmental circumstances, should qualify. In DSM-IV, one personality disorder category – antisocial personality disorder – is defined as applying only over age 18. Below that age there is a 'corresponding diagnostic category', namely conduct disorder.

Since the various categories of personality disorder have been identified in adults, rather than in children, a detailed consideration of them here would be inappropriate. Nevertheless we do encounter, in child psychiatric practice, children whose clinical presentation suggests that they may be developing the characteristics of one or other of the personality disorders seen in adulthood. When this is the case, it is reason to examine carefully any factors in child or family that may be contributing to this development, and to address these in the treatment of the child and the family.

Schizoid personality disorder has been discussed in Chapter 11. Antisocial (DSM-IV) or dissocial (ICD-10) personality disorders – or what used to be called *sociopathic personality* – merit brief consideration here. They are characterized by what ICD-10 calls 'callous unconcern for the feelings of others'; irresponsible attitudes and a lack of regard for society's norms, rules and obligations; relationships which, although they are readily established, are not maintained; very low frustration tolerance with the ready expression of aggression, often through violent behaviour; the lack of the capacity to feel guilt; inability to learn from experience, including attempts at punishment; and a strong propensity to blame others for the behaviours that lead to conflict with society, or to offer rationalizations to explain things away. Incipient signs of these personality problems can be discerned in some children and adolescents seen and treated in child psychiatry clinics and facilities. They are danger signs and usually indicate a need for careful clinical assessment and, often, intensive treatment.

It is well to bear in mind that, while ICD-10 rightly suggests that a diagnosis of personality disorder is seldom appropriate before the age of 16 or 17, some of the characteristics of these conditions may be evident earlier. There is no magic about the age of 18. Indeed much of what child psychiatrists do is designed to intervene when personality development is taking a deviant course, so that adult personality disorders do not develop.

Treatment

The *treatment* of incipient personality disorders often proves challenging, one of the greatest challenges being that of establishing a trusting relationship with the young person. Those whose clinical picture suggests that they may be developing the characteristics of a serious personality disorder, especially a dissocial or borderline one, may arouse therapists' despair, anger, disgust or other negative emotions. These young people are often reluctant or quite unwilling to enter therapy and may need to be treated in residential settings where the environment is tightly structured and cannot be manipulated.

A telling account of what may be involved in the treatment of a personality-disordered adolescent is that of Rossman (1985).

Psychosexual problems

Both ICD-10 and DSM-IV describe *gender identity disorders*. This term is used for the disorders of children who display persistent, severe distress about their assigned sex. They either desire to be, or insist that they really are, of the opposite sex. Such individuals may repudiate the anatomical attributes which define their sex. Onset is before puberty, often well before and the first manifestations are frequently apparent in the pre-school years.

This condition must be distinguished from non-conformity with sex-role stereotypes, which is much more common. To make the diagnosis of gender identity disorder there must be what the ICD-10 manual calls 'a profound disturbance of the normal sense of maleness or femaleness'. Nevertheless, there appears to be a continuum from those who are completely identified with their anatomical sex, to those who completely reject it. What may be mild forms of the same condition, though these certainly do not justify a diagnosis of gender identity disorder, are effeminacy in boys and 'tomboyishness' in girls. Again, in this condition as in so many others, it is essentially arbitrary where one draws the line. The DSM-IV criteria, being more specific, are the more stringent.

In child psychiatric practice, parents who express concern that their sons are overly effeminate are met with more often than those who are worried about masculine behaviours or attitudes in their daughters. Society tends to be more accepting of tomboyish behaviour in girls than of effeminate behaviour in boys. Girls may wear masculine clothes and play boys' games without causing concern, but boys who wear girls' clothes and engage in 'feminine' behaviour are less readily accepted (Williams, *et al.*, 1985).

Causes

Biological, especially genetic, factors and environmental ones combine to produce a child's sense of identity, as was explained in Chapter 1. Just how this happens, and the relative roles of different factors are incompletely understood. Social learning theories have been advanced to explain the process but the child's biological substrate surely limits what social learning can do.

The sexual identity assigned to a child in infancy, and the consequent experience of being raised as a member of that sex, used to be considered the most important factors. This appears to be an over-simplification and the process is nowadays regarded as involving a more complex interaction of factors than was realized. The nature and concentration of the hormones produced as boys and girls grow, approach puberty and become adolescent, differ and play their parts in the process (Green, 1985).

Effeminate boys tend to be overinvolved with their mothers from an early age and for well into middle childhood (Sreenivasan, 1985). This may be a factor in causing the effeminacy but it may also be the result of biologically determined behaviour in the child.

There is less information on the development of 'tomboy' girls but Williams, *et al.* (1985), in a longitudinal study of 50 such girls and a control group of 'nontomboys', found that tomboys are more likely to take their fathers as favoured parent and model, rather than their mothers. Tomboys had less physical contact with their mothers during the first year of life than the 'nontomboy' controls, though father-daughter interaction did not differ between the two groups. These investigators found that the mothers of the tomboys dressed in 'masculine' clothing significantly more than the 'control' mothers. More of them were also reported to have been tomboys themselves as children, suggesting a possible genetic influence.

Description

Sreenivasan (1985) assessed 100 consecutive referrals to a psychiatric clinic of boys aged 6 to 12. She found that 15 showed a high measure of effeminacy, though none met the DSM-III criteria for gender identity disorder and none was referred because of a gender identity problem. There was, however, a relationship between high effeminacy and paranoid (or 'hypersensitive') personality.

Sreenivasan (1985) describes a 'composite picture of the effeminate boy'. He is born to, or adopted by, a woman who sees him as not very manly; is a cuddly baby; clings to his mother as a toddler; and continues to wish to do so. His mother does not discourage this. He sleeps in his mother's bed well into late childhood, even though his father lives at home; has personality traits of hypersensitivity and insecurity; and may develop a neurotic disorder. Antisocial behaviour may develop later when he feels rejected by those who previously accepted his cross-gender activities, and peers stigmatize him. In Sreenivasan's series, only one of the 29 boys living in a traditional nuclear family showed high effeminacy. The presence of the father in the household seemed to be more important in promoting masculine attitudes than the quality of the father-son interaction.

Gender identity disorders, as defined in either of the two diagnostic systems, are much rarer than effeminate boys or tomboy girls. Boys with this condition have a strong and persistent desire to be female or even insist that they are. They may like to dress in girls' clothes, participate in girls' games and play with dolls as girls do. Less commonly, they may disclaim their penis or testes or express the belief they will disappear. Onset of cross-dressing is usually before the fifth birthday.

Girls with gender identity disorders show a desire to be, or believe they are, boys. While they prefer boys' clothing and games, this usually causes less concern.

It appears that extreme boyhood feminity is usually not an isolated phenomenon. It is often accompanied by other behavioural or emotional symptoms, particularly separation anxiety disorder (Bradley, *et al.*, 1980; Coates & Person, 1985).

Treatment

In considering what *treatment* is required in these cases, certain ethical issues need to be considered. These are discussed by Green (1985). It is not always clear what the treatment of children with atypical psychosexual development should aim to do. In severe cases of gender identity disorder it may not be realistic to try to reverse the child's sexual identity; to try might be traumatic or at least less helpful than other approaches. Yet the parents often seek treatment for these children, who may be socially ostracized and suffer much unhappiness, especially the boys.

Psychotherapy for child and parents is usually the treatment employed. It should aim to increase the child's comfort in being anatomically male or female, reduce sex-role behaviours which peers will regard as inappropriate, strengthen the child's relationship and contact with the same-sex parent, and facilitate the child's involvement with a same-sex peer group which will accept him or her. As well as individual therapy with the child and therapy for the parents, behaviour modification, group therapy and family therapy may sometimes be helpful. Whatever treatment is employed, it is important that it conforms to the wishes of the child and parents, and that it is undertaken only once properly informed consent has been obtained.

Outcome

There are limited data on the later *outcome* in children with gender identity problems. Green, *et al.* (1987) reported data derived from a group of 66 families evaluated at a gender identity clinic between 1969 and 1974 and followed up 15 years later. About one-third of the boys who had presented with 'feminine' characteristics could not be traced, so that 44 'previously feminine' (PF) boys were compared with 35 matched controls. During their childhoods the PF boys had played with dress-up dolls, dressed in girls' clothing, adopted girls' roles in play, stated the wish to be girls, primarily had girls as friends and avoided rough-and-tumble play. At follow-up there was found to be a high incidence of homosexual orientation in the PF group and indeed a majority of these boys presented with a bisexual or homosexual orientation as adults. Within the PF group, role-playing as a female, playing with dress-up dolls and having a female peer group were the characteristics with the greatest predictive value. The more these behaviours were reported, the greater was the tendency to a higher rating on homosexual orientation at follow up in adulthood. Green, *et al.* (1987, page 88) comment that:

> 'The development of adult sexual orientation appears most likely to involve interplay among a variety of intervening factors, such as innate features, relationship to parents, medical background, and parental concern over cross-gender behaviour.'

Other psychosexual problems

Various other psychosexual problems are sometimes encountered in young people. They include voyeurism, in which the subject spies on unsuspecting people who are undressing, or naked, or engaging in sexual intercourse; and exhibitionism, the exposing of one's genitals to strangers to achieve sexual excitement. Some children, and especially adolescents, who have been sexually abused later sexually victimize others.

The causes of these problems are usually complex and how they develop is not fully understood but some of these children have had unstable lives and difficult childhood experiences, with long periods of institutional care or deviant rearing. Individual psychotherapy, counselling for the parents, family therapy or behaviour therapy, or some combination of these treatments, may be helpful. The therapy of severe, established cases can be extremely challenging.

Tics and Gilles de la Tourette's syndrome

Tics, sometimes known as habit spasms, are repeated, sudden movements of muscles or groups of muscles, not under voluntary control and serving no obvious purpose. They most often affect the muscles of the face, and eye-blinking tics are common. Various facial contortions may occur and muscle groups in other parts of the body may be affected. The head and neck may be suddenly and briefly moved in one direction or contorted. There may be similar movement of trunk and limbs. The same movements tend to occur repeatedly, in severe cases scores or hundreds of times daily. This contrasts with the involuntary movements seen in the various forms of chorea which are more varied and less predictable. Tics, especially when they involve large movements of trunk or limbs, can be seriously handicapping.

Tics are sometimes subdivided into simple and complex varieties. Simple motor tics include eye-blinking, shoulder-shrugging and grimacing movements of the face. Examples of complex motor tics are hitting one's self and jumping. Examples of simple vocal tics are grunts, sniffing and throat clearing, while complex vocal tics are such things as repeatedly saying words, often socially unacceptable, and sometimes obscene, ones, and the repetition of one's own words or sounds (palilalia). The term *coprolalia* has been used for the uttering of obscenities.

Both ICD-10 and DSM-IV distinguish three main categories of tic disorder.

- Transient tic disorder.
- Chronic motor or vocal tic disorder.
- Combined vocal and multiple motor tic disorder, or Tourette's syndrome (or disorder).

In keeping with its aim to be inclusive, ICD-10 also has two *residual* categories:

- Other tic disorders.
- Tic disorder, unspecified.

Transient tic disorder is the most common form of tic disorder. It is most frequently encountered in the 4- to 5-year-old age range. Tics such as eye-blinking, facial grimacing and head-jerking appear but do not persist for long, often only a few weeks or months. The term *transient tic disorder* is reserved for tics which last for less than a year, though there may be remissions and relapses during the year. In many cases there is only one episode. Mild, occasional tics are common in normally developing young children and the borderline between them and transient tic disorder is not well defined.

Chronic motor or *vocal tics* are characterized by either motor or vocal tics, but not both, lasting more than a year. The tics may be simple or complex, or there may be a combination of the two.

In *Tourette's syndrome*, described in ICD-10 as *combined vocal and multiple motor tic disorder* and in DSM-IV as *Tourette's disorder*, there is a history of both motor and vocal tics, though they need not both be present at the same time. In severe cases there are complex and multiple tics, often with the use of obscene words and phrases. These may be accompanied by obscene gestures (copropraxia).

Prevalence studies have come up with widely differing figures ranging from 2.9 per 10 000 to 59 per 10 000 in child populations (Leckman & Cohen, 1994). What does seem clear is that tic disorders are much more common (probably 5 to 12 times more common) in children than in adults and in males than in females – the ratio having been variously reported between 3:1 and 9:1 (Leckman & Cohen, 1994).

Tourette syndrome is much less common, affecting perhaps 1 in 1000 children (Zahner, *et al.*, 1988), or about half that many according to DSM-IV.

Causes

In the *causation* of tics and especially Tourette's syndrome, genetic factors are important. There is evidence of an autosomal dominant pattern of transmission of Tourette's syndrome, chronic tics and obsessive disorder (Pauls & Leckman, 1986). The concordance rate for Tourette's syndrome has been found to be more than 50% in monozygotic twin pairs, while in dizygotic pairs it is about 10% (Price, *et al.*, 1986), the concordance rates increasing to 77 and 30% respectively if co-twins with chronic motor tics are included.

It seems that tics are more likely to develop in boys with the gene, and obsessive-compulsive disorders in girls. Apparently only some cases of obsessive-compulsive disorder are inherited in this way, and some individuals with Tourett's syndrome (perhaps about 10%) may be phenocopies, that is, non-genetically determined cases.

Other factors than genetic ones no doubt contribute to the development of these conditions, but these have not been clearly delineated. Emotional tension, brain damage, developmental deviation and adverse learning experiences have all been suggested but their roles, if any, are not established. Biochemical theories have also been put forward, and no doubt there are disturbances of brain function in these disorders, but these have not so far developed beyond the hypothesis stage.

Clinical features

The main *clinical features* of these disorders have been outlined above. The onset of tics is usually between the ages of 1 and 15, the peak occurring around 7. Severity varies greatly. Mild cases may present little problem to the child or to others, but in severe cases the symptoms can be seriously handicapping. In addition to obsessive-compulsive disorders, other conditions which may be associated with tic disorders include attention-deficits, hyperactivity, behaviour problems, learning difficulties and sleep problems (Singer & Walkup, 1991). Sleep difficulties seem to be particularly frequent in boys with both Tourette's syndrome and attention-deficit problems (Allen, *et al.*, 1992).

The association with attention-deficit disorders is important. It is not uncommon for tics to develop while children are receiving methylphenidate and other stimulant drugs for their attentional disorder. Whether the stimulant drugs play a part in precipitating, or even causing, the tics, or whether the relationship is simply due to the fact that the two conditions naturally tend to occur together, is not clear.

Treatment

The treatment needed depends on the nature and severity of the tics and on what, if any, associated conditions are present. Children with transient tic disorders, unless these are very severe, probably require no treatment beyond reassuring the parents and child that they are common and are likely to disappear within a year or so. While in some cases the tics prove not to be transient, conditional reassurance is probably justified, as the tics do usually disappear without any specific treatment. Moreover the proportion of young children who go on to develop Tourette's syndrome is quite small. The possibility exists, however, and it is therefore advisable to keep these children under periodic review until the tics have ceased and have been absent for a period of six months or more, if this does happen.

In managing these children and their parents, a supportive attitude, and the relief of any stress the child may be experiencing, are important. Any apparent causes of anxiety should be removed and co-existing psychiatric problems should receive the appropriate treatment.

Although many treatments have been suggested for tic disorders, including individual psychotherapy and behaviour therapy, treatment with certain drugs seems to be the most effective. The mainstays of drug therapy have been the antipsychotic drugs haloperidol and pimozide. Haloperidol is probably the more effective but can have serious side-effects (discussed in Chapter 21). Clonidine, a drug primarily used to control hypertension, is sometimes effective in controlling tics, though usually less so than haloperidol and pimozide. It has the advantage, however, of having fewer serious side-effects.

Various reports have been published, with widely differing results, on the use of members of the tricyclic group of antidepressant drugs, especially when tics and attention-deficit disorders co-exist. Spencer, *et al.* (1993a; 1993b) summarize these and describe a retrospective study, based on chart reviews, that suggests that the tricyclic drug, nortriptyline may be of value when these conditions co-exist. Further studies are clearly needed before definitive statements can be made concerning the role of the tricyclics, if they have one, in these disorders.

The use of the drugs mentioned above is discussed further in Chapter 21.

Outcome

The *outcome* in tic disorders is generally favourable. One study (Corbett, *et al.*, 1969) found that 40% of 100 ticquers who were followed up five years after psychiatric consultation had recovered. Associated anxiety and other neurotic symptoms may persist after the tics have ceased. The outlook in Tourette's syndrome, and especially in severe cases, is less good. The combination of medication with behavioural management often keeps the symptoms in abeyance and in some individuals they remit in due course.

Stuttering

Both ICD-10 and DSM-IV list stuttering as a diagnostic category. Sometimes called stammering, it is the repeated interruption of the flow of speech by repetition, prolongation or blocking of sounds. In the speech of children in the 2- to 4-year-old-age range there are often hesitations and irregularities of the rhythm of speech. This is known as *clutter* and sometimes precedes true stuttering, though more often it gradually disappears and the child then speaks normally.

Stuttering may appear after speech has been normally acquired but the onset is usually before the age of ten. It occurs in about 4% of boys and 2% of girls. About 1% of children continue stuttering in adolescence, more of them being boys than girls. Its causes are not fully understood, but there is often a positive family history and genetic factors may play a part. So also may anxiety and stress (Greiner, *et al.*, 1985). Other psychological factors are also probably involved and some stutterers can sing fluently or speak normally while acting on stage, but stutter in ordinary conversation. Disturbed parent-child relationships may affect the learning of fluent speech.

The severity of stuttering varies from occasional repetition of speech sounds to severe blocking of speech which seriously interferes with communication. Sometimes there are associated movements of the face or other parts of the body coinciding with the repetitions, prolongations or pauses in the flow of speech. Anticipatory anxiety may be present, leading to avoidance behaviour. At first a few letters or sounds may be avoided. Later many places and social situations may be shunned. This can affect the subject's life quite drastically. Stuttering may cause children to become isolated and impair their ability to take part in school activities.

Stuttering is not usually part of a general psychiatric disorder. In most cases emotional factors probably play only a small part in its causation, though anxiety may either complicate or exacerbate the condition.

Treatment

This is usually undertaken by speech therapists and the psychiatric contribution is limited. Techniques designed to relieve anxiety, promote relaxation and encourage self-confidence may help.

Conture (1990, Chapter 3) provides an excellent review of current approaches to the treatment of children who stutter. Remediation, he points out, may involve:

- Environmental modification. This includes sharing information with and counselling parents about what they may or may not be doing to facilitate their child's speech fluency.
- Speech-language modification. This consists of identifying those

speech production strategies the child is using which cause the fluency of speech to be disrupted.

● A combination of the above two approaches.

Conture (1990) advocates the treatment of most young children who stutter in parent-child stuttering groups. He recommends that children who do not improve with group therapy receive indirect or direct individual speech therapy, the degree of 'directness' depending upon the nature of the child's problem, and the child's level of development, and emotional and intellectual awareness of the problem.

Psychotherapy should be reserved for children or families in whom there is associated emotional disorder.

Stuttering is often mild and transient and most children outgrow it by their mid-teens, though in a few cases it persists into adult life.

The two diagnostic systems mentioned above each also have a category for *cluttering*. This is similar to the *clutter* mentioned above. It is primarily a disturbance of the rhythm of speech. Speech is rapid, erratic and lacks the normal rhythm; instead there is irregular production of phrases, groups of words being produced unrelated to the proper grammatical structure of the sentence.

Elective mutism

This is a condition in which the child, though able to talk, refuses to do so in certain situations. DSM-IV has renamed it *selective mutism*.

Prevalence

The *prevalence* of elective/selective mutism depends on the age range studied. Brown & Lloyd (1975) surveyed 6072 five-year-old children starting school in Birmingham, UK. They found that 42 were still not speaking in class after eight weeks in school, a prevalence rate of 7.2 per 1000. During the following four terms the number of mute children fell steadily, so that after 64 weeks only one child remained silent in school. The condition is thus fairly common as an initial reaction to starting school but rare as a persisting problem. Immigrant children were over-represented.

The prevalence in 7-year-olds is probably about 0.8 per 1000 (Kolvin & Fundudis, 1981), but it depends on the diagnostic criteria used. Elective mutism, unlike most child psychiatric disorders, is as common in girls as in boys, possibly a little more common.

Causes

Among the *causes* that have been proposed for elective mutism is a biologically based delay in maturation. Electively mute children are often considered to be unusually shy and a high prevalence of shyness has been reported in their parents. Kolvin & Fundudis (1981) reported several 'subsidiary' patterns of behaviour: 'submissive'; 'sensitive and weepy'; and 'moody, sulky and stubborn'. The last named was the most common. These children tend to be late talking, have speech abnormalities when they do start to talk, and are enuretic and encopretic more often than controls. This condition does not seem to be specially prevalent in any particular socioeconomic group. The increased prevalence in immigrant children suggests, however, that sociocultural factors may play a part.

Elective mutism is probably a complex disorder in which genetic, personality, emotional, family and sociocultural factors all contribute.

Clinical features

The main *clinical feature* is the child's refusal to talk in certain, often most, situations, while talking freely in others – mainly in the home and when in the company of family members or other very familiar figures. These children usually do not talk in a wide range of other situations – school, public places, clinics, doctors' offices and consulting rooms. Brown & Lloyd (1975) found that children who were mute at school showed other behaviour patterns which distinguished them from children who spoke. They were more likely to stop an activity when the teacher approached and to avoid playing with other children. They were also less likely to draw, go to the toilet or approach the teacher's table.

In the doctor's office or therapist's playroom these children often behave as negativistically non-verbally as they do verbally. They may passively decline to sit down or to play when invited to do so. Some will nod or shake (usually shake) their heads in reply to questions, others deny the interviewer even this response. At the same time they are usually looking around the room, apparently taking everything in. They can be extraordinarily stubborn, remaining silent for session after session. One girl who was making good, if non-verbal, progress at school was observed on closed circuit television to be talking freely and in an apparently relaxed way when alone with her family, but as soon as a member of the clinic staff entered she became silent and remained so until that person left.

Various subtypes of elective mutism have been described. Hayden (1980) distinguished 'symbiotic', 'reactive', 'passive aggressive' and 'speech phobic' varieties. Wright, *et al.* (1985) suggested that Hayden's 'symbiotic' and 'reactive' cases are what Kolvin & Fundidus (1981) called, respectively, 'elective' and 'traumatic' mutism. Haydon's 'passive aggressive' group seems rather different, with a later age of onset, often in adolescence.

In clinical practice it is hard to categorize cases of elective mutism. Rather than there being various distinct groupings, it seems that what we deal with is a syndrome which has varying manifestations and which occurs in children from many different types of families. There are, however, some children in which anxiety seems to dominate the clinical picture and others in which negativism does. Whether the various sub-groupings mentioned above reflect anything more than differences in emphasis in the clinical picture is uncertain.

Kolvin & Fundudis (1981) reported a mean IQ of 85 in their 24 elective mutes, while the mean IQ of a speech-retarded comparison group was 95 and that of normal control subjects was 101.

Treatment

Many *treatments* have been proposed for electively mute children. The established, severe case often presents a considerable therapeutic challenge. Treatments that have been suggested include suggestion, persuasion, coercion, psychodynamically oriented play therapy, speech therapy, family therapy and behaviour therapy. Wright, *et al.* (1985), reviewing reports of 81 cases, found that behavioural intervention was used most often (in 27 cases), with *psychodynamic* intervention second in 15. They also reported three cases, all with onset at age three, which presented in the pre-school period and were treated in a diagnostic nursery with good results. They suggested that early treatment may prevent the condition becoming chronic and less responsive to later treatment measures. They thought that important factors contributing to their good results were early intervention, the expectation that the children would speak and the conjoint family work that was done. A problem with such studies, however, is that one does not know what the spontaneous recovery rate would have been without treatment, though we do know that it tends to be quite high.

While many children grow out of their mutism quite quickly, this does not necessarily justify inaction, since some of these children do not do so for a long time. In the case of the child who does not speak on first entering school, especially when there is no evidence of other serious problems in child or family, it is probably reasonable to wait a few months before initiating any attempts at therapy. Many of these children will start speaking during this period.

When treatment is undertaken it seems that a small group setting with speaking peers and adults who expect the child to talk and do not accept the mutism as inevitable, together with family intervention, as described by Wright, *et al.* (1985) is a helpful approach. For older children, combinations of behavioural interventions, family therapy and, in some cases, play therapy may offer the best prospects of success.

Outcome

The *outcome* in elective mutism is generally favourable. The condition is usually self-limiting and total mutism seldom persists into adult life, though in severe cases – a very small minority – it may persist for much of childhood and into early adolescence. Few data are available on the emotional adjustment of these children once they do start to speak, but it seems that they are inclined to be shy, retiring individuals. The outlook is good for the child whose mutism is a reaction to starting school and who has previously communicated normally.

The Kleine-Levin syndrome

This is a disorder of unknown cause, in which there are episodes of disturbed mental function, greatly increased appetite and excessive sleepiness (Billiard, 1989). The episodes last from a few days to several weeks. The onset is usually in adolescence but may occur before puberty (Ferguson, 1986). Psychiatric symptoms reported in these cases include disturbances of mood – depression, unwarranted anxiety or mania – and delusional ideas, including erotic ones, have been reported. No particular treatment methods have been shown to be effective, but the condition usually resolves spontaneously in time.

Epilepsy

While epilepsy is primarily a neurological, rather than a psychiatric, condition it has considerable psychiatric importance for the following reasons:

(a) Epilepsy may have major repercussions in children's lives (Barker, 1993a). Repeatedly losing consciousness or displaying abnormal behaviour in school or other public places may lead others, especially a child's peers, to become frightened, anxious or hostile. Depending on the attitudes of family, friends and others, epileptic children may come to feel imperfect or stigmatized, so that their self-esteem suffers. Anxiety or depression may follow.

(b) Symptoms which are due to epilepsy may be erroneously regarded as psychogenic. Thus *absence seizures*, lapses of consciousness which last 5 to 15 seconds and which may occur hundreds of times a day, may be mistaken for inattention of emotional origin. This applies also to *complex partial seizures*, in which there is an aura (a brief subjective experience the child becomes aware of before the seizure itself commences), then loss of consciousness for, usually, 30 seconds to 2 minutes. There may be automatisms (apparently purposive movements which are not under conscious control) in both these types of seizure but they are more common in the latter (Stores, 1987). Complex partial seizures are due to epileptic discharges in the temporal lobes of the brain and the 'automatic' behaviours, which may include running about, screaming and shouting, aggressive behaviour and temper attacks, may lead to an incorrect diagnosis of conduct disorder.

Non-convulsive status epilepticus is a condition in which epileptic discharges continue for periods which may be as long as several months, but without typical seizures appearing. As well as neurological symptoms such as ataxia (lack of muscular coordination), dysphasia (impaired verbal language function), myoclonic jerks (spontaneous, sudden movements of muscles), and atonic attacks (in which muscle tone is lost), there may be disorientation, fluctuating responsiveness, developmental regression and aggressive behaviour (Manning & Rosenbloom, 1987).

(c) Epileptic seizures and *pseudoepilepsy* may occur in the same individual. The concept of pseudoepilepsy takes in certain manifestations of conversion disorders and dissociative disorders (see Chapter 8) and also behaviours due to other non-epileptic conditions. Distinguishing seizures which are epileptic from those which are not can be difficult. The EEG is useful but recordings taken between epileptic attacks may be normal, unless they are taken immediately after an attack. Detailed study of the circumstances in which the attacks occur and careful observation of the attacks themselves – which often have to be carried out by relatives, teachers and others, and reported to the professionals concerned – are necessary to unravel these complex cases.

Nowadays equipment is available for the continuous monitoring of the EEG while patients go about their activities. The recording of the EEG can be done using a radio transmitter, or by means of a cable running from the child to whom the EEG electrodes are attached to the EEG laboratory. The subject needs to be near the EEG laboratory, which usually means being in hospital. *Ambulatory* recording is also possible at home, in school or elsewhere, using small cassette recorders worn by the subject (Stores,

1985). These devices can help distinguish epilepsy from other types of seizure.

Secondary gain, such as the experience of increased attention and solicitude, or special consideration when family or other activities are planned, may be part of the unconscious motivation behind *pseudoepileptic* seizures, especially when the organically caused ones are controlled by medication. In some instances the child has other emotional problems or there are contributory factors in the functioning of the family system.

(d) *Pseudoepileptic* or *hysterical* seizures may masquerade as epileptic ones in children who do not have epilepsy at all. These children may have had contact with epileptics or have witnessed seizures. Such experiences serve as the unconscious models of disturbed or 'sick' behaviour. These may appear as part of the symptomatology of an anxiety or neurotic disorder. Careful history-taking, a full psychiatric assessment of child and family, EEG examination, perhaps with continuous monitoring, and paediatric consultation usually lead to the correct diagnosis.

(e) Epilepsy may be a complication of certain psychiatric disorders, notably infantile autism and some of the conditions causing disintegrative psychoses.

(f) The side-effects of the drugs used in the treatment of epilepsy include depression, irritability and various forms of behaviour disorder. Phenobarbitone, phenytoin and carbamazepine, all valuable anticonvulsants, are among the drugs that can cause such problems.

In the management of the above clinical situations, close collaboration and communication between psychiatrists, paediatricians and others who may be involved – teachers, psychologists and social workers, for example, are vital if good clinical results are to be obtained. There are few areas in which collaboration of child psychiatrist and paediatrician is more important.

Goodyer (1985) provides a valuable article on the assessment and investigation of seizure disorders. Stores (1987) reminds us that there is no such thing as the *epileptic personality* and points out that 'the typical psychological problems of people with epilepsy are depression and anxiety caused by unhelpful and uninformed social attitudes' (page 90).

The episodic dyscontrol syndrome

This term is sometimes used for individuals who have violent outbursts of anger or rage, usually involving physical aggression. It has been described as occurring in both children and adults. It is probably the same as the *intermittent explosive disorder* of DSM-IV which requires that there be 'discrete episodes of failure to resist aggressive impulses that result in serious assaultive acts or destruction of property. The aggressiveness is grossly out of proportion to any provocation or precipitating psychosocial stressor.' It excludes such behaviour occurring as part of another psychiatric syndrome, such as a psychotic disorder, 'organic personality disorder', conduct disorder or intoxication with a psychoactive substance.

The aetiology of this condition is unclear and its status as a distinct diagnostic entity uncertain. Treatment with the anticonvulsant carbamazepine, or with propanolol, a drug used primarily for the treatment of hypertension, may be helpful.

Chapter 16

Mind–Body Relationships

Both physical and emotional factors play a part in most, maybe even all, illnesses. The division of diseases into those that are *organic* and those that are *non-organic* – or into *physical* and *psychological* categories is, at best, a gross over-simplification and perhaps quite wrong. It is also open to question whether the conceptual division of mind and body makes sense.

The brain, a part of the body, is the organ of the mind. Changes in a person's emotional state inevitably have their correlates in the activities of the brain, whether these are chemical, electrical, physical or structural – in most instances some combination of changes is involved. In an analogous way, changes in the electrolytes in the blood have their correlates in the activity of the kidneys, lungs and other organs and bodily systems.

It is easier to investigate and understand the relationships between, for example, electrolyte levels and renal activity – each of which affects the other – than it is to come to an understanding of the relationship between brain activity and emotional state and behaviour. This is partly because the brain is an immensely complex organ and singularly difficult to study. Nevertheless it is established that there are significant changes in brain chemistry and activity in subjects experiencing different mood states such as depression or mania. Modern imaging techniques and other techno- logical advances are likely to throw more light on this in the coming years, but we already know enough to be sure that any rigid division of mind and body is an artificial and false dichotomy.

The influence of the body on the mind

It is well known that being diagnosed as having a serious or life- threatening disease may have major effects on a person's mental and emotional state. Chronic diseases such as diabetes, cystic fibrosis, asthma, rheumatoid arthritis, congenital heart disease or eczema influence the self-images, development and emotional states of affected children. So also may congenital deformities, dwarfism, cerebral palsy and other physically obvious and handicapping conditions (Barker, 1993a).

In all the above disorders the effect of the bodily condition on the mind can be explained as being mediated by the subject's awareness of the condition, the handicap it causes and the effects it has on the attitudes and behaviour of others. The body can also affect the mind in other ways. Apart from obvious examples such as brain tumours and diseases, many physical illnesses influence people's emotional states, thinking processes and behaviour. In diabetics, for example, fluctuations in the blood sugar level, and the accumulation of ketones in the blood, affect the mental state. Hypoglycaemia from any other causes has effects similar to those seen when diabetics have insulin reactions. Raised or lowered levels of thyroid hormones also lead to changes in the mental state.

These relationships are not necessarily or entirely one-way. The effective severity of a handicap can vary according to the emotional reaction to the handicap. Physical handicaps may be regarded as challenges to be overcome or as permanent limitations which the subject does not feel can be overcome or lessened. Notable examples of people who have overcome serious handicaps include Douglas Bader, who continued flying as a Battle of Britain pilot after having both his legs amputated; and Helen Keller who was remarkably successful in overcoming the dual handicaps of blindness and deafness.

The effects of the mind on the body

Some of the effects of the emotions on bodily function are familiar to all and are subsumed in phrases such as 'scared stiff' and 'shaking with laughter'. When people are frightened or anxious they may lose their appetite or feel the urge to urinate or defecate. Some peptic ulcer patients suffer exacerbations when they are worried or under stress and many other conditions are stress-related in similar ways.

Despite such everyday experiences, familiar to all of us, the extent of the mind's influence on the body is too often overlooked or under-estimated. Rossi (1986a) reminds us of the significance of phenomena such as voodoo deaths and the placebo response. In certain cultures people die because they believe a spell has been cast over them. Similar processes also promote recovery from illnesses. The culture of the western world is that of the vitamin pill, antibiotic, sleeping tablet or cold cure, rather than that of the witchdoctor's spell, but the mechanisms by which each work may be much the same. We know that the prescription of inert 'medication' may promote recovery in 30 to 40% of patients with certain disorders, presumably because their faith in the medication they take is as great as that which people in other cultures have in their traditional healing methods.

Rossi (1986a) reviewed research into mind-body mechansims. There is good evidence that nerve impulses arising in the hypothalamus in response to emotional changes affect the functioning of the autonomic, endocrine and immune systems.

The phenomena of hypnosis also provide compelling evidence of the influence of the mind over the body. There have been many reports of major abdominal, dental and other surgery being carried out under hypnosis without the use of any conventional anaesthetic. Hypnosis has been shown to be of value in pain control, for example that due to burns (Patterson, *et al.*, 1992) and as an adjunct in the treatment of cancer (Walker, 1992). Painless and haemorrhage-free dental extractions can be carried out under hypnosis, even in haemophiliacs, who can be taught to control the blood flow to the dental sockets concerned.

Swirsky-Sacchetti & Margolis (1986) investigated a comprehensive self-hypnosis training program for haemophiliacs. They found that during an 18-week follow-up period the amount of Factor VIII concentrate used to control bleeding by the research subjects was significantly less than that used by control subjects. (Factor VIII is lacking in the blood of these patients.) The authors seemed justified in their claim that self-hypnosis is both an effective and a cost-effective treatment for haemophilia.

Psychosomatic considerations in child psychiatry

What are the implications for child psychiatry of the relationships discussed above? One is that in formulating the cases of child patients, and in treatment planning, consideration should be given to:

- organic factors, whether inborn or acquired,
- emotional/psychological factors,
- family relationships,
- the interplay of all the above three.

We need no longer regard some disorders as *organic*, others *psychological* and yet others *psychosomatic*. In a sense every disorder is psychosomatic, in that both physical and psychological factors are involved in some degree. This applies even to conditions as 'organic' as a fracture of a leg bone. Not only is there inevitably some emotional reaction to such an injury, but the patient's attitude and behaviour can affect the rate of healing. It is also the case that some children are more accident-prone than others and predisposition to injury is greater in some families than in others.

Graham (1985) suggested that one can construct a hierarchy of conditions on the basis of the relative importance of physical and psychological components in their aetiology and treatment. He proposed that, among conditions commonly dealt with by paediatricians, psychological factors might be ranked in the following ascending order of importance: congenital malformations, cancers, metabolic disorders, infections, epilepsy, failures of growth, bronchial asthma, enuresis/encopresis, accidents and emotional/behavioural disorders. This is a more realistic approach than labelling conditions either psychosomatic or not, but it does have the disadvantage that it suggests a static relationship between physical and psychological factors. In reality, the relative importance of these factors varies from child to child and even from time to time and is not simply a question of what the diagnosis is.

As an example of the above, we might take anorexia. This may start as a largely emotional disorder but it may progress to become a mainly physical, and even a fatal one. The causation of other conditions, such as growth failure in infancy and early childhood, varies from child to child. It may be due predominantly to physical disease, such as chronic infection, or predominantly to psychological factors such as severe psychosocial deprivation.

A word of warning about the dangers of linear thinking is in order here. In many, perhaps most, conditions we are dealing with circular processes, rather than with one thing causing another. Consider the example of retentive soiling, discussed in Chapter 14. Retention of faeces may be a reaction to coercive bowel training. This may lead the parents to increase the coerciveness of their efforts to train the child. The reaction of the child may be even more determined retention of faeces. Parental despair may follow, together with demoralization of the child and ostracism of the child by peers. By this time a major physical problem is present – with chronic constipation, psychogenic megacolon and overflow incontinence, requiring both physical treatment measures and, probably, counselling or psychotherapy for child and family.

Many examples could be cited to illustrate the interaction of mind and body. We will now consider asthma, eating disorders and 'factitious illness by proxy'.

Asthma

Bronchial asthma is characterized by paroxysmal attacks of difficulty with breathing. The smaller air passages in the lungs become constricted due to contraction of the muscles in their walls. Secretions accumulate and the walls of the passages swell. The subject has difficulty coughing up the secretions and the lungs tend to get over-filled with air causing the chest cavity to become over-expanded.

The muscles in the walls of the air passages (bronchi and bronchioles) in the lungs are controlled by nerves belonging to the autonomic nervous system – a network of nerves which controls a range of functions not normally under conscious control, heart rate, blood pressure, body temperature, for example. Normally this system of nerves is responsible for ensuring that the physiological processes it controls are adjusted to take care of the person's needs – increasing the supply of blood to muscles and that of air to the lungs, during exercise, for instance. This system also responds to emotional changes. This is a primitive physiological response, deriving from the need the startled animal has for 'fight or flight'. A quick physiological response was important for our phylogenetic ancestors, even if it is not for most of us in the majority of situations we encounter in life today.

Two further factors affect the air passages in the lungs. One is infection; the other is allergy. An allergic reaction is an adverse reaction by the body to a substance which is not harmful to most people. Pollen, dusts and many other substances may provoke such reactions. Among the reactions that may occur is the precipitation of an asthma attack as a result of swelling of the air passage walls and the production of liquid secretions which block those bronchi and bronchioles.

In addition to the factors mentioned above there is a biological substrate necessary for the development of asthma. Only certain individuals are prone to it and many of these have suffered from eczema, a skin disease in the causation of which similar mechanisms are involved. Those who are constitutionally susceptible are liable to react to some combination of infection, allergy and emotional tension by developing an asthma attack. This may lead to heightened anxiety and tension in the child, and perhaps in the parents also, which in turn leads to a worsening of the asthma. A circular process is thus set up.

In addition to considering factors directly involving the child, we need to consider also how the way the functioning of the family system of which the child is part may influence, for better or worse, the child's condition. It has been suggested that certain patterns of family functioning may increase the likelihood of asthma attacks occurring, or their severity. According to Minuchin and his colleagues (1975) symptoms are more likely to arise, in a physiologically vulnerable child, when the family system is characterized by the following transactional patterns:

- enmeshment;
- overprotectiveness;

- rigidity; and
- lack of conflict resolution.

Just how important these family factors are in the causation of asthma is not clear. Enmeshment and overprotective parental attitudes could result from having an asthmatic child. Even if that is so, however, they might still contribute to the maintenance of the asthma.

Mrazek (1986) raised what he called 'two questions for child psychiatry' regarding asthma. One was whether asthmatic children 'suffer a greater incidence and prevalence of psychiatric disturbance'; the other asked what role 'emotional stressors' play in causing asthma, given that there is genetic vulnerability. The second question is hard to answer precisely in the present state of knowledge, but the answer probably varies from child to child. The first, however, seems to make the assumption that mind and body are separate, that a disorder is either psychiatric or physical. But mind and body are not separate and despite the tendency of psychiatrists and specialists in respiratory medicine to practice separately, it is not really the question that needs answering. It also raises the issue of what is meant by *psychiatric disturbance*. Perhaps the writer would define this according to the number of symptoms of anxiety, depression, disturbed conduct and so on, displayed by the child. When these reach a certain number psychiatric disturbance might be said to exist. This is very much the DSM-IV approach but it is based on a false dichotomy.

More important questions than those asked by Mrasek (1986) seem to be, 'Are the emotions ever uninvolved when a child has attacks of asthma?' And, if they are involved, 'How do emotional factors interact with other factors that are operating in each particular case?'

The fundamental question which Mrasek (1986) raises, though he does not ask it, is whether we are to regard psyche and soma, mind and body, separately or as one. Can the psychiatric aspects of the cases of children with asthma, for example, be separated from the somatic ones in any meaningful way? Traditionally, medicine has tried to do this, but the attempt has not been very successful. It is of interest that Ernest Rossi, who has produced a scholarly treatise on mind-body relationships (Rossi, 1986a) is not a physician but a psychologist.

Eating disorders

In few, if any, disorders are physical and emotional factors so inextricably intertwined as in the eating disorders of childhood and adolescence. The most important of these are anorexia nervosa, bulimia, childhood obesity, pica and 'rumination disorder of infancy'. The latter two are discussed in Chapter 17.

Anorexia nervosa and bulimia

While anorexia nervosa and bulimia are distinct conditions, they are related and share some common psychopathology. Both are conditions affecting principally adolescent girls, though they are not confined to girls and can occur before puberty.

The essential feature of *anorexia nervosa* is a profound aversion to food, leading to serious weight loss. Not only do these patients lose weight, but their body images are distorted. This leads them to deny that they are thin, even though they are grossly under weight – even cachectic and near to death.

Other symptoms of anorexia include excessive activity, for example running long distances and other forms of 'working out'; depression; amennorhoea (the absence of menstruation), which is always present in established cases in female adolescent and adult patients; and pre-occupation with food and an interest in preparing it for others, though not in consuming it. Anorexic subjects usually have accurate knowledge of what foods are 'fattening' and carefully avoid them, preferring salads, fruit and other low-calorie items.

In due course the effects of self-starvation come to dominate the clinical picture. The patient becomes weak and lethargic, with slow pulse, low blood pressure, constipation, hirsutism and blue and cold extremities. In severe cases death may occur from heart failure induced by starvation. The levels of luteinizing hormone, follicle stimulating hormone and oestrogens in the blood are all very low.

Both ICD-10 and DSM-IV require that the patient's weight is at least 15% below that which is expected. It also requires that there be avoidance of 'fattening foods' and at least one of: self-induced vomiting; self-induced purging; excessive exercise; and the use of appetite suppressants and/or diuretics. Other requirements are body-image distortion and certain endocrine disturbances. When the onset is before puberty, the normal events of puberty are delayed or fail to occur altogether until recovery.

Associated symptoms include depression, dissatisfaction with life and a poor self-image (Lask & Bryant-Waugh, 1992).

Bulimia nervosa, often referred to simply as bulimia, is characterized by repeated bouts of binge eating, often followed by self-induced vomiting. The characteristics of this condition include a persistent preoccupation with eating, together with an irresistible craving for food to which the patient periodically succumbs. There must also be efforts to counter the fattening effect of the food by one or more of: self-induced vomiting, purgative abuse, and the use of drugs intended to cause weight loss (appetite suppressants, thyroid preparations or diuretics); and a 'morbid dread of fatness'.

Bulimic patients are not always under weight and the condition can sometimes persist for years without even the patient's spouse being aware of it. Some individuals start by having the symptoms of anorexia and later become bulimic.

Hoberman & Kroll-Mensing (1992) review the epidemiology of adolescent eating disorders. The incidence of bulimia may be about 0.7% (0.2% in boys and 1.1% in girls), these figures being derived from a French study (Ledoux, *et al.*, 1991). Widely differing incidence and prevalence figures have been found for both anorexia and bulimia. Much seems to depend on the age range and other demographic characteristics of the population studied. Particularly high prevalence figures have been reported in students of fashion (3.5%) and professional ballet students (8.6%) (Garner & Garfinkel, 1980). A study in Munro County, New York, found an annual incidence of new cases of 0.64 per 100 000 population. Other studies have found prevalence rates in girls aged 10–19 as high as 26.3 per 100 000 (Hoberman & Kroll-Mensing, 1992).

Lask & Bryant-Waugh (1992) have provided a valuable review of the literature on early onset (age 8 to 14) eating disorders. They point out that most of the literature on anorexia nervosa and bulimia relates to older patients, so that the findings do not necessarily apply to this age group in which, they also point out, the prevalence of bulimia is very low. They also make the point that most younger subjects with anorexic symptoms fail to meet the complete diagnostic requirements mentioned above. It may be for this reason that ICD-10 has categories for *atypical anorexia nervosa* and also *atypical bulimia nervosa*. These are to be used in the absence of one or more of the key features but when the individual nevertheless presents 'a fairly typical picture' of the disorder.

Fossen, *et al.* (1987) described 48 children with early onset anorexia nervosa, 35 girls and 13 boys. Of these 23 were pubertal (7 boys and 16 girls), 20 pubescent (6 boys and 14 girls) and 5, all girls, post-pubertal. Youngest children were over-represented and there was a bias towards higher socioeconomic groups. Depression was present in 56% of cases. It seems that the proportion of boys is higher in the early onset group than it is in those with onset during adolescence.

Anorexia nervosa provides fertile ground for the study of mind-body relationships. It seems that, while we do not fully understand its causation, it results from what Lask & Bryant-Waugh (1992) call 'a complex interaction of genetic, biological, personality and family factors'. Social pressures which tend to persuade adolescent girls and young women that it is desirable to be thin seem to play a part. A study of the measurement data of the girls appearing in the centrefold of *Playboy* magazine during the years 1969 to 1978 revealed that the percentage of average weight for height decreased significantly (Garfinkel & Garner, 1982), and there were similar changes in the Miss America contestants, and especially the winners, between 1959 and 1978 (Garner & Garfinkel, 1980).

Fossen, *et al.*, (1987) conceptualized anorexia as 'a distorted and overly focused struggle for self-control and autonomy'. They postulated that the likelihood of parents adopting the role of adversary in the child's struggle for autonomy depends on the age, sex and ordinal position of the child. They continued:

'In our culture parents are more likely to be intrusively involved with and/or overly controlling of girls and youngest children than offspring in complementary categories. In some of these families parents will not withdraw in response to the child's emancipatory stirrings. Given this situation, some children will attempt to resolve the ensuing conflict by focusing the controversy on food and control of intake. This is an effective option only if food consumption is consistently at their discretion – that is, not subject to availability or threatened by the family's financial resources.' (Fossen, *et al.*, 1987, page 117.)

This is an ingenious explanation which accounts for several of the features of anorexia nervosa, though in some cases it seems to be the young person who is, if only at an unconscious level, reluctant to grow up. It is important to realize also that we are dealing with complex circular processes. While in the early stages, psychological and family factors may seem to be of the greatest importance; at a certain point, physical ones come to dominate both the clinical picture and the concerns of those involved, though not necessarily the patient herself.

Treatment

The *treatment* of these young people needs to be what Fundudis (1986) calls *multimodal*. That author illustrates this concept by using the case of an 11½-year-old anorexic girl and suggesting a treatment strategy to deal with each of the patient's problems in an appropriate sequence. In the case of the girl that he used as an illustration, the treatments used included stimulus control, systematic desensitization, cognitive restructuring, relaxation training, family therapy, dyadic therapy, social reinforcement and *vicarious modelling*. In practice the treatment program needs to be tailored to the particular needs of each child and family. Less severe cases may be treated as outpatients but the more severe ones usually require admission to hospital.

The following are some measures which are usually needed, at least in the more severe cases. When there has been serious loss of weight a major initial objective must be to restore the patient's weight to a safe level. This may be difficult.

The establishment of rapport with all concerned in cases of anorexia is of particular importance. Without it, treatment is likely to fail. Even with it, it may not be easy. Young people with anorexia nervosa are usually skilled in manipulating those around them to achieve their own particular ends – notably to maintain their symptoms. They may promise to eat if they do not have to go to hospital, they plead for 'one more chance' (and then for another, and yet another ... and so on), and they tend to be experts in the art of 'divide and rule'. Indeed, Fossen, *et al.* (1987) observed that 'Children with anorexia seem to be particularly adept at creating conflict, not from planned behaviour or malice, but as a habitual way of relating, generalized from family interaction'.

Children and adolescents with anorexia nervosa generally respond best to a firm, accepting, non-punitive but unyielding approach. The adults concerned with their care, that is the parents and the treatment staff, must be united and supportive of each other. This implies that the parents trust and have confidence in the treatment team, especially the physician who is ultimately responsible. It should be made clear to the child that she, or he, must eat. This is not negotiable and if necessary all privileges, including family visits, watching television, listening to the radio, even getting up to go to the toilet, may have to be contingent on eating or, preferably, gaining weight. The environment must be structured so that it is impossible for the child to dispose of food, for example down the toilet, without eating it.

The above requires highly skilled nursing care, close teamwork and frequent contact with and support for the parents. Perhaps in no other branch of the profession are psychiatric nursing skills so necessary. Nurses with expertise and experience in relating to and treating these patients are priceless assets.

Being firm with their daughter and not yielding to her threats, pleadings and guilt-provoking statements ('You hate me', 'You've never loved me', 'I hate you' or 'You just want me to die in this hospital') can be exceedingly hard for parents accustomed to surrendering to such emotional blackmail. So it is that the parents, too, require much skilled support.

In the treatment of patients who have lost a lot of weight and whose growth has become retarded, a high calorie intake is necessary to ensure weight gain and catch-up growth. Close cooperation between psychiatrist and paediatrician pays dividends. Both must agree on the treatment plan. The paediatrician may monitor the child's emotional state, electrolyte balance and diet, prescribe the necessary dietary intake, and advise on the weight gain needed before it is 'safe' for the child to be given certain privileges. At the same time, the psychiatrist coordinates the psychological care and treatment of child and family. It must always be clear who is ultimately responsible for the treatment. It is usually the psychiatrist when the child is in the psychiatric unit and the paediatrician when the child is in the paediatric one. Given skilled management by an experienced team, tube feeding should rarely be needed, though it may sometimes be necessary to define a minimum weight at which it will be initiated.

It is helpful to have target minimum and maximum weights. These patients usually have a great fear of becoming fat and it seems to reassure them to say not only that they must reach a certain weight, for example before they can leave hospital, but also that you will not allow their weight to go above a certain figure.

Once the weight that has been predetermined has been attained, family therapy may commence. It is not appropriate, or practical, to start it while the patient is still seriously underweight and is undergoing an intensive, structured behavioural program as described above. The therapy for the family will depend on the particular dysfunctional interaction patterns that are identified. By the time it starts the parents will probably have learned quite a lot, having observed their formerly controlling and manipulative child's response to the measures used to get her to eat and gain weight. The child, too, may have learned from this experience.

Various drugs, for example chlorpromazine and insulin, have been suggested but they probably have little part to play in treatment, except in the therapy of co-existing conditions. If the patient shows evidence of clinical depression, antidepressant medication may be indicated.

In the treatment of bulimia nervosa, a similar approach is usually needed. Again, a comprehensive, multimodal treatment plan is required, and there are usually found to be issues of control, autonomy, self-image and unresolved family conflict. Issues of genital sexuality may be less prominent, however. Substance abuse is common in bulimics and, when present, needs to be one of the focuses of the treatment plan. As mentioned before, bulimia is considerably less common in early-onset eating disorders than anorexia.

Outcome

The *outcome* in younger anorexic subjects may be better than for cases with onset in mid- or late adolescence. Most anorectics gain weight if treated along the above lines but weight gain, while necessary, is not a sufficient objective. The associated problems, including the family ones, must be tackled also. If a comprehensive multimodal treatment plan, as discussed above, is carried through many patients achieve a good degree of recovery, though there are some who pursue a chronic course or become bulimic. Lask & Bryant-Waugh (1992) conclude, however, that 'the prognosis is unsatisfactory with a high incidence of residual impairment'.

Obesity

Obesity is not in itself a psychiatric disorder and consequently does not appear as a diagnostic category in DSM-IV. ICD-10 however does include under *behavioural syndromes* a category of 'overeating associated with other psychological disturbances'. Just how important a role emotional factors play in the causation of childhood obesity is unclear but various psychosocial situations may contribute to it. It seems that sometimes deprived, rejected children may eat excessively as a compensation for lack of affection. Or a parent who feels guilty – though the guilt may be out of conscious awareness – about harbouring rejecting or other negative feelings towards a child may over-feed the child in an attempt at compensation. Over-feeding may also be motivated by a parent's desire to keep the child in a close and dependent relationship. While some children may rebel and even become anorexic in response to such handling, others accept it and remain obese and emotionally immature. Although clinical experience suggests that such mechanisms may contribute to obesity in some cases, hard data to support these impressions are lacking. Obesity is, as Bandini & Dietz (1992) put it in a useful brief review, 'a multifactorial and complex disease', about which many myths hold sway.

Obesity can also contribute to the development of emotional problems. The obese child may be teased and so come to feel self-conscious or anxious. Battles over diets children are supposed to be on but with which they do not cooperate may lead to tension or open family strife. In some instances, however, the obesity simply becomes the focus of a problem which would have been centred around something else if the child had not been obese.

Factitious illness by proxy

This condition is often referred to as *Munchausen's syndrome by proxy* but Fisher & Mitchell (1992) suggest that the term *factitious illness by proxy* is preferable. DSM-IV includes factitious disorder by proxy in Appendix B, 'Criteria sets and axes provided for further study'.

The essence of this condition is the fabrication of a history and/or the physical signs of an illness in a child, usually by a parent, most often the mother. Meadow (1991) defined it as 'a false illness created by mothers for their children', though a few cases have been reported in which it has been someone other than the mother that has been responsible. Fisher & Mitchell (1992) summarize the features of the condition and provide a comprehensive review of the literature.

Almost any condition may be fabricated, including seizures, infant apnoea, diarrhoea, a variety of neurological disorders, skin diseases, and such chronic illnesses as mental impairment and defects of vision and hearing. Since it is a physical illness that is usually being fabricated, these children generally present to family physicians or, especially, to paediatricians. There is invariably serious and often complex psychopathology in the person, usually the mother, who is responsible and in investigating and addressing this lies the main psychiatric contribution to these cases.

It is unclear whether it is at all common for psychiatric illnesses to be fabricated in similar ways to those in which physical illnesses are, but Fisher & Mitchell (1992) suggest that this is a possibility.

Other disorders

Complex interactions of mind and body characterize many other disorders. Conditions in which these may be especially important include *migraine*; the *periodic syndrome* (attacks of headache, abdominal pain, vomiting and a miserable, whimpering appearance occurring in children in the first year of life); *cyclical vomiting* (a variant of the periodic syndrome); *ulcerative colitis* (an inflammatory condition of the large intestine); and *peptic ulcer*. This list is by no means comprehensive.

Chapter 17

Infant Psychiatry

Although early experiences have long been thought to have important influences on human development, the psychiatry of infancy and early childhood has only recently received much attention. During the last decade, however, it has become a major interest of many of those working in the child mental health field. Among the stimuli responsible for this change were Bowlby's (1951) challenging views on the effects of maternal deprivation, subsequent research on the attachment and bonding processes that affect children early in life, and the work of Thomas & Chess (1977) on the temperaments of infants and young children, and how these differ.

Infant psychiatry, or infant mental health as it is often termed, is now a major subspecialty of child psychiatry. Its current status is documented in the *Handbook of Infant Mental Health* (Zeanah, 1993), which contains contributions by 57 clinicians and researchers in the field.

The relatively late development of interest in the psychiatric study of young children has probably been due, at least in part, to difficulties inherent in the study of this age group. Among these are the following:

(1) In infancy and early childhood we are dealing, to an even greater extent than in later childhood, with development and its disorders, rather than with clearly identifiable psychiatric syndromes. While a developmental viewpoint is useful, indeed usually essential, at any age, in older children and adolescents it becomes possible more often to identify specific syndromes, with their characteristic signs and symptoms. This applies even though many of the disorders of childhood are complex reactions to multiple factors rather than 'disease entities' such as can more readily be identified in other areas of medicine.

When we deal with the disorders of infancy, the borderline between psychiatry and developmental psychology is often unclear.

(2) Neither of the diagnostic schemes currently in use – ICD-10 and DSM-IV – is well suited for use in this period of life. The traditional *medical model* of disease entities may be only marginally relevant when we

are dealing with the, largely interactive, psychiatric problems of early childhood. Although the two diagnostic schemes each have categories for developmental disorders, these are limited to rather specific areas of development. We do not yet have any generally accepted, comprehensive system for categorizing the ways in which the early development of infants may get off course. While both diagnostic schemes have categories for the various degrees of mental retardation, these are crude instruments and are of little value in infancy. Any categories that might be developed will need to take into account not only the young child, but also the interactional processes occurring between child and parents or those substituting for the parents. As Zeanah (1993, page 1) puts it, 'Infants are so dependent upon their environments for the opportunity to develop competently that any discussion of their mental health must include a careful consideration of context'.

(3)   While it is clear that infant psychiatry involves not only the study of infants but also that of infant-adult relationships, it is less clear what the balance between the two should be.

(4)   The assessment of infants and young children demands special skills and the use of techniques different from those needed in assessing older children. Children who have not yet developed speech, or whose development of verbal language is at an early stage, cannot provide the sort of information we seek from older patients. Despite the widely acknowledged importance of non-verbal communication, psychiatrists and physicians depend largely on what their patients tell them in assessing their mental states and disorders. But infants cannot tell us in words how they feel, nor what they are thinking or subjectively experiencing. The infant mental health worker must become skilled in interpreting non-verbal behaviour, the natural means by which infants communicate. In the past this has not been a part of the training of most psychiatrists and other mental health workers.

(5)   The intimate involvement of infants and young children and their families means that the children are very susceptible to tensions and other problems in their families or wherever else they may be living. The emphasis on context therefore needs to be greater than in other areas of psychiatry. The drastic and tragic deterioration of babies placed in impersonal institutions, many years ago documented by Spitz (1946), is testimony to this.

Disorders of infants and young children

Despite the above considerations, a few relatively well defined disorders of infants and young children have been identified. Foremost among these is infantile autism (Rutter & Schopler, 1992). The other *pervasive developmental disorders* (discussed in Chapter 11) are less clear-cut conditions, however. Severe developmental delay can also be distinguished at an early age, as can disorders of motor development. Disorders of speech and language development (Chapter 12), perhaps better described as communication disorders, can also be discerned quite early in life, certainly in the toddler period. The *Handbook of Infant Mental Health* (Zeanah, 1993) also lists regulatory disorders, post-traumatic stress disorder, sleep disorders, failure to thrive and feeding disorders, disorders of attachment, and psychosomatic processes. While these categories depend for their definitions on a mixed bag of concepts, their delineation seems a worthwhile first step towards establishing some sort of order in this difficult field.

Prevalence

There have been few studies of the prevalence of mental health problems in infants in their first year of life, but Richman and her colleagues (1975) surveyed 3-year-old children in a North London borough and found that 7% had moderate or severe behaviour problems and a further 15% has mild problems. There were no significant sex differences in overall prevalence rates, but overactivity and wetting and soiling problems were more frequent in boys and fearfulness in girls.

While surveys of pre-school children do not tell us anything specific about the prevalence of problems in even younger age groups, clinical experience suggests that problems in 3-year-olds do not usually arise *de novo*. They seem often to have been preceded by problems in either the child or, more often, the parent-child relationships, earlier in life.

Assessment of infants and young children

The assessment approaches used with older children require some modification when children in their first year or two are seen. As Emde (1985) points out, the expression of emotion is particularly important in infancy. Infants do not talk. Instead they cry, smile, make cooing noises and, in a variety of ways which the perceptive parent soon learns, communicate fear, anger, sadness, joy, contentment and so on. The observation and interpretation of such communications by the clinician is an essential part of the assessment process.

Even more important than observing the young child is observing the interactions, non-verbal ones especially, between parents and child.

Indeed what is being assessed is not the infant but the infant-in-context – in other words the infant in his or her natural environment, usually the family. Therefore it is important to ensure that both parents are present. Sometimes one parent – most often the father – is reluctant to attend. If this proves to be the case, strenuous efforts to obtain the missing parent's attendance should be made.

The assessment usually begins with an interview with child and parents. If there are other children in the family it is helpful to have them present also, if not at the first meeting, then at a subsequent one. As Hirshberg (1993, page 181) puts it, 'the family interview process presents an opportunity to attend carefully to the sample of interaction between each parent and the baby'. The parents should be encouraged to do whatever they would normally do, for example if their child cries, needs changing or appears hungry. Hirshberg (1993) suggests that the following aspects of the relationship should be considered:

● *The attachment relationship*. This involves looking to see if the infant uses the parents as sources of security and comfort and, if this is the case, how this is achieved. How freely does the infant explore the environment? When the infant seeks comfort from a parent, is this provided and how? Does the child then feel free to resume exploration?

● *Safety and protection*. This is a matter of how vigilant and diligent each parent is about ensuring that the child is safe and properly protected from dangers. Parents may be overprotective as well as neglectful in this area. The child's responses to the parents' protective measures should also be observed.

● *Physiological regulation*. This is a matter of observing how the parents respond to changes in the child's physiological state – hunger, cold, sleepiness, need to become active and so on. Does the parent intervene in an effective way to meet the child's physiological needs or to respond appropriately to the child's attempts to become more or less active?

● *Play*. Opportunity should be provided, if it does not happen naturally, for the parents and child to play together for a time. Are the parents relaxed and at ease with the child? Do they respond appropriately to the infant's signals, understanding what their child wants, and initiating play activities when structure and organization are needed?

● *Teaching and learning*. This is related to play and is a matter of how the parents help the infant learn things. Hirshberg (1993) suggests that, if necessary, the parents may be asked to 'help the baby learn' a task appropriate to the baby's development level. The parents' willingness and ability to do this, and their approach and degree of flexibility should be noted.

● *Power and control.* 'Do the parents present themselves to the infant as calm, confident, and in control ... of the situation ...' or, 'do they appear as passive, overwhelmed, disorganized, or confused, or perhaps tense, even potentially explosive?' (Hirshberg, 1993, page 184).

● *Regulation of emotion.* The expression and communication of emotion, and the regulation of these processes is considered to be 'probably the most important area of relationship functioning' by Hirshberg (1993). The affect surrounding the interactions between child and parents seems to be a key factor in determining how experience is organized and is thought to shape later interactions and relationships. The examiner should observe the overall affective tone as parents and infant interact, how freely emotion is expressed and whether the voice tones, facial expressions, gestures and non-verbal communications are congruent. Differences between the reactions of the two parents, and also their affective relationships with each other should also be noted.

The above observations should be supplemented by questions to the parents about how they function in each of the above areas. It can be helpful to ask each parent to describe how the other reacts in different areas of the infant's life and in different situations, and then to find out whether each agrees with the other's perception. Any differences between their ways of interacting with their child, or their beliefs about child rearing, should be explored.

It is important to observe infants directly in various situations. Gaensbauer & Harmon (1981) described a systematic assessment procedure for use in the age range 9 to 21 months:

(1) A free play period with mother and infant, during which the infant can play either with toys or with the mother.
(2) Approaches to the infant by a stranger and by the mother. This is designed to discover the extent to which the mother is used as a source of security.
(3) Developmental testing using the Bayley Scales of Infant Development.
(4) A separation and reunion sequence involving the mother's departure and return three minutes later.

The authors reported differences in the response to all four experiences when a group of *abused/neglected* children was compared to a control group who had not been abused. The biggest problem with this procedure as described is that it takes no account of the father and his role in the infant's life. Its modification to involve him provides additional useful information.

In addition to the above, a full history of child and family, and a genogram, as set out in Chapter 5, should be obtained. In assessing infants and their families the establishment of rapport, and an empathic, positive and supportive approach are basic requirements for success. Parents bringing their young children for mental health assessment are often both anxious and prone to feeling guilty. They wonder if their infant's problems are their 'fault', yet invariably they prove to have been doing their best, given their knowledge of child-rearing, and their own emotional states and personality resources. Many parents who have difficulty raising young children have themselves been raised in dysfunctional ways and lack a clear sense of just how to approach the parenting task.

Questionnaires for administration to the parents of young children, and to those caring for them in group settings, have been devised. The Behavioural Screening Questionnaire (Richman & Graham, 1971) has been found useful in large scale epidemiological studies. It has been further validated by Earls, *et al.* (1982). It contains 12 items dealing, respectively, with eating, sleeping, soiling, activity level, concentration, attention-seeking/dependence, moods, 'several worries', 'many fears', relationships with siblings/peers, temper tantrums, and 'difficult to manage' behaviour. Each item is scored either 0 (absence of the behaviour), 1 (mild) or 2 (severe).

The Preschool Behaviour Checklist (McGuire & Richman, 1986) has 22 items and is designed for use by the staff in group settings where preschool children receive care. It is intended as a screening instrument and has satisfactory inter-rater reliability, internal consistency and validity. It is not intended to be used in the assessment of individual children, but may have value in directing the attention of staff to children with problems, especially those who are isolated, anxious or withdrawn, who may get overlooked in group settings. Inconsistencies between the ratings of different staff members may draw attention to the differential effects of different management methods.

Common problems of infancy and young children

Temper tantrums

Temper tantrums are normal in toddlers but may become a problem if they are severe and persistent and fail to respond to the parents' commonsense attempts to deal with them. Babies' needs and wants, which are essentially the same, are normally met more or less on demand in early infancy. It is not usually until the second year of life that restrictions begin to be placed on what they may have and do. Such restrictions become necessary when the child starts to walk and can thus explore places and do things which could be dangerous. Tantrums are an understandable reaction to being denied the gratification to which the child has become accustomed.

Whether tantrums continue or escalate depends largely upon the reactions to them of parents and other involved people. Firm but kind limit-setting in a warm, accepting context usually leads to rapid improvement. The tantrums themselves should be ignored as far as possible. Children have tantrums because they want something which is denied them, or because they are not allowed to engage in a particular behaviour. It is important not to defer to their wishes in response to their tantrums. To do so is to ensure that the tantrums will continue. A better response is to allow the tantrum to run its course without special attention being given to the child while it is happening. Once the tantrum has ceased, attention may be given to the child. Consistently applied such a program will ensure that the *tantrum behaviour* is extinguished (though at first it may increase), and that *non-tantrum behaviour* is reinforced.

In practice the management of temper tantrums, especially as children get older, is not always as easy as the above might seem to imply. Physical restraint may be necessary when children, during their tantrums, are doing things dangerous to themselves or others, or are physically damaging or destroying property. Persisting tantrums are most often seen in children living in unstable and chaotic families in which they are handled and responded to inconsistently.

The outcome in children with serious temper tantrum problems depends very much on how secure the relationship with the parents is, and on how far the parents prove able and willing to make appropriate modifications to their own behaviour in response to the tantrums. The child's temperament seems also to be a factor. As we saw in Chapter 2, some children are temperamentally more 'difficult' than others and this, and the *goodness of fit* between the temperaments of the child and those of the parents are also relevant factors.

Sleep problems

Many parents express concerns about the sleep patterns of their infants and young children. Some of these arise simply from lack of knowledge of what is normal. Children's needs for sleep vary and there seem to be temperamental factors affecting the ease with which they are able to settle into regular patterns of sleeping and waking behaviour. Failure to adopt a regular sleeping pattern may also occur in chaotic and disorganized families in which there are no regular bedtimes or bedtime routines.

Failure to sleep, often with crying, is common in babies but normally settles after a few months at most, if the feeding and general care of the infant are satisfactory. Persistence of such problems into the toddler period is fairly common, however, and there seems to be an association between waking at night and other behavioural and temperamental difficulties (Richman, 1985).

Among the specific sleep problems that are encountered in infants and young children are *night terrors*, *nightmares* and *sleepwalking* – which are sometimes known as *parasomnias* – and *sleep apnoea*. The parasomnias do not usually appear until the third year of life or later but will be considered here for convenience. All are more common in boys than girls and they are often isolated symptoms unassociated with other psychiatric or behavioural problems.

Nightmares

These are unpleasant or frightening dreams. They occur during *rapid eye movement* (REM), that is, light sleep. The child does not wake up, nor necessarily become overtly disturbed while having the nightmare, and if woken up reacts normally.

Night terrors

ICD-10 calls these *sleep terrors* and DSM-IV *sleep terror disorder*. They are also sometimes known as *pavor nocturnus*, and occur on waking from 'stage 3 or stage 4' (deep) sleep, usually during the first third of nocturnal sleep. The child wakes up in a frightened, even terrified, state and is inaccessible, not responding when spoken to, nor appearing to see objects or people. Instead he or she appears to be visually or auditorily hallucinated, talking to and looking at people and things not actually present. The child may be difficult to comfort and the period of disturbed behaviour may last up to 15 minutes, occasionally even longer. Eventually the behaviours subside, with or without comfort from an adult, and the child goes back to sleep, awakening in the morning usually with no recollection of the incident. Night terrors are said to occur in up to 3% of toddlers (Clore & Hibel, 1993). In a few cases they persist into the school age years.

Sleepwalking

This also occurs in a state of deep sleep and is closely related to night terrors. Like night terrors, sleepwalking may appear in the course of a childhood febrile illness. The child gets up, usually while in the first third of nocturnal sleep and walks around with a blank, staring facial expression, not responding when people try and communicate with him or her. It is usually difficult to waken the child, but once awake the subject appears normal, perhaps after a short period of disorientation and confusion. Episodes may last from a few minutes to half an hour.

Although all the above parasomnias are listed as disorders in both ICD-10 and DSM-IV, in most of the children who experience them there is no other evidence of a psychiatric problem. The sleep problem is probably best regarded as a transient developmental disturbance. If there is no evidence of any other abnormality, the parents can be reassured. Any associated abnormality should receive the appropriate treatment.

Sleep apnoea syndrome

The *sleep apnoea syndrome* is not classified as a parasomnia. According to Sadeh & Anders (1993) it is the most common organic sleep disorder in young children. Our breathing is under involuntary control for much of the time, including during sleep, but is also subject to voluntary control in the waking state. The essential feature of sleep apnoea is the occurrence of periods of failure to breathe while asleep. These may be due to mechanical obstruction of the airway, for example by enlarged tonsils or adenoids, or as a result of severe obesity, disorders of the control systems in the central nervous system, or to a combination of neurological dysfunction and peripheral problems. When breathing stops, the oxygen level in the blood falls to dangerous levels and the subject wakes up and the voluntary control of breathing takes over. It has been suggested that some cases of *sudden infant death syndrome* (SIDS) may be due to the failure of a child who suffers from sleep apnoea to awaken when the blood oxygen falls to a dangerous level.

Sleep apnoea may occur at any age from infancy upwards. It can cause chronic loss of sleep and consequently daytime sleepiness, chronic fatigue and, in severe cases, intellectual deterioration, depression, personality changes and outbursts of irrational behaviour (Guilleminault, *et al.*, 1976; Sadeh & Anders, 1993).

Treatment

The treatment of the sleep disorders of early childhood requires that close attention be given to the parent-child interactions. When the problem is sleeplessness unassociated with any other disorder, the best approach is probably a behavioural one.

Richman, *et al.* (1985) described the results of such an approach designed to help the child stay in bed quietly without disturbing the parents, and to settle down to sleep without parental attention. Alteration of the parents' responses to the children's night-time behaviour seemed often to lead to rapid resolution of the problem, suggesting that the parents' previous responses had contributed to maintaining the problem. Treatment was in each case developed following a behavioural analysis. Complete or marked improvement occurred in 27 of 35 children treated, but five did not complete treatment, so that the improvement rate in those that did was 90%. At follow-up four months later it was 80%.

Although sleep inducing medications are sometimes prescribed for young children, evidence of their effectiveness, except in the very short term, is lacking. Richman, *et al.* (1985) carried out a double-blind trial of trimeprazine tartrate which, while demonstrating a significant improvement in sleep on the drug, confirmed clinical impressions that benefits are limited and not long-lasting.

In managing the parasomnias any associated emotional disorders or stresses in the family should be addressed first. When there appear to be no associated disorders, little may need to be done beyond reassuring the parents and others concerned that the problem is a developmental one which is likely to lessen and resolve spontaneously over time.

There is some limited evidence that some of the benzodiazepine drugs, such as diazepam, and also the anticonvulsant, carbamazepine, may be of value in the treatment of night terrors and sleepwalking (Green, 1991) but controlled trials of these drugs in such cases have not as yet been reported.

Sadeh & Anders (1993) provide an excellent review of current knowledge in the area of sleep disorders in infancy.

Feeding problems

Appetite and feeding problems in infants may be symptoms of physical disorders or of emotional and relationship problems in the family. In many cases there are elements of both. Children may eat, or be thought by their parents to eat, too little, too much, or the wrong sorts of foods; they may be excessively fussy about what they will eat; or they may try to eat inedible foods (*pica*).

Failure to thrive (FTT)
This is a term often used to describe the condition of infants and young children who show a serious failure to gain weight. FTT is a symptom, not a disorder and, while it may result from failure to eat, many and various other factors may be involved.

ICD-10 lists *feeding disorder of infancy and childhood* and defines it as 'refusal of food and extreme faddiness in the presence of an adequate food supply and a reasonably competent care-giver, and the absence of organic disease'.

Feeding problems often arise in the context of disturbed parent-child relationships. The inexperienced, over-anxious and perhaps immature mother of an infant may fail to respond to her child's cues, and may communicate her anxiety and insecurity to the child in the feeding situation. Some feeding problems miraculously disappear when the child is fed by the grandmother or a nurse. In these cases the problem is not really a feeding one but one of parent-child interaction.

FTT is often attributed to 'deviant care-giving relationships' (Benoit, 1993) and is also often considered to be related to child abuse and/or neglect. In these cases, the parental deficits extend beyond anxiety, insecurity and inexperience in the feeding situation.

Food refusal may in due course become the focus of a battle of wills between parent(s) and child. It sometimes accompanies psychogenic soiling. The parents may have exaggerated ideas about the importance of particular dietary regimes and unrealistic fears about what will happen if the child does not eat what they consider to be enough. Some children, consciously or unconsciously aware of this, seem to choose to strike a blow for independence by declining to eat what the parents wish. There may be numerous food fads, yet such children are usually well nourished.

Management
In the *management* of feeding problems, a general and comprehensive assessment of child and family is first necessary. Particular attention should be paid to the parent-infant relationship, but the stability of the family as a whole, and the general care given the children, are also important considerations. If there are serious problems of family functioning these should be addressed as the first therapeutic priority. Family therapy may be needed or, in the case of serious FTT, the child may need to be removed for a while, perhaps to hospital or foster home.

In other cases, some education of the family about children's nutritional requirements may be needed. Sometimes a consultation with a dietician is helpful. If there are no other serious problems, treatment should address the parent-child relationship issues, especially as they involve the feeding situation. An ordinary, nutritiously balanced diet should be offered on a 'take-it-or-leave-it' basis. If this is done calmly without pressure or exhortations from the parents, children usually select an adequate diet, perhaps after some initial testing of the situation. Unless there are severely dysfunctional parental attitudes or the whole family is very disturbed, the response to such an approach is usually good. It is important to bear in mind, in assessment and treatment, that for many people, perhaps particularly those who have been deprived as children, food has great symbolic significance. For such people, ensuring that their children are properly fed may be a means whereby they are able to feel that they are good, caring parents. This can lead to over-feeding, as well as to feelings of being rejected by their children when the latter refuse the excessive amounts of food they are offered.

Pica of infancy and childhood
The above term is usually ICD-10, whereas DSM-IV uses the simpler term *pica*. Pica is the persistent eating of non-nutritive substances such as paper, soil, paint chippings, wood or cloth. The symptom has many causes, including adverse environmental circumstances, emotional distress and relationship difficulties. While it does occur in intact children of normal intelligence, it is more common in those whose development is distorted, for example by brain damage, autism or mental retardation. Iron deficiency, due to a poor diet, may be present. The condition is sometimes encountered in association with lead poisoning, which itself may be the result of the ingestion of lead-containing materials by the child with pica. Other physical complications may arise due to the ingestion of foreign objects. These complications include intestinal obstruction and perforation.

Associated sleep and behaviour problems are common and the families of children with pica tend to be disorganized and poor. In severe cases admission of the child to hospital and intensive work may be needed. Bicknell (1975) provided a good account of this disorder and is a useful source of further information.

Rumination disorder of infancy
This appears in both ICD-10 and DSM-IV. It consists of the repeated regurgitation of food in the absence of other gastrointestinal symptoms, with failure to gain weight or loss of weight. The age of onset is usually between 3 and 12 months and it has been reported to have a 25% mortality (Benoit, 1993). The behaviour is self-induced and usually occurs when the child is alone. So-called *psychogenic rumination* is considered to be associated with disturbed parent-child (usually mother-child) relationships, while *self-stimulatory rumination* is associated with mental retardation.

Breath-holding spells

These are common in pre-school children. They usually start before age two but seldom before six months. Livingstone (1972) reported a mean age of onset of 12 months and a peak frequency between two and three. They usually cease by age five or six.

Breath-holding spells are usually precipitated by minor upsets or frustrations. They follow crying which increases in intensity until the child appears to be in a state of rage. Breathing then stops, usually in expiration, and cyanosis becomes evident in blueness of the face, especially around the lips. Occasionally the spells lead to a major epileptic seizure but in most instances the child starts to breathe again in half a minute or so and recovery quickly occurs.

The three distinguishing features are a precipitating factor, violent crying, and cyanosis. The spells seem to be used by some children to alarm, or express anger towards, their parents or other adults. They may have similar causes and functions to temper tantrums. The tendency to have them may be reinforced if the parents react by a show of concern or by indulgence. It is better to treat the attacks calmly and with a minimal or no response. The prognosis is good if there is no associated disorder.

Thumbsucking and nailbiting

Both these behaviours are common in young children, though nailbiting in particular is also frequently seen in older children. Thumb and finger sucking are normal behaviours in babies and gradually lessen during the second and subsequent years. Persistent thumb or fingersucking have little psychiatric significant in themselves but may be features of regressive behaviour in children who are anxious or under stress. They often require no treatment but if necessary can usually be stopped by simple reminders, rewards or even sanctions. Occasionally thumb and/or fingersucking become severe, compulsive behaviours associated with rocking or masturbation. Severe thumbsucking can cause dental malocclusion in older children and may merit treatment for that reason.

Nailbiting, like thumbsucking, sometimes appears to be a tension-reducing habit in anxious, tense children. In that case attention should be addressed to the underlying problem. If treatment of any of these symptoms is necessary a behaviour therapy program should be developed.

Separation anxiety and disorders of attachment

As we have seen, a major part of infant psychiatry consists of the study and, often, the modification of parent-child relationships and interactions. The processes whereby infants and young children become emotionally attached to the adults in their lives – or fail to become attached – have therefore been extensively studied. Ainsworth, *et al.* (1978), on the basis of studies of the effects of brief separations and reunions of infants and their mothers, identified three groups of infants:

● *Securely attached infants*, who seek contact with their mothers when under stress, are calmed by this, and explore actively in the presence of their mothers.

● *Anxiously attached infants*, who seem ambivalent towards their mothers, seeking contact but apparently failing to be comforted by it. The anxiously attached infant is chronically anxious in relation to the mother and is unable to use her as a secure base from which to explore unfamiliar situations. These mothers are less responsive to crying and other communications than the mothers of the securely attached infants.

● *Anxious-avoidant infants*, who show avoidant behaviour when reunited with their mothers after a period of separation. They do not seek close contact with their mothers, even in high-stress situations, and seem undisturbed when separated from their mothers. The mothers are rejecting and angry, rebuffing or roughly treating their infants when the latter seek physical proximity. The infants thus learn to avoid seeking proximity. In other situations and with other adults, however, these infants can respond positively to close physical contact.

Main & Solomon (1990) have described a fourth category:

● *Disorganized/disoriented*, in which the child shows attachment behaviour which is interrupted, confused or incomplete.

It seems that for optimal, that is secure, attachment to develop there needs to be sensitive parental care in which the parent is neither too highly involved with the child, nor too uninvolved. The former may produce *avoidant* infants, the latter *anxiously attached* ones.

Infants who are securely attached to specific people in infancy, as opposed to the more general attachments of institutionally reared children, seem to achieve higher levels of self-esteem and autonomous functioning, and generally healthy personality development. Insecure attachment seems to lead to later behaviour problems, poor impulse control, low self-esteem, and difficult relationships with caregivers and peers.

Summarizing the literature on *disorganized* attachment, Zeanah, *et al.* (1993) suggest that this tends to lead to controlling, that is role-reversed, behaviour in middle-class families, and behaviour problems in impoverished families. As well as providing an up-to-date review of the literature on disorders of attachment, these authors also propose that:

'Attachment problems become psychiatric disorders for infants when emotions and behaviours displayed in attachment relationships are so disturbed as to indicate, or substantially to increase the risk for, persistent distress or disability in the infant.' (page 338.)

The above proposal falls short of defining disorders in terms of relationships *between* individuals, rather than as disorders *of* individuals, something for which a case might be made, but it does seem an improvement on current diagnostic schemata. ICD-10 lists only two specific disorders of attachment – *reactive attachment disorder of childhood* and *disinhibited attachment disorder of childhood*. DSM-IV lists only the former. Zeanah, *et al.* (1993, page 339) go on to propose five categories of attachment disorder, listing criteria for each. Their categories are:

- Nonattached attachment disorder.
- Indiscriminate attachment disorder.
- Inhibited attachment disorder.
- Aggressive attachment disorder.
- Role-reversed attachment disorder.

In addition to listing the criteria they propose for these categories, the authors also offer illustrative case histories for each category.

Much work remains to be done in the field of attachment disorders, and also in investigating the relationship between these disorders and emotional, behavioural and personality disorders in later life.

The treatment of infants and young children

Treatment in infant psychiatry is usually directed at the relationship between child and parent(s) or other care-givers, or is designed to improve the functioning of the family system as a whole. A variety of approaches has been suggested and the *Handbook of Infant Mental Health* (Zeanah, 1993) has chapters on preventative interventions designed to enhance parent-infant relationships; family support programs; 'interaction guidance' – which aims to first understand and then treat early infant-care-giver relationship disturbances; and 'infant-parent psychotherapy'.

The provision of the best possible care for infants and young children, whether in their families or in day care, pre-school or institutional (for example, hospital) settings is surely of crucial importance for the future of their mental health, and also for that of the community.

Substantial progress in learning how we may achieve this has been made in recent years but much is yet to be learned, and the application of our knowledge is at an even earlier stage.

Outcome

Many feeding, sleeping and behavioural problems of infancy and early childhood are transient and resolve without any specific treatment. They may be little more than minor upsets in the processes whereby parents and their children learn to adjust to each other and meet each others' needs. The stability of the family unit, the 'goodness of fit' between the temperaments of those concerned, and the parents' maturity and experience of child rearing (including their own experiences as children) all seem to be factors which influence outcome.

Even though many of the problems of infancy and early childhood do prove to be transient, this is by no means true of them all. Behaviour problems in the pre-school years, some of which have been foreshadowed by problems, especially attachment problems, evident as early as the first year of life, are liable to persist into later childhood. Stevenson, *et al.* (1985) followed up 535 children from age three to age eight, and found that behaviour problems at age three were strongly related to behavioural deviance at age eight, especially in boys. Poor language development at age three was also correlated with deviant behaviour at age eight. Lerner, *et al.* (1985), who carried out a smaller scale study, came to similar conclusions.

It seems that aggressive children, withdrawn children, hyperactive children and speech- and language-disordered children in the age range three to five are especially at risk of developing later psychiatric disorders. How far these findings can be traced back to disorders of the first two years, and especially to the first year and the nature of attachments formed then, is not clear. Nevertheless we are beginning to have confirmation of the long-held view that many psychiatric disorders of later life have their origins very early in life.

Chapter 18

Special Problems of Adolescence

The developmental tasks of adolescence were reviewed in Chapter 1. Some of the special considerations which apply in interviewing and assessing adolescents were discussed in Chapter 5, and many of the points made there about the importance of establishing rapport apply with particular force in the adolescent age range. Interviewing adolescents, many of whom come to the psychiatrist reluctantly, is challenging and is discussed further in *Clinical Interviews with Children and Adolescents* (Barker, 1990).

The prevalence of psychiatric disorders in adolescence

Studies of adolescent populations have yielded prevalence rates for psychiatric disorders ranging from 8 to 21%, depending on the criteria used and the populations studied. Most have found higher rates in adolescence than in childhood, but even more striking is the difference in the sex ratio. Among pre-pubertal children, disturbed boys outnumber girls by a margin of about 2 to 1, but as puberty arrives and adolescence proceeds the ratio becomes roughly equal, and in adult life it is reversed. Offord, *et al.* (1987) reported the prevalence of disturbance in boys aged 4 to 11 (19.5%) to be similar to that in boys aged 12 to 16 (18.8%), but the rate in girls in the younger group was 13.5%, while in girls aged 12 to 16 it was 21.8%. Urban rates are higher than rural ones, for adolescents as for younger children.

The pattern of psychiatric disorders changes as childhood gives way to adolescence. Schizophrenia, rare before puberty, becomes more common. Major affective disorders, particularly depression, are also encountered more frequently, while encopresis, enuresis and some developmental disorders become much less common. Much of the change in the sex ratio is due to the increased prevalence of affective disorders, principally depression, in girls. In addition some of the developmental disorders, and encopresis, which affect boys more than girls, have resolved by this time. Suicide, rare before puberty, becomes more frequent; and mania, also rare before puberty, increases in prevalence, though it remains relatively uncommon in early and middle adolescence. Alcohol and drug abuse, and anorexia nervosa, are other conditions which most often make their appearance in adolescence, though the abuse by inhalation of solvents, petrol (gasoline) and like substances often commences before puberty.

It is convenient to consider adolescent disorders under three headings, though subdividing them in this way is somewhat artificial, especially the distinction between categories 2 and 3:

(1) Unresolved childhood disorders.
(2) Disorders related to puberty and adolescence.
(3) Adult-type disorders arising in adolescence.

(1) Unresolved childhood disorders

(a) Conduct disorders

Conduct disorders are often exacerbated with the onset of puberty. The tendency to rebel and reject adult standards which is often encountered in adolescents may accentuate pre-existing antisocial feelings and behaviour. In one study, children who were most aggressive at age 8 to 10 were found to be particularly at risk of becoming violent delinquents (Farrington, 1978). It seems that adolescents who do not have secure relationships with their parents and lack internal controls based on identification with them, are especially at risk of becoming involved in antisocial behaviour.

(b) Anxiety/neurotic disorders

These disorders sometimes improve around puberty, as the biological drives towards independence develop. The support of the young person's peer group, which tends to become more important in the lives of young people during this period of life, may help. In many jurisdictions there are important changes in the school setting at this time. From being in a primary, or elementary school (terminology varies in different parts of the world), with one teacher and, usually, a high degree of supervision, the child may move at puberty to a larger, more impersonal secondary (or 'high') school where more responsibility and independence of decision is required. This may be a helpful experience if enough support over the transition is available – from family, friends and, if needed, school staff. These changed circumstances may help emotionally immature children who have been overdependent on their parents to become more self-reliant.

Sometimes these aids to emotional growth prove insufficient. Faced with the challenges of adolescence, some children seem to lack the emotional resources to cope. Such drives to independence that they experience are not enough, and the young person may seek to fall back into the security and comfort of the family. Such children, realizing unconsciously, if not consciously, their incapacity to fill age-appropriate roles, may become even more anxious, with a worsening of their condition.

School refusal in adolescence may represent a continuation or exacerbation of a problem which existed before puberty, or it may be a symptom appearing for the first time. Even if the onset is in adolescence, however, its origin can often be traced to earlier years. The onset of school refusal is often more gradual in adolescence than it is in middle childhood, with increasing withdrawal and isolation from peers. Symptoms of separation anxiety tend to be less prominent and difficulties in school more so. The problems there, which often concern relationships with peer group or teachers, are such as would not usually be problems for children whose emotional development had been proceeding normally and whose family relationships were secure.

School-refusing adolescents tend to have difficulty expressing aggression and asserting independence in normal ways, difficulties they often seem to share with their parents. The adolescent's desire, conscious or unconscious, to be independent, and awareness of the parental protectiveness which is felt to be preventing this, can cause a build-up of intensely aggressive feelings. These may be expressed by violently angry outbursts under stress in a young person who at other times behaves in a passive and dependent way. In such cases, treatment of the whole family group is often the best approach. If the family is not prepared or able to participate, admission, even briefly, to a residential setting may be helpful in allowing the adolescent to grow up and become more independent. There is evidence that school refusal in adolescence is generally associated with more serious pathology in child and family than is often the case in earlier childhood. It may be accompanied by depressive or conduct disorder symptoms.

(c) Affective disorders
Depressive disorders, suicide and attempted suicide are all more common in adolescents than in younger children. Mania, and bipolar affective disorders, from being rare prior to puberty, become less so in adolescence, and are quite commonly seen in late adolescence. These conditions are discussed more fully in Chapter 10.

(d) Autism and pervasive developmental disorders
The handicaps of children with autism and other pervasive developmental disorders persist into adolescence, and epilepsy is sometimes

added to them. Hyperactivity may lessen and autistic adolescents are often underactive. They lack initiative and drive, and their inappropriate social behaviour and responses, and their lack of empathy for others, isolate them from their non-autistic peers. Consequently they remain more closely dependent on their families and other care-givers than do normal adolescents. At the same time the hormonal and physical changes of puberty, particularly their increase in size and physical strength, can make them more difficult to manage. In some cases assertiveness, often in areas in which this is not appropriate, can present serious problems for their parents. This may lead to institutional placement.

(e) Developmental disorders
Many children with developmental disorders have overcome their speech, language and motor coordination problems, or have learned a lifestyle (for example, typing instead of writing) in which any residual problems do not handicap them. Reading difficulties frequently persist, however, and are common in adolescents with conduct disorders. Impairment of reading skills, which often persists through adolescence into adult life, presents a serious problem to those living in technologically advanced societies.

(f) Attention-deficit disorders and hyperactivity
While hyperactivity often lessens or subsides completely around puberty, the other symptoms of attention-deficit disorder frequently do not. Distractibility, impulsivity and aggressive behaviour may continue, though in some young people these symptoms gradually subside over the years. Low self-esteem, poor school performance and poor peer relationships characterize these adolescents. Some exhibit antisocial behaviour, though different studies have yielded widely varying estimates of how many (Weiss & Hechtman, 1986, Chapter 4).

(2) Disorders related to puberty and adolescence

The emotional, social, psychological and physical changes of adolescence provide the context for some of the disorders occurring at this time of life. The following are relevant issues:

(a) The dependence-independence conflict
Adolescents are neither dependent children nor independent adults. They feel, in varying degrees, the urge to be independent and they are subject to social pressures which foster this. But they are as yet uncertain about how far they can act independently. An evident desire to fall back

on their family for support may alternate with shows of independent, but sometimes ill-judged, decision making. Help and support given by parents may be accepted in off-handed and ungracious ways. Dealing with such behaviour requires much patience, tolerance and under-standing on the part of the parents.

(b) Uncertainties about sexual role and sexual adequacy

The principal physical and emotional changes of puberty may occur as early as 10 or as late as 17 in normally developing young people. Puberty tends to come earlier and to be completed more quickly in girls than in boys, though there is considerable overlap. Consequently some young people feel out of step with their peers, especially if puberty comes late to them. Fears of sexual inadequacy are common during this period.

The upsurge of sexual feelings and activity, and the development of sometimes intense relationships with the opposite sex, may provoke feelings of anxiety and confusion. The young person may wish to enter into relationships, while feeling shy and lacking the necessary confidence. On the other hand some adolescents become involved in sexual activity early. This may lead to unwanted pregnancies which, whether carried to term or aborted, are stressful experiences.

(c) Peer group influences

During adolescence the peer group assumes increasing importance in the life of the young person. Adolescents tend to form groups, sometimes of one sex, sometimes of both sexes, and these provide their members with support in meeting the social and emotional challenges of adolescence. With the support of the group, young people who still lack self-confidence are able to do things they would shy away from if on their own. Adolescent groups may be as small as two or three, but membership may run to as many as 10, 20 or even more. Some remain quite constant, but most change as members leave to join other groups, and others join. One young person may have affiliation with several groups of differing size and type.

The influence of adolescent groups is not always beneficial. Delinquent gangs may have seriously adverse effects on their members. Some young people feel 'different' from other group members, and some are treated differently because of appearance, race or religion. This may lead some members to do rash or daring, but often unwise, things to 'prove' them-selves to the group. Adolescent groups usually demand a fair amount of conformity to their standards and unwritten rules. Inability to meet the group's standards may cause individual members anxiety, or even lead to their rejection from the group.

(d) Discrepancies between individual development and the demands of society

A newspaper cartoon pictures a couple at the box office of a theatre over which there was a sign saying, 'Children under 16 must be accompanied by a parent'. The stylishly dressed couple are explaining to the salesperson that, 'We're under 16 but we're parents.' This sums up rather nicely a dilemma faced by many young people in modern day society. Puberty is occurring earlier (in western countries the average age of the menarche is now about one year earlier than it was 50 years ago), yet many of society's institutions take no cognizance of this. For many young people formal education and financial dependency are increasingly prolonged, and those who choose not to remain in formal education beyond their mid-teens are unable to find rewarding work and a satisfying place in the adult world. This can lead to feelings of defeat and low self-esteem, as well as anger directed at the adult world in general. While these changes have been happening, society's attitudes towards sexual activity in adolescence have been changing. Attitudes seem to have become more permissive, becoming pregnant before marriage is scarcely frowned upon, and many unmarried teenage girls who become pregnant opt to keep and try to care for the children. This confronts them with enormous and often stressful challenges as well, it often seems, as putting the next generation at risk.

(e) Family development problems

Accepting the arrival of adolescence in their children, and making the necessary adjustments in the family system, prove difficult for some families. Attitudes and methods of control which have been appropriate, and have worked well previously, may no longer be effective. A process that should be one of gradual, sensitively monitored handing over of responsibility from parents to child may become instead a battle of wills; or the opposite may happen, the parents relinquishing control and responsibility more quickly than the young person can properly take over.

Adolescent behaviour problems

Conduct and oppositional defiant disorders are at least as common in adolescents as in middle childhood, and the numbers of antisocial activities engaged in by conduct disordered adolescents are probably greater (Shapland, 1978).

Some adolescent conduct disorders are continuations of behaviour patterns established earlier, often much earlier, in childhood. Others have their onset in adolescence. The latter lack the association with reading problems commonly found in cases of earlier onset, and their symptoms and the associated family problems are generally less severe and chronic. They seem sometimes to be no more than exaggerated reactions to some combination of the five challenges of adolescence listed above. The soundness of the parent-child relationship before puberty, and the way the parents react to rebellious behaviour on the part of their child, also affect the severity and persistence of these disorders. Sometimes rebellious and antisocial behaviour seems to have the unconscious aim of provoking the parents to take control on the part of a child who is insecure and afraid of his or her own aggressiveness. In other instances the behaviour appears to be a protest against over-strict demands by the parents. In yet others it is associated with feelings of rootlessness and aimlessness in children who have been deprived of love and emotional security. There may be a background of physical and/or sexual abuse. Children who have been sexually abused are especially prone to act out sexually, or even to become abusers themselves.

Some conduct disorders arise in the context of seriously deviant personality development. A follow up study of Canadian children first assessed in grade 1 (about age 6) and then reassessed at age 14, showed that early disruptive behaviour in boys significantly often led to delinquent behaviour at age 14. There was not necessarily poor school achievement in the intervening period. However poor school achievement in elementary school was often followed by antisocial attitudes and behaviours in adolescence. The findings for girls were less striking. They reported engaging in fewer delinquent activities at age 14 and no relationship was found between early disruptive behaviour and later delinquent behaviour, though poor performance in elementary school did seem to presage antisocial attitudes and behaviour in adolescence.

Thus it seems that conduct disorders in adolescents may be either transient blips in the course of their development, or manifestations of long-standing personality development or, presumably, anything between these two extremes. The reported severity of the behavioural disturbance is, on its own, an inadequate indication of the seriousness of the problem. Adjustment before puberty, indeed as far back as the pre-school years; family stability and parental attitudes; the young person's educational status, especially reading skills; and adjustment in situations in which the parents are not directly involved, all need to be taken into account. The latter include school, peer group and the interview situation with the psychiatrist or other health professional.

It is important to be aware that many adolescents emerge as mentally healthy individuals, adjusting well in society, after going through difficult times during their teenage years. The prevalence of antisocial behaviour is considerably lower in young adults than it is in adolescents, suggesting that this is often a transient phenomenon.

Running away from home is a common problem in adolescents, though it also occurs in younger children. The term applies to leaving or staying away from home, with the intention of staying away for a period of time, in circumstances in which the individual will be missed by those remaining at home. It has been reported that in the USA about 10% of boys and 8.7% of girls have run away at least once (Russell, 1981). The homes of runaways are characterized by high rates of parent child conflict, parental death and divorce, and physical and sexual abuse. Physical abuse was reported by 78% of 199 runaway youths admitted to a shelter for runaways (Farber, *et al.*, 1984). Running away seems sometimes to be the best solution the child can find to escape conflict and/or abuse in the family; in other instances it may be seen as a means of avoiding defeat in the battle for independence from the parents.

Alcohol and drug abuse

In this section the term *drug abuse* will be used to include the abuse of alcohol, except where the context implies otherwise. Alcohol is a powerful mind-altering drug and its use may lead to abuse and dependence. It is often just one of a variety of mind-altering substances used by the drug abuser. Separating it out for special consideration can have unfortunate consequences, its use being regarded as less serious than that of 'real' drugs – as if addiction to alcohol is not as serious as addiction to other mind-altering substances.

Adolescent drug abuse is a serious problem in societies in many parts – perhaps even most parts – of the world. Prevalence rates vary from place to place and from time to time, and are difficult to determine. Different drugs come in and out of fashion, and availability and cost are also factors which help to determine what is used.

During the course of the Ontario Child Health Study, drug use in the population studied was investigated. Of a representative sample of 1302 adolescents aged 12 to 16, 1265 participated (97% of those eligible) (Boyle & Offord, 1986). The prevalence figures found in the 14 to 16 age range, expressed as percentages, are shown in Table 18.1.

'Hard' drugs included amphetamines, other stimulants, psychedelics, heroin and other opiates. The prevalence rates for all drugs except inhalants were much lower in the 12 to 14 age bracket. Inhalants, however, were used by 8.3% of the boys and 9.6% of the girls in the younger group. While there was a tendency for drug use to be more common in girls than boys, only in the case of cigarette smoking was the difference statistically significant. There is a clear progression with age and the mid-teen years are a common time for drug use to commence.

Table 18.1   Prevalence of drug use, in percentages, of subjects aged 14 to 16 years (Ontario Child Health Study).

	Boys	Girls
Tobacco		
Occasional use	31.1	45.6
Regular use	15.8	23.4
Alcohol		
Occasional use	42.5	48.8
Regular use	10.6	15.9
Marijuana	13.3	17.6
'Hard' drugs	5.3	7.5
Inhalants	3.8	4.5

The findings of a study in New York City suggested that the major risk period for initiation into the use of cigarettes, alcohol and marijuana is complete by age 20, and that for illicit drugs other than cocaine by age 21 (Kandel & Logan, 1984).

Daily cigarette use has been found to occur in 15 to 25% of most adolescent populations studied. There is a strong correlation between parental smoking and smoking in the adolescent offspring of the parents. The chances of becoming a teenage smoker are about five times greater in smoking than in non-smoking households.

There tends to be a stepwise progression in drug use. It usually starts with the use of beer or wine, going on to, successively, tobacco and hard liquor, marijuana, and then other illegal drugs such as LSD, tranquillizers, heroin and cocaine. Fortunately relatively few of those that set out on this sequence complete it. In some communities the first initiation into drug abuse is with the use of inhalants.

Kovach & Glickman (1986) suggested that a period of drug use has become a normal feature of adolescence in western society, and that the age of onset of use is around 14. They studied the characteristics of users, defined as those who had used marijuana or alcohol at least once a week for three months, or had used any 'high risk' drug (tranquillizers, barbiturates, sedatives, hallucinogens, phencyclidine or amphetamines) in the past year. Comparing users with those who had not used in the past year, they found that users were:

- more often male;
- more often Caucasian;
- older;
- children who had repeated school grades eight times more often than non-users;

- more involved with family crises and conflicts with parents;
- more likely to be arrested, incarcerated, and convicted of property, drug and weapons offences;
- experiencing less enjoyment and satisfaction in school, and more dislike of and fights with teachers.

The users associated with, and claimed as friends, more drug users than the non-users did, and the prevalence of other behavioural and psychiatric problems was higher. The regular drug users stood out as having more personality and family problems. Vicary & Lerner (1986) reported the results of an extensive longitudinal study. This showed that early parental conflict over child rearing, and harsh and restrictive parenting, were associated with drug use in the teen years.

Table 18.2 lists the principal drugs which adolescents have been reported to use, and some characteristics of each. The list is not exhaustive. Among the other drugs which are sometimes abused by young people are cough syrups containing codeine; compound tablets containing mixtures of analgesics, sedatives, antihistamines and/or caffeine; the anti-emetic dimenhydrinate (Gravol); and various other psychoactive preparations.

Drug users have been divided into experimental, situational (or recreational), and compulsive groups. Most adolescents experiment, at least with alcohol, cigarettes or marijuana, at some stage. A smaller group uses drugs at parties and in particular situations, while an even smaller number become dependent on a drug or, more commonly, drugs. These are the ones who become compulsive users. The factors determining whether a person becomes dependent on a drug are incompletely understood. Social pressures can be important in leading to drug use but probably do not determine who becomes dependent. That may be more a matter of the emotional stability and personality characteristics of the individual. There is a small subgroup of drug users who have serious personality problems or psychiatric conditions such as recurrent depression (Amini, *et al.*, 1976). They often have a history of early deprivation, abuse and/or other adverse rearing experiences. It is among this minority that serious drug abuse, leading to addiction, is likely to occur. There is also some evidence that in some addicts there is a genetic predisposition to addiction to alcohol and perhaps other drugs.

There is a correlation between drug abuse and both delinquency and failure in school, though just how these are causally connected – if they are – is not clear. It may be that common factors lead to all three sets of problems. Other factors which have been found to be associated with drug use are social isolation, low self-esteem, poor relationships with parents, depression, and unconventional beliefs and values concerning

Table 18.2   Some drugs of abuse.

Drug	How used	Main characteristics
Tobacco	Smoked Chewed	Powerfully addictive, but widely advertised and readily available to young people
Alcohol	Drunk as beer, wine and distilled spirits	Causes physical and psychological dependence; widely abused; introduced to children in families
Cannabis products – marijuana, hashish, 'hash oil'	Smoked in cigarettes ('joints') and pipes	Intoxicant and euphoric; causes psychological dependence; relatively cheap; readily available, circulates in schools
Stimulants – amphetamines, 'speed', methylphenidate	Orally Intravenous (I.V.)	Euphoric, cause feelings of well-being; increased energy; may cause psychoses, dependence common, mainly psychological
Hallucinogens – LSD ('acid'), mescaline, phencyclidine (PCP, 'angel dust')	Orally	Altered consciousness, hallucinations, unusual subjective states, psychological dependence
Barbiturates	Orally I.V.	Sedative effect; may be used to counter effects of stimulants; can cause serious dependency
Tranquillisers – especially benzodiazepines ('Valium', 'Halcion', 'Librium')	Orally Rarely I.V.	Lightheadedness, relief of tension; used for 'coming down' after using cocaine, amphetamines and other stimulants; psychological dependence
Narcotics – heroin, morphine, methadone, codeine and related compounds	I.V. Orally	Feelings of well-being, pleasant drowsiness, contentment. Major physical dependence may occur
Cocaine	Inhaled as powder, smoked ('freebasing'), or as 'crack' I.V.	A stimulant, producing great euphoria briefly, and stimulation of heart and other organs. May cause psychotic state and severe psychological dependence
Inhalants – solvents in glue etc., gasoline/petrol	Inhaled, often from plastic bag	Brief euphoria and confusion. Psychological dependence may occur; may cause brain damage

drugs and their use. Individuals may seek to have their felt needs for affiliation, satisfaction of curiosity, altered states of consciousness, recreation, anxiety reduction, and general drive reduction met by the use of drugs, especially in the company of others.

Other disorders related to adolescence

Anxiety/neurotic disorders may arise *de novo* during adolescence and in the causation of some of them the stresses of the adolescent period play a part. Clear-cut obsessive-compulsive, conversion, and dissociative disorders become more common in adolescence, and the same applies to social phobias and agoraphobia. These conditions are described in Chapter 8 and their form in adolescence is little different from that seen before puberty. Dysthymia or, less often, major depression, may arise in the context of difficulties in adolescent adjustment.

Anorexia nervosa, which most often has its onset during adolescence and often seems to be in part a reaction to difficulties in meeting the challenges of this period, is described in Chapter 16.

(3) Adult-type disorders arising in adolescence

Any of the major psychiatric disorders of adult life may arise during adolescence. Both schizophrenia and the major affective disorders (depression, mania and bipolar disorders) become more common as adolescence proceeds.

The onset of schizophrenia may be insidious. Its early symptoms can be hard to distinguish from the shyness, diffidence and vagueness of expression common in anxious adolescents who are feeling unsure of themselves but are not developing schizophrenia. It is important not to make the diagnosis of schizophrenia lightly, since such an error may have unfortunate implications for the subject. The criteria set out in Chapter 13 should be the basis on which the diagnosis is made, though in some cases it is necessary to await developments, while bearing the possibility that the symptoms presented may be harbingers of schizophrenia. Sometimes a period of observation in hospital, away from the family and the peer group, is helpful in clarifying the diagnosis.

Other than conduct disorders, depression is the most common type of major psychiatric disorder occurring in this age period. Its features are described in Chapter 10. Further consideration of suicidal behaviour in adolescence is necessary, however.

Suicidal behaviour in adolescence

Suicide is quite rare before puberty but its incidence increases with the arrival of puberty. Around puberty it is still relatively uncommon, but as the teenage years succeed one another its incidence increases. The suicide rate in North American adolescents has been increasing during the last several decades (Pfeffer, 1991) with rates rising to about 13 per 100 000 in the 15- to 24-year-old-age bracket. This is the rate for reported completed suicides. Suicide attempts and suicidal ideation are much more common. Reports cited by Pfeffer (1991) suggest that in the USA about 9% of adolescents attempt suicide at least once.

Garrison, *et al.* (1991) report a study of suicidal ideation in adolescents. The subjects were 1073 young people whose ages ranged from 11 to 15 at the start of a three-year period of study. *Suicide scores* were obtained on a scale which ranged from 0 to 9, a score of 0 meaning that there was no suicidal ideation and a score of 5 or higher being regarded as high. Each year at least 70% of the subjects had a score of 0, while the proportion with scores of 1 to 3 was between 15 and 20%. The proportion with scores of 5 or higher ranged from 4 to 5.5% during each year, girls having high scores more often than boys. The students also completed three tests designed to assess family adaptability and cohesion, to ascertain whether they had experienced 'undesirable life events', and to explore whether they had symptoms of depression (assessed using the Centre for Epidemiological Studies Depression Scale (CES-D)). High suicide scores were found to be associated with a high incidence of undesirable life events, low perceived family adaptability and cohesion, and high scores on the CES-D scale, the latter being the most consistently associated with suicidal ideation.

The term *parasuicide* is sometimes used for self-injurious behaviours which are not seriously life-threatening. Though these are often referred to as *suicide attempts,* many of those carrying them out have objectives other than to kill themselves, although in borderline cases the distinction between them and serious attempts that fail can be a difficult one. Some *attempts* that fail are very real, the subjects only escaping death because chance discovery of their condition led to the prompt provision of medical treatment, or because of some miscalculation. Others, such as minor overdoses, often of drugs with limited lethal potential, wrist-slashings, and other forms of self-mutilation, often carried out without any attempt to hide the act from others, are not. Such behaviours are usually expressions of distress or attempts to stimulate concern, solicitude or attention, or to achieve some other change in the subject's situation. Nevertheless they may have unintended fatal outcomes. They should always be taken seriously even though the risk of suicide may be slight. They are sure signs that a problem exists.

More adolescent boys than girls commit suicide, sex ratios of over 4 to 1 being reported in the 15 to 19 age range (Shaffer & Fisher, 1981). Attempted suicide, or parasuicide, is more common in girls than boys (Hawton *et al.*, 1982).

The psychiatric assessment of adolescents should always include an evaluation of suicide risk. At some point during the interview, preferably after rapport has been well established, questions such as, 'Have you ever felt life is not worth living any more?' or 'Have you ever wished you were dead?' should be asked. If such questions are answered in the affirmative the young person should be asked when, and under what circumstances, these thoughts have been entertained. How severe and frequent have they been? Are they currently present? If not, when was the last time they were present? Was the subject facing particular stresses at that time? If so, is that stress still continuing or has it been resolved? Is it likely to recur?

The questions above address suicidal ideation. The next ones should address suicidal intent. Examples are, 'Have you ever considered harming yourself in some way?' and 'Have you actually thought seriously about killing yourself?' If such questions are answered in the affirmative, the next step is to ask about suicide plans. Ask, 'How have you thought that you might kill yourself?' or 'What plans do you have for killing yourself?' If the subject has, or has had, specific plans these should be explored. It is important to ascertain how carefully the plans have been laid and how effective they are likely to be if implemented.

Finally, in the assessment of suicide risk, enquiry should be made about any previous attempts at suicide. This involves exploring the precipitating circumstances, the actual events, and the consequences that followed. Was the young person taken to hospital? If so, what treatment was provided? Was he or she admitted? If so, for how long? What was the reaction of the parents, other family members and others involved in the patient's life?

The risk of suicide is greater the deeper the degree of depression that is present, especially when the subject has been getting more and more depressed over a period of time. Suicide is more likely the less communication there is with others. The isolated depressed person is very much at risk, especially when communication channels have recently broken down. If there have been previous suicide attempts, especially serious ones, the risk may be greater. A long history of self-destructive behaviour is particularly serious and is an indicator that in-depth psychiatric investigation, and probably treatment, is needed. Also important are the extent to which parasuicidal behaviour has been intended as a means of communication and whether the communication has been heeded, and responded to helpfully, by those to whom it has been directed. If there has been little impact on the environment, the risk of recurrence may be high.

Most serious of all is a history of determined attempts at suicide, carried out in isolation, especially when accompanied by a strong desire to die.

The treatment of adolescents

The treatment approaches for the main psychiatric disorders from which adolescents may suffer have been outlined in the relevant chapters, and treatment methods are discussed further in Chapter 21. This section will cover some general points about treating adolescents.

Many troubled adolescents are reluctant to accept how troubled they really are. Some, especially those with conduct disorders, are resentful towards authority, and psychiatrists and other mental health professionals are often cast by them in the role of authority figures. Adolescents' negative attitudes towards their parents are sometimes displaced and directed towards their therapists – or at least those who are offering them therapy.

In view of the above considerations, the establishment of rapport and a good, empathic working relationship with the young person is essential to effective treatment. This has been discussed in Chapter 5 and is dealt with in greater depth in *Clinical Interviews with Children and Adolescents* (Barker, 1990). Also important is the clarification of goals. If the therapist's goals are not at least reasonably congruent with those of the young person, success is unlikely. Treatment embarked upon on the basis of the parents' goals, or those of the young person's social worker or probation officer, or the family or youth court judge, will probably be unproductive. We need also to temper the enthusiasm we sometimes feel for making changes *we* believe are desirable, rather than those the adolescent is seeking. Time spent discussing, clarifying and agreeing goals is always well spent. The very fact that the therapist takes a position of wanting to understand the adolescent's wishes, aspirations and view of his or her problems, rather than impose his or her ideas, can be both facilitating and even therapeutic.

Sometimes the picture painted by adolescents of their family situation or of themselves is quite different from that supplied by their parents. They may even deny the existence of any problems, while the parents, and often also their teachers, have a long list of complaints. In such situations family therapy may be the best treatment approach. The points of view of all concerned can then be stated and examined with everyone present, and the differences of opinion, or disputed facts, explored. This is often an essential first step in therapy.

Adolescents who have suffered severe and prolonged deprivation earlier in their lives, especially if this has been combined with physical and/or sexual abuse, tend to be a particularly difficult group to treat. Many of them have great difficulty entering into trusting and intimate relationships, and this can make it hard for them to become involved in a psychotherapeutic relationship. Much testing of the therapist and the relationship, and the passage of a considerable amount of time, are often necessary before progress can be made. A telling account of the treatment of an adolescent girl with such difficulties is that of Rossman (1985).

There are differing views on the place of residential treatment in this age group. In the past, severely disturbed young people have been placed in residential institutions where they might remain for months or even years. The idea behind this approach was that certain adolescents needed to be removed from their dysfunctional families and social settings to more stable care in residential settings. On the whole this did not work out well. Often the effects of living with other young people who were equally – sometimes more – disturbed led to deterioration rather than improvement in the young person's adjustment. Current approaches, which are more short-term and emphasize a *competency* approach, that is, working with the young person and family to build upon strengths, seem to offer more promise (Durrant, 1993).

Medication has an established, if limited place, in the treatment of adolescent psychiatric disorders. Depressed adolescents may derive benefit from antidepressant drugs, and those with schizophrenia are usually given one of the major antipsychotics. Lithium carbonate may be effective in controlling bipolar affective disorders and it may have a part to play also in the treatment of some behaviour disorders. How far medication should be used to control aggressive and antisocial behaviour is a moot point. At best it is only a symptomatic treatment and its use, if it is to be used at all, should probably be confined to crisis situations and very short-term behavioural control while the potential of other measures is explored.

Adolescent drug abuse presents formidable challenges. Most teenage drug abusers and addicts deny that their use of drugs presents a problem. Once regular drug use is established, however, 'kicking' the habit can be difficult, even for the person whose motivation is strong. Those whose motivation is weak or absent, as is the case with many adolescents, are unlikely to stop unless they have an experience such as the death of a friend or family member from an overdose, that causes them to see drug use in a different light. Suffering the psychological craving for drugs and/ or the effects of physical withdrawal is simply not seen as worthwhile by young people in whom drug use has not as yet caused serious problems – or at least problems they are prepared to acknowledge. Since many of these young people are members of disturbed families, a family approach often offers the best chance of success. Engaging families also presents difficulties but Szapocznik, *et al.* (1988) described an approach to adolescent drug abusers and their families which used 'strategic structural-systems' principles to facilitate this. It proved significantly more effective than a more traditional approach to engagement.

It is possible to stop adolescents taking drugs by placing them, whether willingly or not, in treatment centres where drugs are unavailable, but unless they can be meaningfully engaged in treatment while there, the effects tend not to last following discharge. Self-help organizations such as Alcoholics Anonymous and Narcotics Anonymous, while helpful to many adult addicts, tend to be less helpful to adolescents. They are based upon the acceptance by the addict that he or she *is* an alcoholic or addict and has an unmanageable life. This usually involves first reaching a psychological 'bottom' which many young people have not yet done.

In the management of suicidal adolescents any associated depression or other psychiatric disorder should receive appropriate treatment. It is important also to do everything possible to open up communication between these patients and their families, as well as exploring their own communication, relationship and other problems and offering appropriate interventions. A combination of individual and family therapy is often effective in achieving these aims.

When the risk of suicide appears high, admission to an inpatient unit for adolescents may be indicated, though some families prove able to provide satisfactory supervision and a safe environment at home. It is thus sometimes possible to allow the young person to be managed as a daypatient or outpatient even though there is some risk of suicide.

Outcome

It is hard to generalize about the outcome of psychiatric disorders in adolescence. Factors influencing outcome include the type of disorder; the adjustment of the individual prior to puberty; whether there are underlying problems of personality development; the support, or lack of support, available within the adolescent's family; and peer group influences.

While there is a strong association between antisocial behaviour in adolescence and similar behaviour in adult life, and most antisocial adults have shown antisocial behaviour as adolescents, the converse is not true. That is to say, most antisocial adolescents do not become antisocial adults (Robins, 1978). Many antisocial and delinquent youths abandon their antisocial behaviour between the ages of 17 and 20. This seems to be in part the result of a maturational process, often associated with changes in attitudes towards drug use, consciously formulated changes in priorities, and support from girlfriends, boyfriends, siblings and others (Mulvey & LaRosa, 1986).

The outlook in anxiety/neurotic disorders is generally better than that for antisocial ones. Most anxiety disorders do not presage adult problems of the same type, though some do persist. On the other hand, the risk of recurrence of major affective disorders, including bipolar ones, is high.

Schizophrenia has a relatively poor prognosis, though with continued treatment the symptoms may remain well controlled.

Many adolescents who have suffered from attention-deficit hyperactivity disorders are found to be functioning well as adults. Hyperactivity is not usually a continuing problem and one-third to a half become indistinguishable from the normal population (Weiss & Hechtman, 1986). Recent research has however yielded evidence that attention-deficit problems sometimes do persist into adult life, and that they may respond to treatments similar to those that are effective in younger subjects.

Autism and other pervasive developmental disorders usually persist into adult life. Many autistic individuals remain severely handicapped and up to half are eventually admitted to institutions. Others survive in the community with varying degrees of support from family members or others. Only quite a small minority find places in the labour force.

Further information and references on adolescent psychiatric disorders are to be found in *Basic Adolescent Psychiatry* (Steinberg, 1987).

Chapter 19

Psychiatric Disorders in Mentally Retarded Children

Mental retardation is usually defined in terms of both social and intellectual functioning. It is not sufficient to use either criterion alone. If social functioning were to be taken as the sole criterion, those with intelligence in or near the average range might be treated as retarded if their social skills were impaired for other reasons. If assessed intelligence were to be taken as the only criterion, some of those whose intelligence is well below average, but who nevertheless function satisfactorily in society, might be stigmatized, admitted to institutions, or otherwise deprived of opportunities of which they could make use.

It is helpful to take children's levels of intellectual and social functioning into account for several reasons. During their school years, children whose cognitive skills are more limited than those of the majority of children often require special educational arrangements and teaching. Later, their limited vocational skills may result in their requiring special vocational training and, perhaps, sheltered employment. Some may never be able to live independently in the community.

Despite the above considerations, dividing children into those who are mentally retarded and those who are not has disadvantages. Although arbitrary divisions may be made, in reality there is a continuum of functioning and needs from those of intellectually bright children, through those of average intelligence to those who fall, in varying degrees, below the average. For the purpose of providing psychiatric services it is better to consider the psychiatry of all children, whatever their level of cognitive functioning, as a part of the mainstream of child psychiatry. In the past, and in some parts of the world even currently, care for mentally retarded children has been provided separately in hospitals and institutions, often large ones, specifically for the retarded. These were often far from the homes and families of the children and they were administered separately from other child psychiatry services. In many jurisdictions, however, moves away from this pattern of services have been under way, particularly in the years since the Second World War.

The prevalence of psychiatric disorders in the mentally retarded

In the Isle of Wight Study (Rutter, *et al.*, 1970b) it was found that *intellectually retarded* children (defined as those whose IQs on the Wechsler Intelligence Scale for Children were two or more standard deviations below the mean for the population) had psychiatric disorders three to four times more frequently than children in the general population. Among severely retarded children not attending school, psychiatric disorder was found in 50%, compared with about 6.6% in the general child population of the age studied. Psychoses and the 'hyperkinetic syndrome' were proportionally more common than in children of higher intelligence (Rutter, *et al.*, 1970a).

Not only are specific psychiatric disorders more common in children of lower intelligence, but so also are a variety of forms of deviant behaviour. Table 19.1 illustrates this using data from the Isle of Wight findings.

Table 19.1 Symptoms reported in 10- and 11-year-old girls (Isle of Wight survey).

	IQ 120 or more (%)	IQ 79 or less (%)
Poor concentration		
Parents' report	2.6	26.4
Teachers' report	9.1	62.3
Fighting		
Parents' report	1.3	9.9
Teachers' report	2.6	11.0

Corbett (1979), in a study in south-east London, found that there were 140 children aged under 15 with IQs below 50, in a population of 175 000. Of these, 43% showed evidence of behavioural disturbance. Common problems were psychoses (17%), sterotypies and pica (10%), and adjustment disorders (6%); conduct, emotional and hyperkinetic disorders were each present in 4% of these children.

Clinical associations and causes of mental retardation

Some of the causes of mental retardation have been mentioned in Chapters 2 and 11. Genetic factors, physical diseases of the brain, brain injury, and environmental factors can all contribute. The high prevalence of psychiatric disorders in individuals of very low intelligence is probably due chiefly to the brain damage which is usually present in these cases.

The relationship is not however a simple one and other factors may be involved. The following points are relevant in considering the associations of mental retardation:

(1)   There is a relationship between IQ and deviant behaviour in children of normal intelligence as well as in the mentally retarded, intellectually brighter children showing less deviant behaviour. This may be in part because greater intellectual capacity makes social adaptation easier.

(2)   Organic brain damage is more common in children of lower intelligence than in those with IQs in the average range, and it is virtually universal in those with IQs below 50. Many brain damaged children suffer from epilepsy which itself is associated with an increased incidence of psychiatric disorder. Behaviour may improve following hemispherectomy, the surgical removal of the cerebral cortex on one side. This procedure is sometimes carried out when one side of the cortex is badly damaged, in children with infantile hemiplegia. Similar improvement may follow the surgical removal of an epileptogenic focus from the brain, especially if the focus is in one of the temporal lobes. All these observations point to brain damage as a factor that may contribute to the development of behaviour problems.

(3)   Social factors such as depriving, hostile and rejecting parental attitudes may adversely affect both intellectual development and emotional stability. The lack of a warm, nurturing and affirming family environment in which to grow up can have consequences which are even more devastating for the mentally retarded than for children whose cognitive skills are greater. Rejecting attitudes of others, including other children, may have similarly adverse effects.

(4)   The developmental immaturity of retarded children results in their language and other skills comparing unfavourably with those of their peers. These differences, and their delay in achieving motor skills, and in becoming toilet trained, are additional handicaps which may predispose to psychiatric disorder.

(5)   Educational failure is associated with psychiatric disorder. Children of lower intelligence progress more slowly than others, and long-standing failure in school can be a potent factor contributing to the development of psychiatric disorder. Much depends on the quality of the education provided and how well it is adapted to the needs of the particular child.

(6)   Institutionalization can adversely affect both intellectual development and emotional growth. The adverse effects on children of the environment of large impersonal institutions have long been known (Spitz, 1946; King, *et al.*, 1971). Yet in some parts of the world children –

orphans and those who have been abandoned as well as the retarded – are still placed in such settings. We have recently seen disturbing pictures and read of the plight of children in institutions in formerly communist Eastern Europe countries. These have provided graphic reminders of the damage such places can do, even to children with good intellectual potential.

(7) There is little evidence that emotional disorders themselves adversely affect intellectual functioning, though they may impair children's cooperation in psychological testing. High anxiety levels may however impair achievement in school, even though intellectual capacity is unimpaired.

Specific forms of mental retardation

(a) Down's syndrome

This is also known as trisomy-21 because those suffering from it usually have three of the '21' chromosomes instead of the normal pair. Occasionally the additional chromosomal material is attached to another chromosome. About 1 in every 700 children born has this condition, making it a relatively common cause of mental retardation. Older parents, especially older mothers, are at greater risk of having children with the condition and Down's syndrome afflicts about 1 in every 100 children born to women over 40 (Mikkleson, 1981).

Down's syndrome children are usually recognizable at birth. They have marked epicanthic folds (these are vertical folds of skin over the inner angle of the eye), inwardly slanting eyes, small heads, short necks, small and low-set ears, and protruding tongues. There is usually only a single palmar crease and the fifth finger typically curves inwards. Moderate to severe mental retardation is present in nearly all cases, though chromosomal mosaics (individuals in whom some cells contain normal chromosomes and others show trisomy-21) may have near-normal intelligence. About 40% have congenital cardiac abnormalities and there is a high incidence of other congenital defects.

Formerly many Down's children were admitted to institutions early in life, but nowadays they are usually cared for in the community while being provided with specialized schooling. This seems to provide them with their best chance of developing as normally as possible. Many of the behavioural problems seen in the past were probably due largely to the adverse effects of institutional life and experiences.

The verbal skills of Down's syndrome children are more impaired than the non-verbal ones, and few achieve reading skills better than those of an average eight-year-old. They exhibit behaviour problems more often than children of normal intelligence, but apparently less often than other retarded children with comparable intelligence levels and they seem prone to problems of attention (Flint & Yule, 1994).

(b) Phenylketonuria

The genetics of this condition were mentioned in Chapter 2. Phenylketonuria is quite rare, occurring in fewer than 1 in 10000 children. Untreated children are usually, though not invariably, retarded and may be hyperkinetic and display other abnormalities of behaviour. They tend to have light coloured skin and hair, and often have eczema and a characteristic urinary smell.

Early detection can be achieved by the screening of newborns using a simple urine test. Treatment consists of a diet low in phenylalanine during the child's early years. This usually leads to normal or near-normal development.

(c) The fragile X syndrome

This is one of the more common specific conditions causing mental retardation and has been discussed in Chapter 2.

(d) The Lesch-Nyhan syndrome

This rare sex-linked inborn error of purine metabolism is characterized by severe mental retardation, self-mutilation, aggressive behaviour, increased muscle tone, other neurological abnormalities and renal failure (Lesch & Nyhan, 1964; Jankovic, et al., 1988). Symptoms are usually evident during the first year of life and the self-mutilation, consisting of biting the lips, fingers and other parts of the body, usually starts in the pre-school age range.

(e) The Prader–Willi syndrome

In this condition there are sometimes, but not always, chromosome abnormalities. The principal symptoms are mental retardation, obesity, underdevelopment of the gonads and various behavioural problems, most notably insatiable appetite; these children gorge themselves and steal food any way they can, and may also exhibit pica (Prader, et al., 1956; Hall & Smith, 1972; Carpenter, 1989).

(f) Cerebral palsy and related neurological conditions

Some children with cerebral palsy and other syndromes associated with brain damage are mentally retarded, though many are of normal intelligence. The combination of a serious physical handicap with limited intellectual skills provides a particular challenge to those caring for, treating and educating such children. This applies, sometimes with even greater force, to deaf and blind retarded children.

Many other, mostly rare, neurological disorders are associated with mental retardation and may have associated behaviour and other psychiatric syndromes.

Sociocultural retardation

While some specific clinical syndrome or neurological disorder is usually found to be responsible in children with severe retardation, in many mildly retarded children no evidence is found of any medical or neurological disorder. In most of these children some combination of sociocultural deprivation and polygenic inheritance is probably responsible. Naturally the innate, genetically determined intellectual potential of some children falls at the lower end of the normal range, and if such children also lack proper cognitive stimulation and suffer general sociocultural deprivation, a mild degree of mental retardation may result. This may only become apparent when the child starts school and proves to be slow to learn. In their home environments these children may not be regarded as having any particular problems.

Clinical management and treatment

There are two populations of retarded children. The larger one comprises those who are mildly retarded and do not suffer from any specific clinical syndrome or medical problems. A smaller group consists of more seriously handicapped people who either suffer from specific clinical syndromes, including those we have mentioned here and in Chapter 11, or who have major brain damage. The boundary between the former group and the normal population is not a clear-cut one. Whether the mildly retarded are identified as having problems depends on such factors as their personality characteristics, social opportunities, and the educational and vocational opportunities available to them.

Also important in determining whether mildly retarded individuals are regarded as having problems is the nature of the society into which they are born. Such children have more difficulty than children of normal intelligence in adapting to the needs of technologically sophisticated societies and those in which there is a high level of literacy. The Industrial Revolution led to the setting up of many institutions for those mentally retarded individuals for whom no place could be found in the industrial work force. Formerly such people had usually been able to find appropriate niches in the rural, village societies in which they lived. Even today many retarded individuals function well in 'third world' societies. The tasks which fall to many young people in such societies, such as minding cattle, sheep or goats, or carrying water from the river to the homestead, are well within their capabilities. If, however, they needed to acquire reading or mathematical skills to function, they would encounter difficulty.

Nowadays, in many parts of the developed world, the potential of the mildly retarded to become integrated into the mainstream of society is better understood than it used to be. Educational programmes, either in special classes or even in special schools, are provided for children who cannot benefit fully from regular school programmes. Families are given support and sometimes financial assistance to enable them to retain their retarded children in their homes, rather than having them placed in institutions. Employment opportunities still exist for those with practical, rather than academic, skills, and sheltered workshops and factories provide work for some who cannot function in the regular work place.

Assessment

The assessment of the skills and potentials of retarded children is usually carried out by educational psychologists. Educationalists also play a major part in the management of these children, who require skilled and specialized teaching. Social workers may be needed to assist these children and their families in overcoming the social adjustment problems they often experience. Family physicians, paediatricians, neurologists and speech therapists all have contributions to make in the management of retarded children, especially in the assessment and treatment of the most severely retarded. Psychiatric skills are required mainly in the management of the emotional and behavioural problems which are often present. Ideally the management of retarded children should be a multidisciplinary undertaking, with contributions from all the above professional groups.

As with other disorders, a comprehensive assessment of the child in the context of his or her family, school and neighbourhood should first be undertaken. In each case the following should be considered in planning a management strategy:

• the medical and biological status of the child;
• the stability of the family and its capacity to provide needed cognitive stimulation and to promote the child's self-esteem;

- the educational status of the child;
- any emotional and/or behavioural problems the child presents.

In many developed countries centres have been established for the early detection, assessment and remediation of developmental delays and problems. These are usually staffed by teams made up of professionals from the disciplines mentioned above. A careful appraisal of each child's developmental and learning problems, perceptual deficits, emotional status and social background leads to a plan of action by one or more members of the team.

Treatment methods

The treatment of emotional and behavioural problems in mentally retarded children follows the same general lines as the treatment of such problems in children of higher intelligence, but some special considerations apply. The following approaches may all be of value.

(a) Behaviour therapy

This is widely used in the treatment of the behavioural problems of the mentally retarded (Yule & Carr, 1980; Crnic & Reid, 1989). Learning theory, upon which behaviour therapy is based, applies as much to the behaviour of retarded children as it does to that of other children. Retarded children tend to learn more slowly, however, so that a greater number of behavioural trials may be needed to achieve similar results. Suitable programmes can promote toilet training, the extinction of such behaviours as temper tantrums, rocking and head banging, the acquisition of motor and speech and language skills and other therapeutic aims.

(b) Other individual therapies

Action-oriented, rather than talking therapies, are particularly suitable for use with retarded children. These include role playing, from which people can often learn more than they can from the verbal discussion and explanation of things; the prescription of tasks and rituals, which may have metaphorical significance (Barker, 1985); and play therapy in its various forms. In using any of these methods the level of cognitive functioning of the child must be taken into account, and the activity matched to this.

(c) Family therapy

Many of the problems of retarded children and adolescents are intimately grounded in their family systems. Family therapy approaches are as applicable to families containing retarded members as they are to other families. Retarded family members of any age often participate enthusiastically in the various action and other special techniques that may be used during family therapy (Barker, 1992, Chapter 11).

(d) Medication

The indications for the use of psychotropic drugs in retarded children are similar to those for other disturbed children. Epilepsy, if present, should be controlled by the use of anticonvulsants. Hyperactivity may respond to methylphenidate or amphetamines. If those drugs prove ineffective, haloperidol or phenothiazine drugs may be helpful.

In the treatment of children who display seriously aggressive and disruptive behaviour, structured and individualized behavioural management programmes are to be preferred as the first therapeutic choice, but medication can be helpful. Phenothiazine drugs such as thioridazine are sometimes of real value but their prolonged use is to be avoided as far as possible. As well as the risk of side-effects with prolonged use, most of the drugs which are effective in controlling aggressive behaviour are prone to produce a degree of sedation which can impair learning – already a problem for these children.

(e) Residential care

Institutional care is necessary for some children, including most of the very severely retarded, such as those who are doubly incontinent and are incapable of the basics of self care. Whether it is needed for a particular child depends on a complex number of factors including the degree of retardation present, the severity of any associated physical handicaps (which are common in the severely retarded), and the capacity of the child's family to provide the care needed. When residential care is required, it should be in small, well staffed units as near as possible to the child's family. Only a small minority of the most severely retarded require the full facilities of a hospital. Most are better placed in small hostels or group homes.

Other management considerations

In dealing with intellectually handicapped children a middle course has to be steered between asking too much of them and asking too little.

Facing such children with tasks, for example in school, which are beyond them can be emotionally damaging. It may lead to needless anxiety, even despair and depression, as well as to a lowering of self-esteem. On the other hand, asking too little, as may happen in a large hospital ward or institution, may mean that the child's potential is not realized.

The assessment of developmentally retarded children should be a continuing process. Their progress, including their responses to the education, treatment or other help they may be receiving, should be monitored regularly. Management plans invariably need to be modified from time to time, and sometimes new ones are needed, when earlier ones have either achieved their objectives or have proved unsuccessful.

Continuity of care is also important. Retarded children often find change difficult, and the care of these individuals should be undertaken as a long-term commitment. The needs of the family must always be kept in mind. It is possible for the attention given a handicapped child to have adverse effects on the care of other children in the family. For the parents, the presence in the family of a seriously retarded child, especially one who also has behavioural or emotional problems, can prove a severe emotional strain and may affect the stability of their marriage.

Outcome

Clinical experience suggests that psychiatric disorders in retarded children respond to treatment in much the same way as similar disorders in other children. It is necessary, however, to distinguish the symptoms and behaviours due to superimposed psychiatric disorders from those due to the child's cognitive delays. Retarded children can suffer from depressive or anxiety disorders, they may develop adjustment disorders or psychotic ones or any of the other conditions discussed elsewhere in this book. While their limited verbal and cognitive skills often dictate the use of non-verbal rather than verbal treatment approaches, therapy should not be withheld because of their intellectual handicap.

While we have no effective treatments for many of the conditions responsible for severe retardation (phenylketonuria being a notable exception), the adverse sociocultural circumstances of many more mildly retarded children can often be ameliorated through the provision of appropriate educational, social and recreational programmes. Professional help often needs to be directed to these children's families, since they are in the best position to stimulate their children's development and help them achieve the best possible level of functioning.

The development of retarded children, like that of other children, depends very much on the general care and the cognitive and other stimulation they receive. Given suitable care, stable family backgrounds, and appropriate treatment of any superimposed psychiatric problems, most mildly retarded children are able to make a satisfactory adjustment in society. Their intellectual limitations do, however, complicate their care, management and education, and place constraints on the ultimate outcomes that may be expected. Sometimes the biggest limiting factor, though, is that imposed by parents, therapists and other professionals, and even the children themselves, who too often take an unduly gloomy view of what these children can achieve.

Chapter 20

Child Abuse and Neglect

While child abuse and neglect are not in themselves psychiatric disorders, they are encountered so frequently in the families of emotionally and behaviourally disturbed children that they merit a chapter in this book. All who work with disturbed children need to be ever alert for evidence that abuse, in one or more of its various forms, has played, or is playing, a part in causing the emotional or behavioural problems with which they are presented.

Background

Child abuse and neglect are not new phenomena. Lynch (1985) pointed out that they are referred to in literature dating back as far as the second century AD. The London Society for the Prevention of Cruelty to Children dealt with 762 cases in the three years following its founding in 1884. These comprised assaults (333), starvations (81), dangerous neglect (130), desertions (30), cruel exposure to excite sympathy (70), 'other wrongs' (116), and deaths (25). The society took 132 cases, many 'almost incredible', to court, and there were 120 convictions (Lynch, 1985). Charles Dickens described graphically, in several of his novels, the plight of many children in Victorian days.

For many years there seemed to be a lack of communication and understanding between those dealing with and interested in abusive situations in the community (such as statutory and voluntary child welfare agencies and novelists like Dickens), and the medical and allied professions. The former saw abuse and neglect as major social problems. The latter for many years largely overlooked their medical aspects. A contributory factor, at least as far as sexual abuse is concerned, may have been Sigmund Freud's conclusion, which was not based on valid research, that the past sexual abuses reported by many of his patients were fantasies rather than historical facts.

Then, in 1946, Caffey, a radiologist, described cases of multiple fractures of the long bones of children, in association with subdural haematomas (bleeding under the *dural* membrane surrounding the brain). He suggested that the fractures were due to inflicted trauma, and it has since been established that physically abused children often show radiological evidence of old fractures. Kempe, *et al.* (1962) coined the term *battered child syndrome*. This seemed to capture the imagination of the medical and related professions and led to increased interest in and recognition of what is sometimes called *non-accidental injury* (Scott, 1977) or, more often nowadays, just *child abuse*.

In addition to abuse causing physical injury, other forms are recognized. These include neglect, which seems to have existed from time immemorial, and sexual and emotional abuse.

Child abuse, in its many and various forms, is important to child psychiatrists because of its role in the aetiology of psychiatric disorders and self-esteem and other problems in children. It is frequently found to be associated with other problems in these children's families.

Incidence

There are wide variations in the reported incidence of child abuse and neglect. While this is no doubt due in part to real differences in the incidence in different populations, other important factors are differences in the definition of abuse and neglect, and variations in the methods used to estimate incidence. In some parts of the world children are systematically exploited in ways that can scarcely be called anything else but abuse. I refer to such practices as the use of young children in the 'sweat shops' of some third world countries, and the selling of young girls, some not even in their teens, by their parents, to work as prostitutes in the brothels of certain countries. Moreover the ruthless exploitation of children in such ways is not confined to the third world. Consider this Canadian newspaper report:

'Judge Peter Leveque said it was clear from the sickening testimony he heard that the 16-year-old girl was as much a victim of this child prostitution ring as were the 12-year-old and two 13-year-old girls she controlled.

But Leveque said the 16-year-old's tough plight in life doesn't excuse her from the torment she inflicted on the three girls when they were raped by an Asian gang or forced to have sex with dozens of other customers.' (*Calgary Herald*, 1993.)

Incidentally the cavalier attitude society and its legal fraternity take to cases such as the above is reflected in the fact that, at the time the above report was published, the 26-year-old man alleged to be the brains behind the child prostitution ring had been freed on bail and, not too surprisingly, had failed to appear in court on the required date.

Cases such as the above, though unfortunately not rare, are only a small part of the child abuse and neglect spectrum. Much abuse, and most neglect, occurs in the family. Even when the actual acts of abuse do not occur in the family setting, the children may have suffered a lack of proper care within their families.

In the USA, studies of children aged 3 to 17 have found rates of physical abuse varying between 19 and 36 per thousand. In the case of sexual abuse, MacFarlane & Waterman (1986) have estimated that there are between 100 000 and 500 000 new cases per year in the USA. Because most of the abuse of children occurs within the family, obtaining complete data is virtually impossible. Much abuse is hidden from the outside world. Sometimes it only comes to light many years later, when adults report it retrospectively. Recent years have also seen the late reporting of abuse that occurred many years earlier in children's institutions.

Physical and sexual abuse of children involve the commission of specific acts, whereas neglect and emotional abuse are less easy to define, though no less real. Problems of definition are even greater in these areas. How many times does a parent have to call a child 'stupid' or 'good for nothing' for it to constitute emotional abuse? There is no easy answer to such questions, and to complicate the matter further, much depends on the non-verbal messages that accompany such statements. There are many ways of saying, 'That was a stupid thing to do' – some light-hearted and jocular, others angry and demeaning.

Despite these difficulties, however, there is little doubt that abuse of all types is common and that it is a major issue for child psychiatrists and their colleagues.

The causes of child abuse

The aetiology of child abuse is complex. As Schmidt & Eldridge (1986, page 269) put it:

'Child maltreatment is a multiply-determined phenomenon that does not lend itself to definitive explanations. The parent, the child, the circumstances, and the environment all contribute to the occurrence of maltreatment.'

(a) Parental factors

Many adults who abuse children have themselves been abused as children. Those who have grown up in abusive homes tend to have identified with a model of parenthood which encompasses the use of violence. They may see physical punishment as the preferred way of dealing with undesired behaviour in children. On the other hand, abuse is not inevitably transmitted from one generation to the next. Many factors may diminish the likelihood of this happening (Kaufman & Zigler, 1987).

Adults who abuse children are often found to have serious personality problems. They may lack adequate impulse control. In their role as parents, they may have difficulty showing love in affectionate, caring ways. Abuse may occur when the perpetrator is under the influence of alcohol or other drugs, which may further impair impulse control.

Neglectful and abusive parents often have problems in other areas of their lives. Their social and vocational skills may be poor, their intelligence below average, and they may have difficulty with the instrumental tasks of everyday living. It seems that the greater the stress parents face, the greater the risk that the limit of their frustration tolerance will be reached and they will abuse their children. While abuse often occurs in families experiencing difficulty coping with the instrumental task of daily living, it is also encountered in families with good incomes and middle-class respectability, though perhaps less frequently.

The neglect of children is often but one of a number of problems in seriously dysfunctional families. There is often serious psychopathology in the parent or parents – often only one is present. The parent(s) may be addicted to alcohol or other drugs, they may be depressed or they may have serious personality disorders.

(b) Child factors

We have seen that children vary greatly in their temperaments. Some are easier to rear than others and sometimes there is a serious clash of temperaments between child and parents – or other adults. Some children find that they only get parental attention when they behave in provocative ways, so that they learn patterns of behaviour which stimulate their abusively inclined parents to acts of violence, emotional abuse or even incest.

Abused children often seem to have poor self-images. They may consider themselves worthy of no more than the treatment they receive, though this may be a consequence of abuse as well as a contributory factor. Children with handicaps or disabilities or various sorts may be at increased risk of abuse. In individual cases this sometimes seems to be the case, but it is not clear how far this is generally true (White, *et al.*, 1987).

(c) Interactional, family and social factors

Child maltreatment seems sometimes to have its origins in the early relationship between parent and child, that is the period during which attachment is normally developed and consolidated. Disorders of attachment may increase the chances of abuse occurring (Schmidt & Eldridge, 1986).

Various other family problems may be found in association with child abuse. For example, Oliver & Buchanan (1979) described an extended family network in which there was an established pattern of abuse. Starting with a mentally retarded young woman and the six men she successively lived with, these authors studied her children and their descendants. In all, 40 members of the family, and their spouses or partners, were investigated. There was revealed a tragic saga, transmitted from generation to generation, of physical neglect, assaults on the children with hammers and knives, incest, prostitution (sometimes taught to the children by the parents), burns causing persistent poker marks, bites, beatings, and hair pullings. While families as dysfunctional as this one are mercifully relatively uncommon, they do exist, and there are many others with problems that differ only in degree.

Child abuse is not confined to families and children living at home. It may occur in correctional and other residential institutions, schools, daycare centres, courts, child care agencies, welfare departments and other settings. Children suffer grievously as a result of wars and civil unrest (Garbarino, *et al.*, 1991). As this is written there are no doubt millions of suffering children in Bosnia, Angola, Burundi, the Sudan and Azerbaijan – to name just a few of the world's current trouble spots. Difficult as it is for many parents to provide optimal care for their children in countries where there are peace and reasonable social and other resources, the tasks facing parents in the less developed parts of the world, and those where there is a state of war, are often overwhelming.

Clinical considerations

In only a minority of cases do families come asking for help because they are abusing their children. Physically abused children are often brought to hospital emergency departments, perhaps with a story that they have fallen downstairs, out of bed or against an item of furniture or household appliance. The tales told by parents can be detailed and imaginative, but they are usually inconsistent and nearly always incompatible with the nature of the child's injuries. Moreover, a full and careful examination of the child usually reveals evidence of previous injury.

Suspected child abuse is sometimes reported to child welfare agencies by neighbours or relatives, who may have heard the child screaming in pain or have observed injuries. Other cases come to notice at school, in daycare centres or during routine physical examinations. The injuries may consist of bruising of any degree of severity, fractures, injury to internal organs, perhaps with internal bleeding, intracranial haemorrhage with consequent damage to the brain, or loss of vision due to eye injuries. Fatal injuries are sometimes inflicted.

Physical abuse may or may not be associated with neglect or emotional abuse. Abused children may be malnourished and ill-cared for. Medical attention may not be sought when it is needed. Both physical and psychological development may be adversely affected. Yet some physically abused children appear to be generally well cared for; in such cases satisfactory general care may be interrupted by episodes of rage during which the child is injured. Some abusing parents display offhand, uncaring attitudes and show a lack of concern about their child's condition. They may be reluctant to accept admission to hospital or investigation for their child, and may have been to many different hospitals. Evidence may emerge of such other family problems as marital conflict, or the abuse of alcohol or other drugs.

Abused children tend to have difficulty enjoying themselves, behaviour problems, withdrawal, oppositional behaviour, hypervigilance, compulsive behaviour, pseudo-adult manner, and learning problems at school (Martin & Beezley, 1977). Low self-esteem seems to characterize both these children and their mothers (Oates, et al. 1985; Oates & Forrest, 1985). In infants, language development may be delayed (Allen & Wasserman, 1985). Abused children may appear fearful towards their parents, perhaps getting upset when they hear father returning home; and they may show 'reversed caring' by anxiously looking out for their parents' needs, offering mother one of her cigarettes and so on. In severe cases of neglect, the child may appear obviously ill-cared for, dirty, under-nourished or even dehydrated.

Sexual abuse may occur in the absence of other forms of abuse or neglect and can continue for long periods undetected. The sexual abuse of girls occurs more frequently than that of boys. It may consist of anything from fondling of the child's breasts or genitals to vaginal or anal intercourse. Another form of sexual abuse is the sexual exploitation of children in pornographic movies, videotapes and photographs. The abuser is often someone known to the child, frequently a family member. Parents, step-parents and foster parents are responsible in many instances. The incest taboo which operates in many natural families seems often to be less strong in reconstituted families, a situation which may lead to stepfather-stepdaughter incest. Sexual abuse by someone outside the family or the family's intimate circle tends to be reported sooner and thus often comes to attention more quickly.

Apart from physical signs of damage in the genital area and evidence of sexually acquired disease, sexual abuse may be suspected if the child shows seductive behaviour, sexual knowledge inappropriate for his or her age, severe psychosomatic or acting-out behaviour (especially non-epileptic seizures or running away), or sexually precocious behaviour. Self-destructive behaviour in the absence of other stress, or pregnancy in the early teen years, especially if the father is not named, are other ways in which sexual behaviour may present.

Ghent, *et al.* (1985) provided useful guidelines in detecting physical and sexual abuse.

Emotional abuse

Many children's emotional and other psychological needs are not adequately met in their families. How severe the family's failure to meet its children's needs must be to justify use of the term *emotional abuse* is an arbitrary judgement, although extreme cases are readily identified. The term could be applied to many children with psychiatric disorders.

In many jurisdictions laws have been enacted defining emotional abuse. These aim to provide a legal basis for intervention in cases in which there is no obvious physical abuse or neglect but there is gross failure to meet children's psychological needs. An example of such legislation is contained in the Child Welfare Act of the Canadian province of Alberta (Government of Alberta, 1984). This uses the term *emotional injury* rather than abuse. It states that a child is emotionally injured:

(i) if there is substantial and observable impairment of the child's mental or emotional functioning that is evidenced by a mental or behavioural disorder, including anxiety, depression, withdrawal, aggression or delayed development, and

(ii) there are reasonable and probable grounds to believe that the emotional injury is the result of
  (a) rejection,
  (b) deprivation of affection or cognitive stimulation,
  (c) exposure to domestic violence or severe domestic disharmony, or
  (d) inappropriate criticism, threats, humiliation, accusations or expectations of or towards the child, or
  (e) the mental or emotional condition of the guardian of the child or chronic alcohol or drug abuse by anyone living in the same residence as the child.

Garbarino, *et al.* (1986) use the term *psychologically battered child*. They define five forms of *psychically destructive* behaviour:

- *Rejecting:* the adult refuses to acknowledge the child's worth and the legitimacy of the child's needs.
- *Isolating:* the child is cut off by the adult from normal social experiences, prevented from forming friendships and made to believe the world is capricious and hostile.
- *Ignoring:* the adult deprives the child of needed stimulation and fails to respond in suitable ways, stifling emotional growth and intellectual development.
- *Corrupting:* the child is 'mis-socialized', being stimulated to engage in destructive antisocial behaviour and reinforced in such deviant behaviour.

Garbarino and his co-authors (1986) provide examples of how each of the above types of behaviour by adults may affect children at different stages of development. In extreme cases the syndrome of *non-organic failure to thrive* may develop (Bullard, *et al.*, 1967). *Deprivation dwarfism* is another term that has been used for growth failure related to adverse rearing experiences, though in this syndrome the failure to grow is usually due at least as much to the provision of insufficient food as to emotional abuse.

In most instances of emotional abuse the child's growth and physical condition are within normal limits, but there are problems of psychological development and of emotional and behavioural adjustment. These often include poor self-esteem, unresolved anger or almost any of the psychiatric syndromes described elsewhere in this book, the main exceptions being those of predominantly organic origin. Conduct disorders, chronic anxiety disorders, and academic failure are common consequences, and as the children grow older some come to meet the criteria for personality disorders.

Many parents who fail to meet their children's emotional needs have themselves experienced poor parenting as children. Covitz (1986) refers to emotional abuse as the 'family curse', handed down from generation to generation. He points out that it is what the parents are and do, rather than what they tell their children, that are important. He describes three 'abusive styles of parenting'. He labels these 'the inadequate parent', 'the devouring parent' and 'the tyrannical parent'. Later in his book he suggests various approaches to breaking the intergenerational cycle of emotional abuse. Many children's behavioural, emotional or physical symptoms may be seen as danger signals – signs that their needs are not being met and opportunities for intervention.

Assessment and treatment

Abused children and their families should be assessed and treated using the principles and approaches set out elsewhere in this book. There are however certain special points to be borne in mind in dealing with these families. Mature clinical judgement and a patient, painstaking and empathic approach are essential. These families tend to be especially defensive. They are often aware that they may face criminal charges and risk having their children removed from their care against their wishes.

A physical examination should be carried out when physical or sexual abuse is suspected. It should include examination of the genitals, and radiological and other special investigations as indicated.

In most jurisdictions the law requires that established or suspected child abuse be reported to the appropriate authorities. It is usually best to deal with the statutory child welfare agency, the staff of which can then involve the police as necessary.

Once it is established that abuse has occurred, the child welfare agency staff are responsible for taking any immediate steps to assure the safety and welfare of the child. They must decide whether to remove the child from the care of the parents or guardians. Admission to hospital and medical or surgical treatment may be necessary. Meanwhile investigation of the family is carried out, if the abuse has been intrafamilial, usually by a social worker from the child welfare agency. At this stage psychiatric help may be sought, either for the whole family or for one or more of its members.

Evidence of abuse, or reason to suspect it, may emerge during the psychiatric assessment or treatment of child or family. In many jurisdictions the person discovering or suspecting the abuse has a legal obligation to report the facts or suspicions to the appropriate agency. In that case I explain to the family members my legal obligations and assure them of my willingness to continue to offer them help. If the family chooses to remain in treatment with me, I can sometimes act as its advocate in its dealings with the child welfare agency.

In working with abusive families it is important to adopt an empathic, non-punitive attitude, however distressing you may find the situations that come to your attention. It can be hard to remain objective and non-judgemental when one is faced with parents or others who have gravely injured or sexually abused a child. Nevertheless it is unhelpful for us to express the anger or outrage we may feel when confronted with such situations. To do so militates against forming effective therapeutic relationships. It is important also not to get emotionally over involved. Many child abusers are plausible, attractive, even charming people. We may come to feel sorry for them because of the hard and deprived lives they have led, or because they themselves have been subject to abuse as children. Like abused children, their principal need is for skilled treatment rather than sympathy, however. They may be expert at manipulating social agencies and authority figures, for example by suggesting that their behaviour and attitudes are changing, thus pleasing the therapist, when in reality they have not changed significantly. The naive therapist can easily be deceived.

It is not necessarily helpful to extract a confession from parents or other adults who have abused children. Sometimes it is enough to tell them that the child's injuries are not compatible with the story given. Investigation and treatment can then proceed on the basis of an unspoken understanding on the part of the adult(s) concerned that the issue is one of abuse, not accidental injury. Securing convictions and applying penalties are the work of the courts and the judiciary, not the helping professions.

The situation is usually rather different when a child has been abused by someone outside the family. In such cases the family is usually united in condemnation of the perpetrator and cooperates actively in the investigation of the case and the treatment the abused child requires. There can nevertheless be major emotional repercussions in the family. The parents may feel guilt, which may be denied, for allowing their child to get into the situation in which the abuse occurred. Sometimes pre-existing family problems are brought to light by an episode of abuse by an outsider – for example inadequate supervision of the children, parental disagreement about the limits to be set to the children's behaviours or activities, or inadequate nurturance which may have led to children seeking nurturance from others who may then exploit them by abusing them.

Many sexually abused children are quite young. Mian, *et al.* (1986) reported that one-third of such children presenting to an acute care hospital were aged 6 or less. In investigating possible sexual abuse, especially in young children, the use of 'anatomically correct' dolls has been advocated. While this procedure was initially greeted with great enthusiasm by many working in the field, it seems that it has not proved as useful as it was initially hoped it would be. The child is interviewed in a playroom containing, among other items, a series of dolls representing adults and children of both sexes. During the interview the child is given the opportunity to play with the dolls and talk about them. White, *et al.* (1986) described a procedure for the use of these dolls. It consists of five parts:

- Identification of the dolls by sex and name.
- Assessment of the child's knowledge of the body parts, sexual and non-sexual, by name and function.

- 'Private part knowledge'.
- 'Abuse evaluation', consisting of asking the child about being touched, hurt, having secrets, receiving threats, and other items which might indicate sexual abuse.
- 'Abuse elaboration', in which any 'positive answers' to the questions in the previous stage are followed up.

The treatment needed by abused children and their families depends on the type and duration of the abuse, and whether the abuse is intrafamilial or is committed by a stranger. Therapy for the whole family may be needed when the abuse is intrafamilial; in such cases there often prove to be serious family system problems. Individual therapy (Jones, 1986) or group therapy may be needed by children who have been abused, especially when there has been a long-standing incestuous relationship with a parent. Group therapy, in which children are treated along with others who have been similarly abused, can often be more helpful than individual therapy. The support and acceptance by others who have had similar experiences can be particularly comforting to many abused subjects. The group can often provide a safe and secure situation in which to talk about difficult and emotionally painful subjects – subjects these children often cannot talk comfortably about in other contexts.

Many abusive parents are also in need of psychiatric help. They may prove to have any of a variety of problems, including personality disorders, anxiety disorders, alcoholism or the effects of drug abuse.

When the abuser is someone outside the family, the main need may be for individual or group therapy for the child. The parents may need guidance on how to deal with the child and help in dealing with their own feelings.

The treatment of abusive families should be a multidisciplinary process. Close cooperation between whoever is providing therapy for the family members and the staff of the child welfare agency, especially the social worker dealing with the family, greatly improves the chances of success. The police and the courts may also be involved, and sometimes the possibility of legal action against abusive parents or other relatives is retained – prosecution not being immediately undertaken – with the objective of increasing the family members' motivation for treatment. This may be achieved by postponing court proceedings, or sentencing, while the effects of therapy, and the family's or the parents' involvement in treatment, are monitored. Alternatively an abusing adult may be placed on probation with a condition that he or she undergoes treatment. It is generally preferable to have a situation in which the family enters therapy voluntarily and willingly. Unfortunately many families do not do this.

Sometimes it is not possible to ensure that the situation in the home is safe, so that it becomes necessary to remove the abused child(ren) from the home. This may be temporary, while treatment is instituted or, if treatment is refused or fails, it may be permanent. In cases of parent-child (it is most often father-daughter or stepfather-daughter) incest it may be more appropriate for the parent to leave, perhaps to go to a treatment setting. In any event, a well planned long-term programme of treatment and rehabilitation for all involved in the abuse should be developed and carried through. Frequent episodes of removal of abused or neglected children, with their periodic return, as happens all too frequently in many jurisdictions, should be avoided.

In cases in which abuse is primarily or predominantly emotional, the main need is to rectify the underlying family problems, using appropriate family therapy or other techniques.

The treatment of abused children and their families is often a long and difficult process, requiring skilled personnel, close cooperation between therapist(s) and agencies, and careful long-term planning. Prevention is much to be preferred, and there is reason to believe that a preventative health service for young children and their families, with frequent visits by nurses and other workers is helpful (Wynn, 1974).

Outcome

A wide variety of physical consequences may result from child abuse (Barker, 1993c). These include permanent mental retardation, blindness, cerebral palsy and other physical injuries and deformities. The psychological consequences are harder to define but a poor self-image, personality and behaviour problems, and delayed development in various areas of functioning are among them. In many cases it is difficult to separate the effects of physical or sexual abuse from those of the other family problems which are often found to exist. Children are rarely abused in healthy, well-functioning families, and factors other than the abuse *per se* probably contribute to the poor outcomes reported in many studies (Lynch, 1978; Hensey, *et al.*, 1983; Oates, 1984).

Elmer (1986) found, in a comparative study of three groups of infants, two of them abused, that the effects of socioeconomic status were more marked than those of abuse. Oates (1984) compared the personality development of abused children with controls matched for age, sex, ethnic group and social class. On follow-up several years later, the abused children were found to have fewer friends, lower self-esteem, and more behavioural disturbance, and to be less ambitious than the children in the control group.

Sexual abuse can lead to problems of psychosexual adjustment later in life. It seems to be associated with runaway behaviour, anxiety and suicidal behaviour in adolescence (McCormack, *et al.*, 1986).

Chapter 21

The Treatment of Child Psychiatric Disorders

The diagnostic formulation made after child and family have been assessed should be the basis of the treatment plan. The formulation should be kept under review and modified as new information comes to light – as it often does in the course of treatment – and as therapeutic goals are achieved. The range of treatment measures that may be required includes the following:

- Individual psychotherapy.
- Therapy or counselling for the parents.
- Family therapy.
- Group therapy for children or parents.
- Behaviour therapy.
- Pharmacotherapy.
- Hypnotherapy.
- Daypatient treatment.
- Inpatient treatment.
- Alternative families.
- Educational measures.
- Speech therapy.
- Other environmental change, including removal from parental care.

This list is not exhaustive and some disturbed children have other special needs – motor coordination problems, for example, which need to be addressed in therapy. Because most child psychiatric disorders have multiple causes, it is often necessary to use more than one treatment.

Setting treatment goals

The goals of treatment should be determined and agreed by therapist(s) and client(s) before therapy starts. It is helpful to have agreement, at least in general terms, on how things will be when treatment is success-fully completed. When children, especially younger ones, are the main objects of concern, it will usually be the parents who are mainly involved in this, but older children, and especially adolescents, should also be involved as much as possible. At the same time we must bear in mind that many psychiatric disorders cause impaired judgement. Depressed individuals, for example, often have little or no hope for the future, so that it can be difficult for them to engage constructively in treatment planning.

In planning treatment it is helpful to take into account the points discussed in the section on 'defining the desired outcome' in Chapter 5.

Individual psychotherapy

The essence of individual psychotherapy is the development of a relationship between therapist and patient (or client), in the context of which change in some aspect of the patient's mental state and/or behaviour is promoted. Every contact between child (or indeed a client of any age) and therapist has the potential to be of therapeutic value, though such contacts can also be anti-therapeutic.

There are many schools of psychotherapy (Zeig and Munion, 1990), and great differences between some of them, but it is not possible here to do more than outline some general principles. Psychotherapy can only be learned 'on the job' and with supervision from an experienced therapist. The following points are relevant, even if psychotherapy is not the primary treatment being used:

(1) Start by accepting your child patients as they are. Whether a child's symptoms are expressions of anxiety, depression or hostility, disapproving or judgemental attitudes are likely to worsen the situation, rather than improve it. Acceptance of children as they are does not imply approval of all they do or feel. Indeed child and therapist are often able to agree on aspects of the child's behaviour, feelings or attitudes that need to change.

(2) Remember that children rarely come for treatment of their own accord. They are brought by others who are worried or concerned about them, or perhaps angry with them. They may arrive with the expectation that they will meet someone who is going to have similar feelings for them. Some parents, though nowadays mercifully few, even present the visit to the psychiatrist as a sort of punishment, or tell their children to expect 'a good talking to'. In such cases the therapist may have to work hard to gain the child's confidence, a process which may take several, even many, interviews.

(3)   Do not plunge straight into a discussion of the presenting problems or symptoms, unless these are brought up by the child.

(4)   Concentrate initially on achieving an understanding of the child's feelings and point of view. It is only when there is such understanding between child and therapist that free communication, such as is a prerequisite to successful treatment, becomes possible. The child should come to see the therapist as someone who is concerned about him or her. This will not necessarily prevent the expression of angry or other negative feelings, in fact it will facilitate the expression of such feelings when these need expression. The experience of giving vent to negative feelings, or revealing 'bad' things about oneself and not being rejected, lectured, blamed or criticized as a result, can itself be therapeutic.

(5)   Remember that, while free expression of feelings is to be encouraged, limits have to be set in the psychotherapeutic setting, as in other situations. For example, physically hurting the therapist, dangerous activities like playing with live electrical fittings, or damaging the fabric of the room and its furnishings and equipment cannot be allowed. It is a good plan to outline the limits of permissible behaviour at the start of treatment. Limits should be imposed on the basis of 'I can't allow you to do that', and with an explanation of the reason why the behaviour is unacceptable. The child's desire to carry out the activity should however be acknowledged and accepted.

(6)   Tell the child about the confidential nature of the interview, and explain the limits to that confidentially. Essentially these extend to reporting any suspected abuse or neglect to the appropriate authorities and to telling someone, usually the parents, if the child expresses something as serious as the desire or intention to commit suicide. I do not usually mention the possibility of the subpoena of records and reports by courts, unless the case is one in which legal proceedings are under way or are likely.

Before embarking on psychotherapy it is necessary to have a plan and to be clear what the treatment is aiming to achieve. These aims should have been set out in the diagnostic formulation.

Psychotherapy may aim to do anything from providing *support*, which usually aims to help the patient cope better with current stressful circumstances, to psychoanalysis which aims to bring about radical change in the patient's emotional reactions and relationships. Supportive psychotherapy may be appropriate when a child faces an acute or severe stress which is likely to subside in the course of time, for example the illness or admission to hospital of a parent or the grief reaction following a bereavement. It may also be needed when a child faces continuous stress which cannot easily be removed, though ideally treatment would lead to elimination of the stress.

Psychoanalysis, in its classical form, involves intensive, long-term treatment, often with therapy sessions occurring as often as five days a week over a period of many months or even years. It is a highly specialized treatment requiring long and rigorous training, and an analysis of the trainee therapist. The objective of the treatment is to explore fully the patient's unconscious life and fantasies, dealing with any problems that are found in the context of the relationship between patient and therapist – the *transference* relationship. Partly because of the great amount of time it takes, and the consequent expense, and also because few, if any, trained analysts are available in many communities, psychoanalysis is not widely used. Child analysis is a particularly specialized field in which Anna Freud (1966; 1972) and Melanie Klein (1932) were pioneers. Although their methods are used by only a very small number of those treating disturbed children, their work is of considerable theoretical interest and has helped in the understanding of children's problems.

The techniques used in the different types of psychotherapy vary widely, depending on the theoretical orientation of the therapist, the treatment goals and the patient's age. Some therapists make extensive use of verbal interpretations of the child's play and statements, while others make little or no use of such interpretation. Some therapists take on a more active role than others. As a general rule, the younger the child, the more the therapy uses play, and such other non-verbal activities as drawing, painting and modelling. Nevertheless some children as young as three or four talk freely. How freely they communicate depends on their level of cognitive, especially language, development and their emotional state.

Common to all forms of psychotherapy with children are:

- The development of a working relationship with the child.
- An appraisal of the feelings and ideas the child expresses in the context of the relationship.
- The use of the relationship to help resolve the child's problems.

How can psychotherapy help children? The first level of help is the simple process of accepting the child's feelings. We all tend to feel better after we have spoken to an accepting and understanding person about things that are worrying us or which are sources of anger or shame for us. This applies equally to disturbed children. It accounts for the considerable improvement that sometimes follows a single interview, even one carried out primarily for diagnostic purposes. For some children it is a new experience to be listened to and given the full attention of an accepting and non-critical adult. When such children discover that what they say does not appear to shock, create anxiety or provoke expressions of outrage in the interviewer, this can be a considerable relief to them.

In many cases it is not sufficient for children just to express their feelings and have them acknowledged and accepted by the therapist. There has also to be emotional interchange between therapist and child. The aim is to help make the child's problems and conflicts manifest – which often involves putting them into words and helping the child understand them, not just or even mainly intellectually, but at a deeper emotional level. Interpretations, if they are used, are usually left until the meaning of a child's play or talk is clear. It is inadvisable to offer speculative interpretations, though incorrect ones are often ignored or rejected.

All the principles outlined above are derived from the psychodynamic view of psychiatric disorders. With the possible exception of supportive therapy, they all aim to use the therapist/child relationship as the context – perhaps metaphor would be a better word – for the resolution of the repressed conflicts which are held to be responsible for the child's symptoms. This is the essence of the methods of such therapists as Allen (1942), Maclay (1970) and Adams (1982).

The wide variety of approaches which are practised under the rubric of *psychotherapy* is illustrated in *What is Psychotherapy?* (Zeig & Munion, 1990). In this book 81 therapists of different schools describe their varied approaches, and offer their definitions of psychotherapy.

What the different psychotherapies have in common may be the process of 'reframing' – or changing the perceived meaning of something (Barker, 1994). It may be a symptom, a repetitive behaviour pattern, or a belief system that is reframed. A type of reframing which is often clinically useful is *positive connotation*. This redefines the intent behind a behaviour. For example, the behaviour of a parent who physically abuses a child might be reframed as being a well-intentioned attempt to discipline the child and eliminate the antisocial behaviour in which the child has been engaging. While the parent's actions are not condoned, their intent is. Therapy then becomes a matter of finding better, socially acceptable ways of achieving the same ends.

Developmental reframing (Coppersmith, 1981) is the re-interpretation of behaviours as characteristic of a different developmental stage than that to which they have been regarded as belonging. Thus the behaviour of the angry, self-centred adolescent boy who is reacting to frustration with displays of temper may be reframed as immature – as being more like that of the toddler who has a tantrum when he does not get his way. The behaviour is thus interpreted as not being that of a 'bad' boy but as being that of one who has not yet grown up.

Various 'strategic' therapy techniques, many of them developed by family therapists, may be used with individuals, including children and adolescents. Examples are the use of paradox, pioneered by Frankl (1960). This can be useful for patients whose problems worsen as they struggle to resist or counter symptoms of which they wish to be rid. Frankl encouraged his patients to bring on or increase their symptoms, but often in a humorous context and always in ways which enabled them to distance themselves from the symptoms. Rapid change sometimes results (Barker, 1981; Weeks & L'Abate, 1982).

Metaphorical approaches, especially the use of stories with metaphorical meanings, may be particularly useful in treating children, who often enjoy being told or read stories. Metaphors may be constructed to serve a variety of therapeutic objectives, for example reframing problem behaviours, helping people to recognize that they have within them resources of which they have been unaware, and suggesting solutions to challenges patients face – solutions they might not consider if they were presented directly. (For more information on the use of metaphors in psychotherapy see Barker, 1985; Wallas, 1985; and Mills & Crowley, 1986).

The work of Milton Erickson (Haley, 1973; Rosen, 1982; O'Hanlon & Hexum, 1990), one of the most creative of psychotherapists, is replete with demonstrations of the use of innovative strategic methods.

While therapy can only be learned by means of supervised clinical work, background reading can be helpful. In addition to the references mentioned above, *Play Therapy* (Landreth, 1982), which contains contributions by 31 authors, and *Psychotherapy with Adolescent Girls* (Lamb, 1986) are good sources of information. Rossman (1985) provides a good description of what therapy with a severely disturbed adolescent may involve.

Therapy and counselling with parents

It is seldom sufficient to provide psychotherapy, or any other treatment, for the child and to leave the parents uninvolved. The parents – or whoever the child lives with if it is not the parents – are enormously important in a child's life. The environment they offer their children, and what they do in response to problems their children develop, are crucial factors in determining outcome.

The initial formulation may reveal factors in the family which are responsible for or are maintaining the problem behaviours for which professional help is sought. There may be a need for counselling of the parents concerning their child's disorder and its treatment – often referred to as *casework* – or for psychotherapy for the parents themselves.

In parent counselling, or casework, the 'emphasis is clearly on the child as patient' (Kraemer, 1987). The aim is to enable the parents to understand the child's problems, the factors which have led to them, and those that are contributing to their continuation. This will include the parts the parents have played, although it is important to avoid suggesting that the parents are to blame for their child's problems. Many parents feel more than enough guilt about having a 'problem' child without the therapist making it any worse. It is important to keep the parents actively involved, emphasizing that they have key roles in the child's treatment and rehabilitation. There is a potential danger, especially when treatment extends over a long period and involves treatments that focus on the child, that the parents may get, or feel, left out. They may begin to leave it to the therapist to 'fix' the child who, they expect, will in due course be returned to them, rather like a car that has been repaired. The danger of this happening is greatest when the child is in residential treatment.

Kraemer (1987) describes the caseworker as 'educator, adviser, supporter, manager and, sometimes, psychotherapist'. The child's relationship with the parents is the main focus of the work. The past history of the child and family relationships, past and current, may be discussed. Casework may also include the promotion of environmental change, for example by mobilizing community resources (play groups, daycare centres, youth groups and the like), and community workers (youth leaders, school counsellors, credit counsellors and so forth) when a family is in need of such help.

Parent management training (PMT), which may be a part, even the main part, of the work done by a caseworker has been defined as comprising 'procedures in which a parent or parents are trained to interact differently with their child' (Kazdin, 1991, page 191).

The main features of PMT are summarized by Kazdin (1991, pages 191–195) who also reviews the literature and gives some clinical illustrations. Behaviour problems are considered to be inadvertently developed and maintained by 'maladaptive parent-child interactions'. The main features of PMT, as described by Kazdin (1991) are:

- Treatment primarily carried out with the parents, who implement in the home the procedures taught them.
- The parents are taught to identify, define and observe problem behaviours in new ways.
- The treatment is based on social learning principles and includes positive reinforcement, 'mild punishment' (such as 'time out from reinforcement' or loss of privileges), negotiation, and contingency contracting.
- The therapy sessions themselves allow the parents to see how the

techniques are implemented and to practise them, as well as to review the changes that have occurred in the home.

PMT uses many of the techniques of behaviour therapy. These are discussed briefly in a later section of this chapter and more fully in Murdoch & Barker (1991).

The borderline between casework and psychotherapy is ill-defined but it is crossed when therapy starts to focus on the parent or parents and their emotional problems or mental states. The parents of disturbed children often prove to have psychiatric problems of their own. Depression is common and may seriously affect parenting. Many parents have themselves had difficult childhoods; past abuse may have left emotional scars and personality problems which may need to be addressed as part of the overall treatment plan.

The relevance of the parents' psychiatric problems to the child's disorder will vary but in many instances they appear to be significant factors in the genesis and/or maintenance of the child's problems. In any event resolution or alleviation of the parents' disorders is likely to be of benefit to the family as a whole, as well as to the children in it. The skills required for casework or parent management training are different from those required for individual psychotherapy, so that sometimes referral of a parent to a different therapist is advisable in order that the parent's own disorder can be addressed. In some cases treatments other than psychotherapy, for example antidepressant drug treatment, may be needed.

Occasionally, the main focus of treatment will be on the parent(s) and the child will be involved in therapy little or not at all. These are cases in which, although the child's symptoms are presented initially as the main problem, investigation of the case reveals that these are secondary to psychiatric problems in the parent(s). For example, a child's behaviour may seem intolerably bad to a severely depressed parent, although objectively the child may appear to be doing nothing out of the ordinary. Once the parent's depression has resolved, the 'problem' may have disappeared.

Kraemer (1987) provides an overview of the respective places of casework and psychotherapy in working with the parents of disturbed children.

Family therapy

As we have seen in earlier chapters, the emotional and behavioural problems of many children arise in the context of problems in the way their families function. This observation has led to the extensive use of family therapy in the treatment of children's disorders.

In family therapy, the family group is the focus of the treatment. The particular symptoms or problems of individual members are regarded as functions of the way the family members interact – in other words of the *family system*. Although one member of the family is usually presented as the *identified patient*, the family therapist tends not to address that member's problems directly but rather to look at the family system as a whole, in the expectation that when healthier family functioning is established the individual members' problems will have resolved, or at least have been alleviated.

In the years since the family therapy movement started – that is to say since the late 1950s – many theoretical frameworks for treating families have been developed and many schools of family therapy have emerged. The subject has become too big to be dealt with adequately here, but the companion volume *Basic Family Therapy* (Barker, 1992) both summarizes (in Chapter 1) the development of this approach, and in later chapters outlines the main schools of family therapy, and provides an overview of the current state of the field.

One of the many schemes for understanding families and how they function is the Family Categories Schema (Steinhauer, *et al.* 1984). This is similar to the McMaster Model of Family Functioning (Epstein, *et al.*, 1978). The Family Categories Schema considers family functioning along six dimensions:

(1)   task accomplishment, which is similar to the McMaster model's 'problem solving',
(2)   role performance,
(3)   communication (which includes the communication of affect),
(4)   affective involvement,
(5)   control,
(6)   values and norms.

These closely related schemes for understanding family functioning are but two among many. Their main value is in helping identify the areas in which families are experiencing difficulties, so that therapeutic attention may be directed where it is needed.

Task accomplishment

This covers what are termed basic, developmental and crisis tasks. The basic tasks are the provision for the family members of the essentials of life – food, shelter, clothing and health care. In modern industrial society the provision of formal education also qualifies as a basic task. Families which fail to provide these essentials for survival in society are generally the most dysfunctional of all.

Developmental tasks are those that must be performed to ensure the healthy development of the members of the family. As the life cycle unfolds, the tasks facing the family change; the care and environment needed by an infant differ greatly from those needed by an adolescent. The well functioning family makes the necessary adjustments as the children grow up and the parents age. Failure to make these adjustments can cause difficulties for particular family members, or indeed for all of them.

Crisis tasks are those with which families are faced when unexpected or unusual events occur. Examples are the death or serious illness of a family member, job loss, natural disaster, loss of the family home through fire or foreclosure, and migration from one culture to another. The family's capacity to adapt to such events is a measure of its health and resilience.

The McMaster Model distinguishes between instrumental problems, such as the provision of food and shelter, and affective ones, for example dealing with hostility between family members.

Family roles

These have been defined as 'prescribed and repetitive behaviours involving a set of reciprocal activities with other family members' (Steinhauer, *et al.*, 1984). In any family there are many roles to be played and the therapist is interested in whether all the necessary roles are suitably allocated in a way that ensures proper functioning of the family. In most families roles are not allocated in a formal way. They develop rather as patterns of behaviour which become habitual. Sometimes, in some families, it becomes necessary to carry out a formal assignment of roles, such as deciding who will do the shopping, mow the lawn, bath the baby, feed the cat, or whatever else needs to be done.

The family therapist is interested both in how appropriate the allocation of roles in the family is, and how easily it is accomplished. Is it a source of conflict or does it happen smoothly and without serious arguments?

The McMaster model distinguishes *necessary* family functions – the provision of material resources, nurturance and support of family members, life-skill development and the maintenance and management of the family system – from *other* functions. The latter are those unique to each family, such as idealizing or 'scapegoating' a family member. Disturbed family members are often found to be playing 'idiosyncratic' roles. In addition to the scapegoat role, other idiosyncratic roles include that of parental child, sick member, handicapped member, disturbed or 'crazy' member and 'family angel'.

Communication problems

These are exceedingly common in the families of disturbed children. Critical aspects of communication, both verbal and non-verbal, are the clarity, directness and sufficiency of the communications sent by family members to each other, and the availability and openness of those to whom communications are addressed. Communication may be affective (the expression of feelings), instrumental (related to the ongoing activities of everyday life) or neither affective not instrumental (for example, the expression of opinions on works of art or music).

Important also is whether the non-verbal and verbal messages being exchanged are congruent. If they are not, as is often the case in troubled families, confusion can result. Helping family members improve their communication skills and practices is a large part of the work needed by many families during therapy.

Affective involvement

This refers to the 'degree and quality of the family members' interest and concern for each other (Steinhauer, et al., 1984). Ideally the emotional needs of family members are met within the family system, but this is not always so.

Most family assessment models make a distinction between families in which the members, or some of them, are over-involved emotionally with each other (often called *enmeshment*), and those in which there is a lack of sufficient emotional involvement, or *disengagement*. A range of degrees of involvement can be discerned:

- *Uninvolved:* the family members live rather 'like strangers in a boarding house'.
- *Interest (or involvement) devoid of feelings:* such involvement as there is may arise out of a sense of duty.
- *Narcissistic involvement:* this is based on a felt wish to bolster one's own feelings of self-worth rather than from real concern for the other person or people.
- *Empathic involvement:* this is based on a true understanding of the needs of those with whom one is involved and results in behaviours which meet those needs.
- *Enmeshment:* this is excessive, intrusive involvement which can

hamper a child's growing up and work against the attainment of autonomy.

The above is an over-simplification. In reality there is an infinite variety of categories of involvement which can, in many different ways, be either nurturant or destructive.

Control

This refers to the influence family members have over each other. The models we are considering distinguish rigid, flexible, *laissez-faire* and chaotic styles of control. Rigid control is high on predictability and low on constructiveness and adaptability. It may work for the day to day maintenance functions of the family, but is less effective when developmental tasks are confronted or change is required.

Flexible styles of control are predictable but constructive and can adapt to changed circumstances. *Laissez-faire* styles are fairly predictable but low on constructiveness. Basically, 'anything goes'. Inertia, indecision, poor task accomplishment and poor role allocation and communication are characteristic of these styles.

Chaotic control styles are low in both predictability and constructiveness. Control switches from rigid to flexible to *laissez-faire*, so that no-one knows what to expect next. Changes occur according to the whim or mood of family members, or sometimes in response to the use of alcohol or other drugs.

'Control' in this context does not refer simply to the parents' methods of controlling the behaviour of their children. It refers to all behaviours in any members of the family which have an influence on the behaviour of other family members, for example how one marital partner influences the behaviour of the other, and how the children's behaviours influence the parents, as well as how each child, by various means both non-verbal and verbal, influences the behaviours of the other children in the family.

Values and norms

This is a category unique to the Process Model. It refers to the family's values on both major issues such as abortion, women's roles in society, whether it is acceptable to smoke marijuana or the existence of God, and such more minor matters as children's bedtimes, who should wash the dishes, and how much responsibility children of different ages should be given for household chores.

The family therapist's task, once the problems in the family have been identified, is to assist the family in making the needed changes in their mode of functioning. In many instances, the successful achievement of this task is accompanied by a reduction or the elimination of the symptomatic behaviour of family members.

While the focus of family therapy is the family group rather than any of the individual members, this does not necessarily mean that all members of the family are seen at each therapy session. In many instances they are, but changes in family systems can often be brought about by seeing family subsystems, for example the parents, the children or even single family members, separately. The essential point that makes it family therapy is that it is the functioning of the system – the way the family members interrelate and communicate – that is addressed, not the mental states or psychopathology of individual family members. The expectation, often realized, is that appropriate changes in the family system will lead to the resolution or amelioration of the presenting problems.

In family therapy the therapist first joins the family – that is, enters into communication and establishes rapport with its members. This is usually done in the course of one or more meetings with the whole family group. This leads to an assessment of the way the family functions, using one of the models briefly described above or one of the many other models that are available. (Several of these are discussed in *Basic Family Therapy* (Barker, 1992)). Interventions are then offered to the family, based on an understanding of how it functions and what may promote the desired changes.

Many methods of intervening in families are available. In practice, which is used depends in part on the theoretical orientation of the therapist, and it seems that many different strategies can be successful, even in the same case. Interventions may be either direct or indirect, the latter often being referred to as 'strategic'.

Direct interventions offer the family alternative ways of functioning, usually by means of straightforward injunctions to do things differently or in a different sequence. With some families this can be effective and an adequate treatment, but in many it is insufficient and a strategy needs to be employed to promote change in a more subtle and, usually, indirect way.

Strategic methods of therapy, which may be used with individuals as well as with families, include reframing and positive connotation (Barker, 1994); metaphorical communication (Barker, 1985); the giving of paradoxical directives (Weeks & L'Abate, 1982); prescribing of rituals and tasks (Imber-Black, *et al.*, 1988); declaring therapeutic impotence; prescribing interminable therapy (Palazzoli, *et al.*, 1978); employing humour (Sutcliffe, *et al.*, 1985); using a consultation group as a *Greek chorus* (Papp, 1980); offering split opinions as to the best course of action; and staging a debate about the family in front of it (Scheinberg, 1985). Further information about these therapeutic methods and their indications is to be found in *Basic Family Therapy* (Barker, 1992) and other family therapy texts. In learning to use them supervised experience is essential.

Group therapy

Both parents and children may be treated in groups. While there are various approaches to group treatment, all aim to enable the members of the group to help each other. They do this both through their interaction with each other and the modelling they can provide for each other. The active, outgoing child can act as a model for the quiet, inhibited one and *vice versa*. Group therapy may have particular value for children who have difficulty with peer group relationships.

Many different approaches to group therapy may be employed. Groups have been used in the treatment of children from the pre-school age period up to adolescence (Cramer-Azima, 1991). When working with groups of younger children, the use of play is emphasized, whereas with adolescents discussion predominates, with the problems of individual members often being addressed quite directly. In all forms of group therapy the therapist or therapists (two therapists are often involved, especially with larger groups) have important roles in facilitating constructive and helpful interchange between the group members. Cramer-Azima (1991) provides a helpful overview of the use of group treatment with children and adolescents.

Parent groups can sometimes achieve many of the aims of individual casework, but often more effectively and economically. The focus of the group is usually on children's problem behaviours and their management. The emphasis is on finding solutions rather than on apportioning blame or elucidating causes. Social learning theory principles and behaviour therapy techniques can be useful in this process (Philipp, 1979). Input and ideas may be offered by the group leader but an important part of the process is the interaction between the parents as they engage in problem-solving discussions as a group. Each brings his or her experience of dealing with various problems, successfully or unsuccessfully, and compares this with the experience of other group members. Such groups also provide mutual support for their members. It can be helpful for parents to know that they are not alone in their difficulties and that others have problems coping with difficult or disturbed behaviours displayed by their children. They may, in the process, acquire a new perspective on the problems of their own children.

Behaviour therapy

Behaviour therapy, based on the principles of learning theory, aims to achieve precise therapeutic goals, either the elimination of symptoms or the development of desired behaviours. Behaviour therapists are not concerned with interpreting the meaning of problem behaviours, nor with promoting insight into their psychodynamics. They believe that problem behaviours, like most other behaviours, are learned and can be eliminated or replaced by desired behaviours through the provision of new learning experiences. Behaviour therapy techniques now have an assured place in child psychiatry. The treatment is often located in the child's natural environment – home, school or treatment centre – rather than in the clinic or therapist's office.

Before behaviour therapy can be started an assessment, which includes a behavioural analysis, is necessary. The circumstances, or *contingencies* controlling the current behaviours must be defined. It is important also to distinguish between skill deficits and performance deficits.

A skill deficit is something the subject is unable to do. A performance deficit is the failure, or perhaps refusal, to perform a task that the subject is capable of carrying out. Thus a boy who does not tie his shoe laces either may not know how to do this, or may simply be refusing to do it. Clearly, the treatment of the two conditions will differ. The child who is not able to tie shoe laces must be taught how to do this, if the task is to be accomplished. The child who can tie shoe laces but, for whatever reason, fails to do so when the laces need to be tied needs a different approach. This will either reward the child in some way for carrying out the task or, perhaps, 'punish' the child for failing to do so. Generally speaking, rewards are preferred, and are more effective, than punishments.

Although early work in the behaviour therapy field emphasized motor functions, nowadays behaviour therapists define behaviour more widely, including emotional responses, cognitive processes, and physiological activities.

The main techniques of behaviour therapy are operant and respondent conditioning, modelling and cognitive behaviour therapy, otherwise known as social learning therapy.

Operant and respondent, or *classical*, conditioning are concerned with altering the circumstances following (in operant conditioning) or preceding (in respondent conditioning) the behaviour concerned. The latter is the same basic process that Pavlov used in his famous experiment with dogs. These were taught to salivate when a bell was rung, by providing them with food in association with the ringing of the bell. In due course they salivated to the sound of the bell, even in the absence of food.

Another example of respondent conditioning is the process of *systematic desensitization*. This is often an effective treatment for phobias. The preliminary behavioural analysis consists of a study of the circumstances in which the fear is present. These are then placed in order in a hierarchy according to the severity of the fear in each situation.

As a first step in the treatment proper, the patient is taught relaxation – that is, the reduction of muscle tension throughout the body. Once this has been achieved the phobic object is presented in mild form, that is one at the bottom of the hierarchy that has been established. This might consist of presenting a small, monochrome picture of the phobic object, or even asking the child to imagine it. There is then a gradual, planned increase in the intensity of the stimulus, based on the hierarchy previously determined. A small, monochrome picture might lead to a larger one, then a coloured one, then a film of the object, then viewing the object itself from a distance, and so on. The rate of increase in the intensity of the stimulus is such as to enable the patient to maintain a state of relaxation. The therapist does not proceed to the next stage until the patient is perfectly at ease in the current one.

In the treatment of specific phobias, for example of water, snakes, dogs or other animals, systematic desensitization is usually effective. It may also be used for phobias of specific situations, for example heights, closed spaces, open spaces, or travelling on buses or aeroplanes.

Operant conditioning is the planned modification of behaviours through manipulation of the consequences perceived as controlling them. If every time a girl touches something hot, she suffers a painful burn, she will soon stop touching that particular object. If whenever the girl helps her mother with a household task, she gets a smile or a hug from her mother, this will probably increase the likelihood of her helping her mother – assuming that smiles and hugs are reinforcing for her.

The above example illustrates the principle of reinforcement. There is no limit to the number of possible reinforcers. They may be material items such as sweets but social ones, like smiles, attention, or words of praise or thanks have advantages. In some situations *token economy* systems are useful. The children acquire tokens for certain specific behaviours, and in some systems lose them for others. The tokens are redeemable later for rewards such as money, toys, privileges like watching television or playing video games. Such programs may be used in the child's home and in schools and institutions of various types. They lend themselves well to the treatment of groups of children.

Behaviours learned through operant conditioning may be lost as a result of non-reinforcement. If a door which in the past has always opened readily is then locked, people will at first try it to see if it will open, as it has done in the past, when they want to get to what is on the other side.

But if they find it locked every time they try it, they will in due course stop bothering to try it. In behaviour therapy language, the behaviour has been extinguished by non-reinforcement. This procedure may be used to eliminate unwanted children's behaviours, for example temper tantrums which, if consistently ignored usually subside, sometimes after an initial increase. This is because the attention they have previously received is no longer being provided in response to the tantrums.

Operant methods have been used to treat many children's problems including aggressive behaviours, obsessive-compulsive symptoms, anorexia nervosa, tics, speech and language disorders and enuresis. They have also been used to promote attendance at school and the development of social skills.

Modelling is the process whereby the subject observes a behaviour, or series of behaviours, of another person and imitates them. Normally developing children learn much through observing the behaviour of parents, other family members, and peers and adults they have contact with in other situations. In many situations the best way to teach another person to do something is to demonstrate the procedure. Parents sometimes fail to realize that their behaviours powerfully influence the behaviours of their children. Thus the parent who smokes may tell the child not to smoke, but such injunctions are usually much less effective than the modelling they provide by smoking themselves.

Cognitive-behaviour therapy, sometimes called just *cognitive therapy*, is based on three premises:

(1)   cognitive activity affects behaviour,
(2)   cognitive activity may be monitored and altered,
(3)   desired behaviour change may be brought about as a result of cognitive change (Dobson, 1988).

Although cognitive therapy is the most recent addition to the behaviour therapy field, it has been the subject of extensive study and research and there is a vast literature on it. It is discussed further in *Basic Behaviour Therapy* (Murdoch & Barker, 1991, particularly Chapter 6), which also provides a guide to the relevant literature on the subject. Its essence, however, is teaching those being treated to think about things differently, so that their behaviour changes.

Other behavioural treatments have also been proposed. For example, in treating obsessive-compulsive rituals, *response prevention*, the active restriction of the rituals, has been found to be of value. It seems that if the rituals are consistently prevented, the urge to carry them out eventually disappears (Stanley, 1980).

Patterson (1976; 1982) has been a pioneer in the development of learning theory-based treatments for children with severe behaviour problems. He has observed high levels of *coercive behaviour* in these families, each member trying to get the others to do as he or she wishes them to do by the use of some form of aggression. One person will make a coercive attack on another who would then retaliate with aversive behaviour designed to terminate the attack. Whenever coercive (that is, aggressive) behaviour succeeds in terminating another's coercive attack that behaviour is reinforced, so that over time the severity of each behaviour increases. Patterson's research has demonstrated that careful behavioural analysis, followed by appropriate interventions can reverse such processes.

Hypnosis and hypnotherapy

Hypnosis does not seem to be used very extensively in the treatment of child psychiatric disorders but there is evidence to suggest that it has a place. Hypnosis has received many definitions, but in its essence is a state in which the subject's attention is focused upon inner ideas, relations and feelings. In a state of hypnosis the subject's awareness of and attention to other stimuli is reduced. In the deepest trance states the individual becomes unaware of what is going on in the immediate environment, or indeed of where he or she actually is (Watkins, 1987, Chapter 7).

Hypnosis is best induced in the context of an intense rapport between therapist and patient. Self-hypnosis is a similar state which the subject enters without the assistance of a therapist present at the time. It is usually first taught to the patient by a therapist. As attention becomes increasingly focused, various *hypnotic phenomena* may appear. These included the release of inhibitions, reduced capacity for volitional activity, heightened susceptibility to suggestion, arm levitation, catalepsy (the prolonged maintenance of a rigid posture), ideomotor activity (involuntary movements and actions), dissociation, time distortion, age regression, 'positive' and 'negative' hallucinations ('negative' ones being the inability to see things which are actually there), amnesia and hyperamnesia. Many of these appear only in states of moderate to deep trance.

The state of trance, which is the essence of hypnosis, is a commonplace one. All of us focus our attention on particular things from time to time – a day dream or a story with which we become deeply engrossed. As we do so we are often in a state of light trance, a state not basically different from that induced by the clinical hypnotherapist. In trance, our awareness of certain things is heightened and that of others is decreased, those on which our attention is not focused being ignored, even though we may be distantly aware of them. Many of us have had the experience of driving somewhere and having no memory of the journey on arrival at our destination. This is an example of an everyday trance.

Children are generally good hypnotic subjects, at least once they have reached middle childhood. Brown & Fromm (1986) point out that they live naturally for much of the time in a world of imagery. The hypnotherapist may use this characteristic to advantage in the treatment of many disorders.

The following are among the uses hypnotherapy may have in the treatment of disturbed children:

(1)   It may help children gain access to emotional and other mental states which are more conducive to adaptive behaviour. States they have experienced in the past can often be recalled and put to use in the hypnotic state.

(2)   It may promote access to material which is not currently available at the conscious level. Such *repressed* or *state-dependent* material may be responsible for anxiety, phobic or other symptoms. Hypnosis may help make it available so that it can be dealt with in psychotherapy.

(3)   It may enable patients to obtain access to resources of which they are consciously unaware. We have seen how important the acquisition of a good measure of self-esteem is as children develop. Most children (and adults too) are unaware, at the conscious level, of many of their capabilities and have forgotten or repressed the memory of many of their past achievements. In trance they can become aware of these things, so that their views of themselves are modified and, often, improved.

(4)   It facilitates mind-body communication (Rossi, 1986a). Thus it may help promote physiological changes, for example to blood pressure, body temperature, bleeding (Swirsky-Sachetti & Margolis, 1986), healing of wounds and burns, enuresis (Edwards & van der Spuy, 1985) and nausea.

(5)   It can assist in the control of anxiety, often through some of the processes mentioned in paragraphs (1), (2), and (3) above.

(6)   It can assist in pain control (Barber, 1982).

(7)   It can help diminish or remove abnormal repetitive behaviours.

(8)   It may be a helpful adjunct in the treatment of various other disorders, for example 'learning difficulties; behaviour disorders; temper tantrums; hair pulling; nail biting; prolonged thumb sucking; phobic reactions, including school phobias, needle phobias and animal phobias; shyness; and drug abuse' (Brown & Fromm, 1986). The strength of the scientific evidence for the value of hypnosis in the treatment of these

disorders varies. In practice, much seems to depend on the skill of the therapist and the specific approach used.

In none of the above conditions is hypnosis a panacea. Inducing trance in itself has little therapeutic value beyond facilitating – usually – a state of relaxation. Moreover, it is seldom sufficient simply to offer suggestions that the symptoms will improve. More important is the making of new associations and gaining access to psychological resources.

Hypnosis does not provide a means of 'mind control' but rather a heightened state of responsiveness and trust between patient and thera- pist. The hypnotherapist then leads the patient to become involved in a past experience or previous learning situation that may be of benefit in the present situation. For example, a child oncology patient receiving chemotherapy may be enabled to re-experience in trance, during the procedure, a previous enjoyable trip to a farm. This may lead to reduced nausea and enhanced feelings of well-being.

A difficulty with hypnotherapy is that the susceptibility of individuals to hypnosis varies. Some achieve trance, especially its deeper forms, more easily than others. Nevertheless it can be successfully applied in a large proportion of the population, especially once a high level of trust and rapport has been established.

Hypnosis and Hypnotherapy with Children (Gardner & Olness, 1981) describe in detail techniques which can be used in hypnotic work with children. Other accounts are to be found in Crasilneck & Hall (1985) and Brown & Fromm (1986).

Pharmacotherapy

Psychoactive drugs have a limited but established place in the treatment of certain child and adolescent psychiatric disorders. Usually they are but one component of a comprehensive treatment plan which takes into account all the relevant family and other factors which are having an impact on the child's condition.

Drugs for children with attention deficit-hyperactivity disorders (ADHD)

The group of child psychiatric conditions for which drug treatment is most widely used are the *hyperkinetic disorders* of ICD-10 and the *attention- deficit/hyperactivity disorders* of DSM-IV. Many of these children, whether their most prominent symptom is hyperactivity or a short attention span, benefit – sometimes dramatically – from the administration of stimulant drugs. Several of these are available. The one most used in North America is methylphenidate (widely known by its proprietary name 'Ritalin'). Alternative stimulant drugs are dexamphetamine and pemoline.

Methylphenidate is unusual in that it has a very short half-life (the time it takes for the blood level to fall to half its original value) of only two to three hours (Gualtieri, *et al.*, 1982). This means that the drug has to be taken every three to four hours to maintain an adequate blood level. While this does have certain disadvantages, it also enables dosage to be adjusted quite finely to meet the needs of each particular child, for example in providing control of symptoms during the school day. It also makes possible the assessment of the value of the treatment by comparing ratings of the child's activity level and behaviour on days when the drug is administered with those on days when it is not being taken.

When there is doubt about whether the drug is having a significant therapeutic effect, a *double blind* trial may be carried out, the child being given active methylphenidate tablets on some days and 'placebo' medication – that is tablets with similar appearance which do not contain the drug – on others. Ratings of the child's behaviour are made by observers who do not know which days the child is on the active medication and which on the placebo tablets. Various rating scales are available to assess children's behaviour and response. The most commonly used is that developed by Conners (1969). This is a simple one-page questionnaire with 12 questions that are to be answered on a four-point scale. It takes little time to complete and can be used by teachers, parents, residential care staff and any others who have contact with these children.

Hyperactivity and short attention span tend to be most troublesome in the school situation. When this is the case, it is often sufficient to confine the use of medication to school days and to use it to cover just the hours the child is in school. A dose given about half an hour before the start of school and another at midday, on school days only, may be all that is needed. In some cases, though, the hyperactivity and problems with attention cause difficulties at home or in other activities – scouts, brownies, church attendance and so forth – so that the drug may be needed to cover these situations. A sustained release preparation of methylphenidate is also available.

Amphetamine compounds and pemoline are stimulant drugs which may be effective in children who do not respond to methylphenidate. Their longer duration of action means that their effectiveness cannot be assessed by comparing children's behaviour on successive days on and off medication. Various other drugs have been reported to be effective, including the tricyclic antidepressants, clonidine and antipsychotic drugs such as haloperidol and the phenothiazine group of drugs.

Imipramine, a tricyclic drug, has been quite extensively studied as a treatment for attention-deficit hyperactivity disorders but seems to be less effective than the stimulant drugs (Green, 1991). It can diminish hyper-active behaviour and may improve performance on tests of attention (Taylor, 1986b).

The pharmacological treatment of children who have both ADHD and tics or Tourette's syndrome presents difficulties since the stimulant drugs are inclined to exacerbate tics, and the antipsychotics are of limited value for attention-deficit problems. This has led to the search for alternatives, particularly among the tricyclic drugs. Spencer, *et al.* (1993a; 1993b) report the results in a series of 33 children treated with the tricyclic drug desipramine, 30 of them having the combination of a tic disorder and ADHD. This was a retrospective report of an uncontrolled study, but there was significant improvement in the chronic tic disorder in 82% of cases and of the ADHD in 80%. No major adverse effects were encoun-tered in the course of a follow-up period which extended for an average of 16 months.

Clonidine, a drug originally marketed as a treatment for hypertension, has been reported to be of value in the treatment of attention-deficit hyperactivity disorders (Hunt, *et al.*, 1990). Although it seems to be effective in reducing many of the symptoms of ADHD, it appears not to reduce distractibility. Hunt (1987) suggested that an additional small dose of methylphenidate, if added to the clonidine, may improve response, particularly distractibility. Clonidine has the additional merit that it is sometimes effective in the treatment of tic disorders. It therefore has the potential to be of value in children who have both tics and ADHD.

Table 21.1 lists the principal drugs that may be of value in the treatment of hyperactive/ADHD children, with their usual dose ranges and main adverse effects.

Drug treatment of affective disorders

The role of drugs in the treatment of depression in children and adoles-cents is not firmly established, though it seems that these drugs are less effective than they are in adults. While there have been reports of favourable responses to tricyclic antidepressant drugs in both children and adolescents, and clinical experience suggests that they may some-times be of value, support from properly designed controlled studies is lacking. Such controlled studies that have been carried out have usually found no difference between the response to the antidepressant and that to the placebo (Ambrosini, *et al.*, 1993a). It may nevertheless be that there is a small group within the total population of depressed children who do respond to these drugs, but perhaps not a big enough group to have a statistically significant effect when the trial includes a large number of non-responders.

Table 21.1   Drug doses and adverse effects.

Drug	Dose	Principal adverse effects
Stimulants (for hyperactive children)		
		Excitement
		Sleeplessness
Methylphenidate	0.25–1.0 mg/kg/24 hr ⎫	Loss of appetite
		Growth failure
Dexamphetamine	0.2–0.5 mg/kg/24 hr ⎬	Palpitations
		Headache
Pemoline	0.5–2.0 mg/kg/24 hr ⎭	Abdominal cramps
		Drug dependence (rare in hyperactive children)
Phenothiazine drugs		
		Drowsiness
		Tremor
Chlorpromazine ⎫	1–3 mg/kg/24 hr ⎫	Muscle rigidity and spasms
⎬	(night sedative dose	Precipitation of epilepsy
Thioridazine ⎭	up to 3 mg/kg) ⎪	Jaundice
	⎬	Blood dyscrasias
Fluphenazine	0.05–0.25 mg/kg/24 hr ⎪	Urinary retention and incontinence
Perphenazine	0.15–0.3 mg/kg/24 hr ⎭	Skin rashes (chlorpromazine may cause photosensitive skin reactions)
		Painful muscle spasms
Haloperidol	0.025–0.3 mg/kg/24 hr ⎬	Muscle rigidity and tremor
		Drowsiness
		Depression
Benzodiazepines (for over-fives)		
Diazepam	2–5 mg 2 or 3 times daily ⎫	Drowsiness
	⎬	Skin rashes
Chlordiazepoxide	5–10 mg 2 or 3 times daily ⎭	Muscle tenderness or weakness
Clonidine	2–5 g/kg/day ⎫	Drowsiness
	⎬	Low blood pressure
		Exacerbation or emergence of depression in predisposed patients

Notes: (1) The above doses are guides only. Dosage should be individualized according to response.

(2) Long-term administration of phenothiazines or haloperidol may cause 'tardive dyskinesia' (A syndrome of rhythmical involuntary movements of the tongue, face, mouth or jaw).

(3) Muscle spasms and tremor caused by phenothiazines or haloperidol may be countered by 'anti-Parkinsonian' drugs such as benzhexol (1–5 mg twice daily).

The tricyclic drug that has been most extensively investigated in depressed children is imipramine (see Table 21.2). Its absorption is variable in children and its use requires careful monitoring with, if possible, periodic estimations of the blood level. Blood levels between 125 and 250 ng/ml have been recommended as effective and safe (Preskorn, *et al.*, 1989). Side effects are quite common and adverse cardiac reactions, which can even be fatal, have been reported. There is some suggestion, in the literature summarized by Green (1991), that tricyclic antidepressants may be less effective in adolescents than in children. Because of the possibility of cardiac side-effects – specifically conduction problems – it may be advisable to carry out electrocardiographic (ECG) studies before starting tricyclic medication, to rule out congenital conduction defects, and when increases in the dose are made. Boulos & Kutcher (1992) suggest that the following ECG changes should lead to discontinuation of treatment or a reduction of the dose:

- a PR interval greater than 0.18 (under ten years of age) or 0.20 (over ten years).
- A QRS interval greater than 0.12 seconds, or 50% over the baseline level.
- A corrected QT level greater than 0.48 seconds.
- Resting heart rate greater that 110/minute in under ten-year-olds, or greater than 100/minute in those over ten.
- Resting blood pressure greater than 140/90 in those of under ten or greater than 150/95, or persistently greater than 140/85 in children over ten.

Caution may be especially appropriate when the tricyclic desipramine is used, as occasional cases of sudden death of patients on this medication have been reported.

There is even less information on the place of other antidepressants in children. Monoamine oxidase inhibitors probably are of some value in children but their side-effects and dangers have prevented their widespread use. The use of the newer selective, reversible inhibitors of monoamine oxidase, such as meclobamide, in children has not so far been the subject of any reported research as this is written. These drugs cannot therefore at present be recommended for use in this age range, despite their apparent value in adults.

Despite the lack of evidence that antidepressants are superior to placebo, Ambrosini, *et al.* (1993a, page 4) suggest that 'if a depressed youth is either not amenable or unresponsive to nonpharmacological interventions while maintaining functional impairment in school, social or family domains [antidepressant] treatment is warranted'. These authors suggest that the choice of antidepressant should be based upon the side-effect profiles of the various drugs available. Thus among the tricyclic drugs, amitriptyline, which causes a degree of sedation may be used when there are sleep problems and nortriptyline, which is less sedating, if there is a need to minimize daytime sedation.

A number of newer antidepressant drugs have become available in recent years but there has been rather little research into their use in adolescents and, especially, children. Nevertheless Ambrosini, *et al.* (1993a) suggest that fluoxetine and sertraline – drugs which inhibit the uptake of the neurotransmitter serotonin in the brain – should be used in suicidal patients and those with impulsive tendencies, since these drugs are less dangerous when overdoses are taken.

Manic states in young people are treated along the same lines as with adults. In the acute phase the administration of an antipsychotic drug, usually haloperidol or a phenothiazine such as chlorpromazine or thioridazine, may be required (see Table 21.1) to control the manic behaviour. These drugs are usually given orally but if necessary they can be administered by intramuscular injection.

Table 21.2   Doses and adverse effects of tricyclic drugs and lithium.

Drug	Dose	Principal adverse effects
Imipramine Amitriptyline	1.5–5 mg/kg/24	Arrhythmias, blood pressure changes and other cardiac disorders Dry mouth Difficulty with visual accommodation Tremor Precipitation of epileptic seizures
Imipramine (for enuresis)	10–50 mg at bedtime	Jaundice and blood disorders (both rare) Psychosis Drowsiness (amitriptyline)
Lithium carbonate	600–1200 mg per day (depending on blood levels)	Tremor Anorexia, nausea Abdominal discomfort Thirst, polyuria Goitre Fatigue, weakness

Note: The absorption and metabolism of tricyclic antidepressants by children is very variable. If possible blood levels should be checked regularly.

Lithium carbonate is often effective in the treatment of bipolar disorders and may be used in the maintenance of adolescents with this disorder. Given in doses which maintain a blood level of 0.8 to 1.2 milliequivalents/litre, it leads to a reduction or cessation of attacks of mania and depression in perhaps 80% of cases (Hassenyeh and Davidson, 1980). In addition to its use in the treatment of mood disorders, lithium may be of value in some severely aggressive adolescents, especially when there is accompanying explosive effect. The uses of lithium in young people and the various possible adverse effects and necessary precautions are well summarized by Green (1991, pages 143–56).

Anxiety/neurotic disorders

Drugs have quite a limited role in the treatment of anxiety disorders in children and adolescents. In treating these disorders the emphasis is usually on addressing the circumstances thought to contribute to the anxiety the young person is experiencing. Thus family and/or individual psychotherapy, casework with parents, and intervention in school if the child's situation there is anxiety-provoking, tend to be the first line treatments. Occasionally the short-term use of a benzodiazepine tranquillizer, such as diazepam or chlordiazepoxide, may be indicated to tide a child over an acutely stressful experience, but this should be limited to a few days at most, while other measures are instituted or take effect.

The tricyclic antidepressants may have a significant role in the treatment of some anxiety disorders, particularly obsessive-compulsive disorders (OCD). Ambrosini, *et al.* (1993b), reviewing the use of these drugs in conditions other than major affective disorders, suggest that they may be 'more appropriately viewed as broad spectrum pharmacotherapeutics', since they have been found to be of value in enuresis and bulimia nervosa as well as with OCD. Although early reports suggested that imipramine was of value in the treatment of separation anxiety manifesting itself as school refusal, this work has not been confirmed in later studies (Ambrosini, *et al.*, 1993b). On the other hand, clomipramine has been shown to be of value in the treatment of obsessive-compulsive disorders. Administered in doses of up to 3 mg/kg/day, this drug appears to be significantly superior to placebo (De Vaaugh-Geiss, *et al.*, 1992).

Other uses of the tricyclic antidepressants are in reducing the frequency of bedwetting, and in the treatment of bulimia. Whether imipramine's effects on bedwetting are sufficient to justify its use is open to question, since it only leads to completely dry nights in 10 to 20% of cases. It may be of more value in reducing the frequency of binge eating in bulimia, at least in the short term. What place these drugs have in the longer-term treatment of bulimia is uncertain (Ambrosini, *et al.*, 1993b).

Schizophrenia

The drug treatment of schizophrenia occurring in children and adolescents follows the same general lines as in adult patients.

'Antipsychotic drugs' such as haloperidol and the phenothiazine drugs (examples are chlorpromazine, thioridazine and perphenazine) may be effective, though they may be less so in children than in adults. They should be part of a comprehensive treatment plan involving the family and the wider environment of the child. Dosage is summarized in Table 21.1. Unfortunately these drugs are liable to produce a number of adverse side effects. These include acute dystonic reactions (painful spasms of groups of muscles); Parkinsonism (tremor, rigidity of muscles, drooling and expressionless face); akathisia (motor restlessness); neuroleptic malignant syndrome (a combination of tremor, abnormal movements, akathisia, hypertonia of the muscles, hypertension, fever, sweating, altered consciousness and even coma and death (Latz & McCracken, 1992)); agranulocytosis (reduction of the white blood cells with consequent susceptibility to infections); tardive dyskinesia (see Table 21.1); and undue sedation. Despite these potential problems these drugs are of value and many children receiving them do not suffer serious adverse effects.

Among the newer antipsychotic drugs which may be of value in the treatment of schizophrenia are thiothixene, chlorprothixene, loxapine and clozapine. None has been widely studied in children and clozapine in particular is prone to cause a number of serious adverse effects. Chlorprothixene has been approved by the United States Federal Drug Administration for use in children over the age of six and is administered in doses of 10 to 25 mg three or four times daily. These newer drugs should only be used after review of the current relevant literature and discussion with a consultant familiar with their use.

Other conditions

The place of drug treatment in the management of *behaviour disorders* is limited, except when there is an associated hyperkinetic or attention-deficit hyperactivity disorder. The latter may respond to treatment as outlined above. Many behaviour disorders are of complex aetiology and are reactive to family and other environmental circumstances, as we saw in Chapter 6. The management plan should address the underlying and associated factors rather than using pharmacological means to tackle what are usually but symptoms of family systems and other problems. Exceptions may be children in whom the behaviour problems are related to brain damage or abnormality. Some such children, especially some of the more severely retarded, remain aggressive and difficult to manage even when handled in optimal fashion. Treatment with phenothiazine drugs, generally in smaller doses than are used for psychotic disorders, may be helpful. The dose of these drugs can sometimes be reduced by simultaneously administering a benzodiazepine drug such as lorazepam.

There have been reports that fenfluramine may improve the functioning of some mentally retarded children. Aman, *et al.* (1993) reported a double-blind, placebo-controlled, crossover trial of fenfluramine and methylphenidate in a group of non-autistic mentally subnormal children who were also hyperactive and/or inattentive. When the response to these drugs was compared with that to placebo, significant improvements in attention, decreased activity level, and enhanced mood were found, based on the ratings of examiners who observed the children.

No drugs have been shown to affect the course of *pervasive developmental disorders*, though medication may sometimes be helpful in controlling particular symptoms. Antipsychotic drugs may produce improvement in some symptoms but it is questionable whether their regular use is justified in view of the risk of adverse effects. Drugs which have been suggested as possible treatments for autistic children include fenfluramine and naltrexone, but convincing evidence that either of them is effective is currently lacking. (See Green (1991) for a summary of the research on these compounds.)

Several drugs are available that may be effective in treating *tics* and *Tourette's syndrome*. These include haloperidol, clonidine and pimozide. In view of the possible side-effects of haloperidol it may be better to assess the response to each of the other two first. Pimozide may be given in doses up to 0.2 mg/kg/day. While it can cause side-effects similar to those of haloperidol they are usually milder. Clonidine may also be effective. Dosage should start at about 1 µg/kg/day and may be increased gradually as high as 6 µg/kg/day if necessary and if there are no untoward side-effects – chiefly drowsiness or lowered blood pressure.

Sleeplessness should not usually be treated with drugs. It is often a manifestation of anxiety and/or problems in parent/child relationships. Treatment should address the underlying problems that usually exist. If medication is to be used it should be, at most, a short-term measure to tide over a crisis, and use should rarely, if ever, extend beyond two weeks. Behavioural methods and counselling for the parents are probably more appropriate in most cases (Richman, *et al.*, 1985; Richman, 1985).

General points about drug treatment

Caution is advisable in the use of medication to treat behavioural and emotional disorders in children. While drugs may suppress symptoms, their effects may mask underlying problems, for example family relationship difficulties. They may also convey the message that the problem lies within the child who is being given the drug, whereas disturbed children are often reacting to factors in their environment. This does not apply in all cases, however, and in some conditions medical/biological factors are important, examples being schizophrenia, Tourette's syndrome and some hyperkinetic and affective disorders. But in many behavioural disorders this is not so and the use of drugs may lead those concerned with the child's care to take an unrealistic view of the problems.

Many of these drugs can have serious side-effects. All psychoactive drugs can be lethal if taken in overdoses, and this risk is particularly great in the case of the tricyclics, the phenothiazines and haloperidol. It is important therefore to warn the families of children for whom psychoactive drugs are prescribed, that they should always be kept in a secure place and the child's access to them controlled.

It seems that the patterns of psychoactive medication use in children vary greatly. According to Taylor (1985), stimulant drugs are used 'very extensively in the United States and very seldom in Britain'. A study of the prescription of psychoactive drugs in the Canadian province of Saskatchewan revealed a pattern of use differing substantially from that suggested in this chapter, minor tranquillizers (mainly the benzodiazepines), sedatives and hypnotics being the most frequently prescribed. Stimulants were prescribed less than might have been expected (Quinn, 1986).

Inpatient and residential treatment

Inpatient treatment usually refers to treatment in a hospital unit for disturbed children, and *residential treatment* to that provided in other specialized centres. The latter tend to be longer-term units than those in hospitals, but there are exceptions to this. Some hospital units have treated children as inpatients for periods as long as a year, occasionally longer, and some non-hospital units offer short-term admission. In many jurisdictions, however, recent years have seen substantial reductions in the usual length of stay. These have often been dictated by fiscal restraint but there has also been a re-examination of the basic philosophy underlying the treatment approaches in these centres. There is nowadays more emphasis on day treatment and work in families' homes, with the aim of empowering parents to meet their children's needs, rather than on removing children to other settings where professionals undertake these tasks.

Hospital and non-hospital treatment centres differ in other respects. Hospitals are usually directed by psychiatrists and take a more medical approach, while other centres may be directed by psychologists, social workers or other mental health professionals. Nevertheless the two types of treatment facility share many features and treat similar types of clinical problems.

Children may be admitted to units of either of the above two types primarily for assessment or for treatment, though separation of the two functions is somewhat artificial. Children may be admitted for *assessment* for the following reasons:

● Because the case in unusually complex and intensive observation and investigation beyond what is possible as an outpatient or even a day-patient is needed. This applies especially when there is doubt about the relative roles of suspected organic factors and of psychological and family factors in the aetiology of a child's problems. In such cases investigation in a hospital unit by a team of specialists may clarify the situation.

● Because there is doubt about how far a child's symptoms are being maintained by the current dynamics at home or, in certain cases, in the school and/or wider social environment. Observing whether symptoms persist, worsen or improve away from home may help resolve such issues.

● Because the child lives at a great distance from the centre, making repeated outpatient visits impractical. This is more commonly the case in North America, with its vast rural and thinly populated areas, than in more thickly populated European countries.

Admission for treatment

The main indications for admission for *treatment* are:

● Because the child's behaviour is so disturbed as to make treatment or even care elsewhere difficult or impossible. This applies to some children with very severe conduct disorders, especially those complicated by severe hyperactivity or extremely impulsive behaviour, and also to some with schizophrenia and other psychoses.

● Because of danger to the child or others if the child remains at home.

This applies to many suicidal young people, to a few who are a danger to others, and to most severe cases of anorexia nervosa, that is those in whom there has been a dangerous degree of weight loss.

• Because the child's environmental circumstances are very unfavourable and efforts to ameliorate the situation have failed. In many such cases, however, removal to an alternative long-term living situation, rather than admission to hospital, may be what is needed.

Adverse circumstances which may justify admission include an unstable home with gross marital strife, other serious family systems problems; severe parental rejection of the child; parental alcoholism or drug addiction; and serious emotional deprivation or abuse. In such cases, admission may be helpful if it seems likely, or at least possible, that more can be done to alter the adverse conditions in which the child has been living during a period of inpatient or residential treatment. It is sometimes possible to do more to help the family, and promote improvement in parents' attitudes and handling of their children, while the latter are temporarily out of the home. Work with the parents, some of which may be done in the child's inpatient setting where appropriate child management techniques can be taught and modelled, may be carried on while the parents are temporarily relieved of the constant irritant of the child's disturbed behaviour in the home. In due course, it may be possible to return a less disturbed child to a better functioning family. Treatment may then be successfully continued on an outpatient or daypatient basis.

When admission for inpatient or residential treatment is being considered, the situation in the family, or in the group home, foster home or other setting in which the child is living, should be carefully examined. Requests for admission are sometimes disguised attempts by parents or others to get rid of an unwanted child. When this is the motivation behind the request, admission of the child is not usually the best response. Sometimes the child whose admission is requested is the family scapegoat. In such cases the best response may be to offer family therapy, with the aim of promoting changes in the family system such that the scapegoating will cease.

Many inpatient units admit children for short periods of just a few weeks during which intensive assessment and short-term treatment are carried out. This leads to the development of a long-term plan of treatment to be continued after discharge. This is often a plan based on outpatient or perhaps daypatient attendance, though occasionally transfer to a longer-term residential unit may be recommended.

Following admission to the inpatient unit, an assessment process along the lines suggested in Chapter 5, will usually be carried out. Such additional physical investigations as are indicated will be undertaken, and consultation with other specialists will be sought as required. An important part of the assessment is observing how the child responds to different management strategies and regimes. The best way to assess how a child will respond to a treatment program is to implement it and observe the results.

Hospital units are usually staffed by nurses and child care workers. These *front line* staff are part of a larger team. This usually includes psychiatrists, psychologists, social workers, occupational therapists, speech therapists, teachers and others. A key feature of the treatment is the general emotional environment or *milieu* of the unit. An emotionally warm, relaxed atmosphere is much to be desired. However difficult and disturbed their behaviour may be, the children should be met with accepting attitudes and responses, rather than the rejecting and hostile ones they may have experienced previously. Along with acceptance should go firm, calmly applied limit-setting; this is as necessary in residential settings as in other therapeutic situations. Children's current clinical states and behaviours are accepted, while work proceeds to resolve the child's emotional and/or behavioural difficulties. The treatment staff work with child and parents to achieve this.

Many models of residential treatment exist but in all a comprehensive plan to address the child's and the parents' problems is required. This involves the use of a variety of therapy modes. As a background for them all there is usually a program of behavioural management – that is to say, the unit is structured to reinforce desired behaviour and extinguish antisocial and other undesired behaviours. In a sense this is no different from what parents normally do as they raise their children, encouraging socially desired behaviour and discouraging that which is not desired. What *is* different is the degree of intensity of the behavioural program that is required, since many behaviourally disturbed children have a long history of behavioural problems and are well set in their ways.

To the basic behavioural management program are added such additional treatments as are needed. These may include individual and/or group psychotherapy, behaviour therapy addressing specific items of behaviour, occupational and recreational therapy, speech therapy, special educational measures, and pharmacotherapy. In most cases family therapy and/or counselling for the parents are important parts of the treatment plan. Parents, as well as children and adolescents, can often with advantage be treated in groups. Active involvement of the family is important. Children who are left in residential units to be 'fixed', while their parents go about their business relieved of responsibility for their child seldom do well.

Ney & Mulvihill (1985) described an interesting 12-week treatment concept. During the first two weeks the child and family are assessed comprehensively as outpatients. This is followed by a five-week period of intensive, multimodal inpatient treatment, and then by a five-week follow-up period. All children are admitted for 5 weeks, no more and no less, but they can be re-admitted for a further five weeks at any time after the follow-up period. These authors also describe 44 treatment techniques designed to deal with a range of symptoms. They offer comprehensive treatment programs for child abuse, anorexia, autism, depression, encopresis, firesetting, incest, school refusal, weight control and conversion reactions.

Other sources of information on inpatient and residential treatment are to be found in Barker (1982), Schaefer & Swanson (1988), Lewis & Summerville (1991) and Durrant (1993). The possible drawbacks and potential dangers of residential treatment, and means of lessening these, are discussed by Barker (1988).

Day treatment

Treatment in a daypatient unit can provide many of the benefits of inpatient treatment without completely removing the child from home and family, and at less expense. In daypatient units children can spend substantial parts of their waking hours in a therapeutic milieu and can receive comprehensive, multimodal therapy, much as inpatients do.

Most day treatment programs operate five days a week and the children attend from 8 or 9 AM until about 4 or 5 PM, though hours vary. In most units treatment tends to be organized around the school day, with active involvement of the family. Some programs offer half-day programmes for younger children and in some there is the option of having children attend less often than five days a week. It is often possible to have staffing that is more consistent in day treatment units than in inpatient ones. In the latter the need to provide staffing at nights and days off for staff means that the staff present vary from time to time. In daypatient units the staff members' working hours usually approximate to those of the children's attendance.

While day treatment relieves parents and other family members of some of the strain of caring for their disturbed child, it also ensures that contact between child and family is not lost and that the family does not come to deny the existence of the problems. The latter is an ever-present danger in residential treatment. In the ordered environment of the residential unit the child's behaviour may become more settled, while at home the family becomes used to being without the disturbed child and begins to forget about, or repress memories of, how things were.

Day treatment may be of particular value when the child's problems are selectively manifest at school, adjustment at home being relatively satisfactory. Most day treatment units have teachers on their staff, so that the educational problems and needs of the children can be met while they attend as daypatients.

Day treatment may be contraindicated for:

- children who are dangerous to themselves or others;
- children whose parents or other caretakers are themselves severely disturbed, dangerous and/or abusive;
- children with a physical illness or handicap which necessitates round-the-clock care;
- children whose cases can be adequately managed in an outpatient setting.

Day treatment may be of short or long duration, extending from a week or two up to a period of many months or even several years. In most cases a period of a few weeks or, at most, months is sufficient, especially if the family is in active treatment at the same time. Many day treatment services are located in centres where there are also inpatient and outpatient services. Day treatment may then be one phase in a program of treatment which also includes outpatient and inpatient therapy.

Further reading on day treatment is available in Zimet & Farley (1985), Pruitt & Kiser (1991), and Zimet (1993).

Alternatives to residential treatment

Sometimes, rather than being admitted to inpatient or residential treatment centres, children are placed in alternative families. These may be foster parents who are given additional support and training, and usually also extra remuneration, so that they can provide for the care and treatment needs of disturbed children. Such arrangements are seen as approximating more closely to the child's normal environment. Early examples of such programs were the *parent-therapist* program in Hamilton, Ontario; the Kent Family Placement Project (Hazel, 1977) and the *family care program* in Toronto, Ontario (Barker, *et al.*, 1978). The latter program provided weekend care for children in residential treatment when the parents were unavailable or unable to provide care, as well as, in many cases, a home for the child to live in upon discharge from residential treatment. Subsequent years have seen a substantial expansion of these programs in many jurisdictions.

It is possible to make most of the services provided for children in residential treatment available also to the children in these *alternative family* settings – for example the diagnostic and therapeutic expertise of psychiatrists, psychologists, social workers, child care workers, speech therapists and so forth.

Educational measures

Since many disturbed children have educational problems, for example the reading difficulties often associated with conduct disorders, educational help often needs to be part of the total management plan. This may consist of remedial teaching, changes in the educational methods being used, transfer to a more suitable class or school, or some combination of these things.

In many jurisdictions special classes or even schools are provided for children with psychiatric disorders, learning disorders or behaviour problems. The various British Education Acts have long recognized *maladjustment* as one of several categories of handicap which may necessitate special education. Local education authorities are required to provide special education for maladjusted children. Some of these children's special needs are provided for in residential schools run, in the UK, either by education authorities or privately. The development of schools for maladjusted children was reviewed by Bridgland (1971).

In the USA, the arrangements for the education of disturbed children are more varied. There are some schools, mainly privately run, that specialize in the education of disturbed children, but these are often available only to children whose families can afford to pay the fees, which are often high. Most school boards, however, provide special, small classes for disturbed children and for those with learning difficulties.

While special schools and classes are helpful for some disturbed children, most are educated in ordinary schools and classes. Many educational, emotional and behavioural problems can be satisfactorily dealt with in such settings, using when necessary the services of educational psychologists, remedial teachers, speech therapists and other specialists. In *Help Starts Here* Kolvin and his colleagues (1981) described various methods of intervening in ordinary schools to provide help for disturbed children. These were:

- a *behaviour modification* approach,
- a nurturing approach, using *teacher-aides*,

- parent counselling-teacher education,
- group therapy for the children.

The progress of children using each of these approaches was compared with that of a control group of untreated 'at risk' children. All the approaches proved to be of some value, though short-term results often differed from long-term outcome, the latter being better in some instances. The book offers much of value to anyone planning intervention in schools with the objective of treating or forestalling psychiatric problems in the children. Smith (1990) provides a brief discussion of approaches to the management of disturbed children in both ordinary and special schools. Another source of information, with contributions from a broad range of authors, is *The Management of Behaviour in Schools* (Varma, 1993).

Speech and language therapy

Since speech and language disorders are often associated with psychiatric disorders in children, comprehensive treatment plans often need to include speech therapy. Speech therapists, sometimes known as speech pathologists, are able to contribute much to the treatment of developmental language disorders, as well as to the remediation of disorders of articulation. Improvement in a child's speech and language skills often contributes to the resolution of a variety of emotional and behavioural problems. Speech therapy is crucial in the treatment of children with severe communication disorders, including the pervasive developmental disorders, such as autism.

Removal from parental care

Some disturbed children are found to be living in severely dysfunctional families in which their basic emotional, and sometimes even their physical, needs are not being met. They may have experienced, or still be experiencing, physical, sexual or emotional abuse, or they may be subject to neglect. They may also face any combination of these problems. When such situations come to light, the first need, once the immediate safety of the child is assured, is to help the family care adequately for their child(ren). This is not always successful. In some cases the parents seem to lack the motivation needed to make the necessary changes. In others, problems such as the chronic abuse of alcohol and/or other drugs prevent change; in yet others the marital relationship is grossly unstable, and sometimes, if it proves impossible to achieve a more stable situation, all attempts to help the parents to provide adequate care for their children fail. In these circumstances, removal of the child(ren) from the home may be the only way to ensure the children's well-being and to provide them with the treatment and care they need. In all developed countries there are child welfare agencies which exist to provide help and, if necessary, alternative care for such children.

Many child welfare agencies are government-run but some are non-governmental agencies. In the UK the principal non-governmental agencies are the National Society for the Prevention of Cruelty to Children, the National Children's Home, and Barnardos. The latter also has branches in other countries, including some African ones.

Sometimes parents are aware that they are unable to care properly for their children and are willing, when it is necessary, to relinquish care to the child welfare authorities. If the parents' consent and active cooperation can be obtained, this is much to be desired. Sometimes, however, this proves impossible. In such cases legal action under the relevant child welfare legislation becomes necessary, although adversarial legal proceedings should be avoided if possible. The current British Children Act is summarized in Appendix A, but all developed countries have legislation allowing intervention by the child welfare authorities under such circumstances. In the United States and Canada, child welfare is a responsibility of, respectively, the states and the provinces.

Children who have had to be removed from their families because of neglect or abuse often show evidence of retarded or abnormal psychological development. They may display serious behaviour problems, emotional difficulties, low-self esteem, disorders of development, educational difficulties, or any combination of these problems. It is not surprising that child welfare authorities often have difficulty meeting the needs these children have for love, security, and the rebuilding of their shattered self-esteem. In attempting both to assess such children's needs and, when indicated, to plan treatment for them, psychiatric help may be sought. These can be some of the most challenging clinical problems with which child psychiatrists are asked to deal.

The substitute environment provided for these children is usually either a foster home or a group home (often called a *children's home* in the UK). The large impersonal orphanages, which themselves were sometimes called children's homes, of the past have now been replaced by smaller homes, usually ordinary houses in which children are cared for in much the same way as in other families. One or other of the house parents may have employment outside the family. Many group homes are run by married couples, usually with some help from other, perhaps part-time, staff who may be resident or non-resident. The trend from large impersonal institutions has also affected the care of mentally handicapped children, many of whom used to be cared for in large, impersonal institutions, often understaffed and poorly equipped to stimulate the development of their inmates. Unfortunately these changes are not universal and the institutional care provided to the mentally handicapped – and to some deprived, neglected and disturbed children – in some countries, generally the less developed ones, is of a poor standard.

Psychiatrists have much to contribute to the decision making processes which are necessary in the management of children in care. An excellent and comprehensive discussion of these issues is to be found in *The Least Detrimental Alternative: A Systematic Guide to Case Planning and Decision Making for Children in Care* (Steinhauer, 1991).

The care and treatment of antisocial young people, especially those who have committed serious criminal acts present great challenges. In most jurisdictions there are residential institutions for the more serious offenders, and in some of these treatment for those with psychiatric problems is provided. There is a wide variety of institutions for such young people, some progressive and humane, others primarily custodial and/or punitive.

Child psychiatric consultation and liaison

There are many more disturbed children in the community than can be treated by the available numbers of psychiatrists and other child mental health professionals, and it seems likely that this will always be the case. Much can, however, be done to help these children by providing consultation to those caring for them. Such consultation is an important part of the work of child psychiatrists and their colleagues. Psychiatrists may give guidance to the staff of group homes, institutions and schools, and also to foster parents and child welfare social workers, about how the needs of the children in their care may best be met. In the course of this work they may assess children to determine their psychiatric status and care and treatment needs, but the primary function of the consultant is not to do direct work with the children or their families, but to work with and through those looking after the children and working with the families.

Psychiatric liaison, as opposed to consultation, work addresses not the needs of particular children but those of the agencies, institutions and care-givers dealing with children. It is concerned with program issues such as the development and improvement of the milieu and the fostering of the skills of staff. Psychiatric liaison work can also have important applications in the prevention of psychiatric disorders.

Chapter 22

Prevention of Child Psychiatric Disorders

It is obviously preferable to prevent disorders rather than to wait until they are established and then treat them. Three types of prevention are distinguished (Caplan, 1964):

(1) *Primary prevention.* This consists of planned measures designed to reduce the incidence of specific disorders in a population not currently suffering from those disorders. An example is the preventive immunization of healthy individuals against infectious diseases.

(2) *Secondary prevention.* This aims at early diagnosis and case finding, followed by intervention to bring the disorder under control as quickly as possible, thus minimizing the impact on those affected.

(3) *Tertiary prevention.* This consists of measures taken once a disorder is established. It aims to limit the effects of the disorder, to prevent it getting worse and to give support to afflicted individuals and/or their families.

Definitions

(1) *Epidemiology.* This is concerned with the incidence, prevalence and distribution of disorders in communities. It is a basic tool in the development of primary prevention measures. By means of epidemiological studies, it is possible both to establish a baseline – essential if the effectiveness of preventive measures is to be known – and to identify risk factors.

(2) *Risk factors.* These are circumstances that make the development of a disorder more likely.

(3) *Incidence.* This is the number of new cases occurring in a defined population in a specified time period.

(4) *Duration.* This is the length of time a disorder persists, that is the period from the time of onset until recovery or death.

(5) *Prevalence.* This is a measure of the number of cases of a disorder present at a given time in a specified population. It is a function of two independent variables – incidence and duration.

(6) *Intervening variables.* In the present context, these are the factors that determine whether individuals at risk do or do not develop the disorder in question. No risk factor leads to the disorder in 100% of those experiencing it. In any epidemic, some individuals will escape. Primary prevention aims to alter the environment so that more individuals escape.

Primary prevention

A landmark in the development of preventive psychiatry was the publication of *Principles of Preventive Psychiatry* (Caplan, 1964). The same author later provided an account of how primary prevention may be achieved in child psychiatry (Caplan, 1980).

Risk factors and primary prevention

(a) *Genetic factors.* The role of genetic factors in causing child psychiatric disorders was discussed in Chapter 2. Recent advances in genetics and the discovery of the location of the genes responsible for a number of disorders, hold out the promise that we may be able to prevent many genetically determined disorders. Genetic counselling for members of families in which heritable disorders have occurred, and particularly for parents who have had a child with a possibly genetically caused disorder, can prevent the birth of children with certain disorders.

(b) *Pregnancy risk factors.* These include toxaemia of pregnancy (a condition in which there is fluid retention and raised blood pressure, sometimes leading to convulsions), and various infections which may be passed from mother to fetus. Examples of the latter are rubella, syphilis, toxoplasmosis (a disease due to the protozoon *Toxoplasma gondii*), and acquired immune deficiency disease (AIDS). Poor nutrition of the mother can also adversely affect the development of the fetus as can the use of a variety of drugs and the abuse of alcohol.

Good antenatal care greatly reduces the risk of damage to the fetus, or its delayed development. It involves the provision of advice about nutrition, general health and lifestyle issues as well as monitoring physical health and treating any conditions which are discovered. Congenital syphilis and the mental retardation and other abnormalities that may be caused by rubella early in pregnancy are rare nowadays when there is good antenatal care. Women approaching child-bearing age who have not had rubella should be immunized against it. A pregnant woman with HIV antibodies, who may not be ill with AIDS, has about a 50% chance of infecting her child. It is important, therefore, that such women are informed of the risk before they make the decision to embark on a pregnancy.

(c)   *Birth trauma*. The brain can suffer damage during birth, and injury to other parts of the body may also occur. Good obstetric care reduces the risk of such injuries.

(d)   *Prematurity and other neonatal problems*. These may cause brain damage and they may have indirect effects resulting from the prolonged separation of parents and child which occurs when a newborn child is treated for a long period in a special care unit. This may disrupt the parent-child bonding process.

(e)   *Accidents in and outside the home*. These are common causes of neurological and other injuries which may in turn predispose children to the development of psychiatric disorders or mental retardation. Many factors can reduce the incidence of accidents. These include the proper supervision of children in and out of the home; taking care to make the home 'child proof' by ensuring children do not have access to dangerous objects such as matches, knives and guns; the use of child restraints in motor vehicles; and teaching children about road safety and other precautions they can take to prevent injury.

(f)   *Poisons*. Poisoning by lead and other toxic chemical substances in the environment can put children at risk of developmental problems and psychiatric disorders. Exposure to radioactive material is another ever-present possibility today. Secondhand smoke from cigarettes and other smoking materials – also known as sidesmoke – is another example of a toxic substance that can adversely affect children's development.

(g)   *Physical illness*. Illnesses, especially those affecting the central nervous system, may place children at risk of developing psychiatric disorders (Barker, 1993a). The risks are greater for children who are ill repeatedly and are admitted many times to hospital.

(h)   *Deprivation, ill treatment and neglect*. Children may be deprived of a variety of things they require for their healthy development. The rates of psychiatric disorders, mental retardation and failure to learn at school have all been found to be greater in culturally deprived homes than in better endowed ones. The failure to provide children with proper food, clothing, shelter and medical care can also contribute to developmental delay and other problems. In some families the culture is one of ill treatment and neglect, which has often been the experience of the parents when they were children (Oliver, 1988).

(i) *Family disruption and disharmony.* Children from dysfunctional families generally have higher rates of emotional and behavioural disorders than those from better functioning families. Oliver (1988) suggests that there is scope for much improvement in the help given to such families and to the children in them. He points out that all branches of psychiatry, medicine, sociology, education and the law are involved with these children. He recommends the linking of 'the fields of work of child psychiatry, paediatrics, mental handicap, community health, special education, social work, and child protection' in dealing with these families (Oliver, 1988, page 552).

(j) *Parental illness.* This is a particularly serious risk factor when both parents suffer from mental illness; also when the parental disorders are serious and prolonged.

(k) *Early school failure.* This is often associated with specific learning disorders, hyperkinesis and neurological problems.

(l) *The experience of being in the care of a child welfare agency.* This is discussed further below.

(m) *Large family size.*

(n) *Father absence.*

This list is by no means exhaustive. In each case there is evidence to support the listing, though the precise mechanisms by which some of the factors lead to increased risk are not completely understood. Other risk factors, as yet undetermined, no doubt exist.

Protective factors and primary prevention

Protective factors are the converse of risk factors. They reduce the likelihood of a disorder appearing. The World Health Organization (1977b) listed the following:

(a) *Sex.* Girls appear to be less susceptible to psychosocial stress in childhood than boys.

(b) *Temperament.* An adaptable temperament, or an 'easy' one as described by Thomas & Chess (1977), seems to protect against the effects of deprivation and disadvantage.

(c)   *Isolated nature of stress*. Even chronic stresses, if isolated, tend to cause little damage but multiple stresses interact to potentiate the adverse results of each.

(d)   *Coping skills*. There is evidence that children can acquire the skills to cope with a variety of stressful circumstances. For example, children who are used to brief, happy separation experiences such as short stays with friends or relatives cope better with hospital admission.

(e)   *A good relationship with one parent*. This helps protect against the adverse effects which may result when a child is brought up in a discordant, unhappy home.

(f)   *Success or good experiences outside the home*. Good schooling, for example, or success in sports, can help mitigate the effects of a bad home environment.

(g)   *Improved family circumstances*. Later years spent in a harmonious family setting seem to lessen the effects of earlier adverse circumstances.

The concept of invulnerability

It has been observed, for example by Rutter (1979), that some children are able to survive gross deprivation and severe psychosocial stress without developing psychiatric disorders. Precisely what makes some children less vulnerable than others is not fully understood. The study of such resilience is fraught with difficulty and resilience is not a unitary characteristic (Luthar, 1993).

Werner & Smith (1982) carried out a longitudinal study of 698 children living on the Hawaiian island of Kauai. They point out that:

'From an epidemiological point of view, these children were at high risk, since they were born and reared in chronic poverty, exposed to higher than average rates of prematurity and perinatal stress, and reared by mothers with little formal education.' (Werner & Smith, 1982, page 153.)

The children were followed from birth into adult life, with less than a 10% drop-out rate. Some of them triumphed strikingly over adversity, becoming competent and autonomous young adults.

What distinguished the resilient high-risk children? They:

● had few serious illnesses in their first two decades, and recovered quickly from those they had;

- were perceived to be *very active* and *socially responsive* as infants;
- showed advanced self-help skills and adequate sensorimotor and language development in the second year of life;
- had adequate problem-solving and communication skills and age-appropriate perceptual-motor development in middle childhood; and
- as late adolescents had a more internal locus of control, a better self-concept, and a more nurturant, responsible, achievement orientated attitude towards life than their less successful peers.

Environmental factors associated with resiliency and stress resistance included:

- the age of the opposite sex parent (younger mothers for resilient boys and older fathers for resilient girls);
- four or fewer children in the family;
- a spacing of more than two years between the child and the next-born sibling;
- the presence and number of 'alternate care-takers' (father, grand-parents, older siblings) available to the mother within the household;
- the amount of attention given to the child by the primary care taker(s) in infancy;
- the availability of a sibling as caretaker or confidant in childhood;
- the cumulative number of chronic stressful life events experiences in childhood and adolescence.

Other factors that emerged were the mother's workload; the cohesiveness of the family; and whether there was an informal multigenerational network of kin and friends in adolescence.

Although these families were materially poor, a strong emotional bond was typically forged between infant and primary caretaker in the first year of life.

'The physical robustness of the resilient children, their high activity level, and their social responsiveness were recognized by the caregivers and elicited a great deal of attention. There was little prolonged separation of the infants from their mothers and no prolonged bond disruption during the first year of life. The strong attachment that resulted appears to have been a secure base for the development of self-help skills and autonomy noted among these children in their second year of life.

Though many of their mothers worked for extended periods and were major contributors to family subsistence, the children had support from alternate caretakers, such as grandmothers or older sisters, to whom they became attached.' (Werner & Smith, 1982, pages 155–6.)

Primary prevention methods

Offord (1987) divided primary prevention programs into:

- milestone programs, which restrict their efforts to children at particular ages or developmental levels;
- high-risk programs, which aim to prevent disorders in groups believed to be at above-average risk for the disorder; and
- community-wide programs.

Epidemiological data, together with evidence concerning risk factors, intervening variables and protective factors, make it possible for primary prevention plans to be made.

Milestone programmes

Examples of these are the 'Head Start' centres which were established in the USA in the mid-1960s. By the mid-1980s there were 9400 of these centres serving some 500 000 children supported by funding from the federal government of $1 billion (Parker, *et al.*, 1987). The aim of these centres was to provide intensive cognitive and emotional stimulation for pre-school children and their families. While they resulted in spurts in the children's development, the longer-term results were not striking. One study suggested that the mothers derived benefit, experiencing fewer psychological symptoms, increased feelings of mastery and increased satisfaction with the quality of life:

'For some of these mothers, burdened by having to care for a number of small children, living in poor quality housing, and unable to further their own career aspirations, Head Start seemed to be a haven. The benefits they received from their involvement appeared to have alleviated the symptoms of distress they were experiencing.' (Parker, *et al.*, 1987, pages 230/31).

Offord (1987) reviewed *milestone* prevention measures which have been suggested for school-age children. *Affective education* aims to promote awareness and acceptance in children of the ways in which feelings, attitudes and behaviours influence inter-personal behaviour (Baskin &

Hess, 1980). Offord (1987) concluded, however, that the results have been disappointing. His conclusions regarding the value of teaching children problem-solving skills, another proposed means of promoting better emotional and social adjustment, are similar. More hopeful approaches may be measures to prevent unwanted pregnancies in teenagers. These often occur in adolescents living in disadvantaged circumstances and carry increased risk of psychosocial disadvantage for both the teenagers concerned and their progeny.

High-risk programmes

Children who may be at specially high risk include those who are admitted to hospital; those suffering from chronic illnesses; those who have experienced a death in the family; those with very low birth weights; those treated in special care units in the neonatal period; and children admitted to the care of child welfare agencies. Children living in families in which there has been child abuse or neglect, either in the current family or the previous generation, are also at risk (Oliver, 1988).

Preventive measures have been suggested for all of the above groups. For example, Caplan (1980) suggests that positive steps can be taken to help children cope with crises such as admission to hospital. He advocated *anticipatory guidance* and *preventive intervention*. The former consists of explaining and discussing the upcoming crisis and the feelings and experiences the subjects are likely to encounter. This is best done in groups. Preventive intervention consists of guidance given to children and their families, focused on the here-and-now. The children are helped to understand what is happening, to find solutions to problems, counter blame of self and others, and maintain hope and find outside help – from extended family members, friends and professional care-givers. These measures may enhance children's coping skills, so that what might have been an emotionally damaging experience can become a growth-promoting one. There is evidence that measures such as the above may be effective in reducing the adverse effects of admission to hospital (Byrne & Cadman, 1987).

Children with chronic physical illnesses are a high-risk group, though how best to reduce the risk is not entirely clear. A helpful review of the field is that of Cadman, *et al.* (1987).

An important high-risk group consists of children who are or have been in the care of child welfare authorities. Such children have often been subject to neglect and/or abuse before being taken into care, and the task of meeting their, often great, needs in a fully adequate fashion may defeat the child welfare agencies attempting to deal with them. Not infrequently they are moved from placement to placement, as one living situation after another breaks down. The task of looking after these often angry, difficult and insecure young people is a daunting one. Another hazard some children face is that of being shuffled between the care of their parents and that of the agency as courts make dispositions, new information comes to light, and the parents are given further opportunities to learn and practise the skills needed to care for their children. Psychiatrists can assist child welfare agencies by offering advice as to the needs of parti- cular children, and – even more important – providing input in the planning of services, with the aim of ensuring that these have the best chance of meeting these children's many needs.

Children whose parents are admitted to hospital for psychiatric reasons are another high risk group (Shachnow, 1987). As well as losing their parents for a time, they may have already have been in an unstable environment because of the psychiatric problems of their parent(s). Attention to their emotional needs at this time may prevent them from developing disorders of their own.

Steinhauer (1984; 1991) provides a psychiatrist's perspective on the needs of children in care and how these may be met. He suggests way of preventing *drift* (the all-too-common process whereby children admitted to care languish in temporary placements for extended periods); mini- mizing emergency placements; and providing effective casework for the children and their families.

Many self-help groups provide support for individuals and families with particular problems. These range from groups for the families of children with cystic fibrosis or diabetes, to programs such as 'Alateen', which assists teenagers who have alcoholic parents.

The concept of high risk can also be applied to communities. In the UK, attempts have been made to work at the community level in areas in which there is a high prevalence of child and family problems. This has been called *intermediate treatment* (Leissner, et al., 1977). It involves the use of various social work techniques, but especially community work. This seeks to promote 'the participation of the parents and adults of the neighbourhood in the planning of services to children and youth, while fostering the involvement of the youngsters in the life of their community' (Leissner, et al., 1977). The idea is to apply these methods in 'areas of deprivation', with the objective of achieving both primary and secondary prevention.

Community-wide measures

Many characteristics of the communities in which children live have their effects. Good obstetric and neonatal care can prevent many of the ill-effects that result from brain damage. The removal of lead from the environment and the control of infectious diseases by immunization and other public health programmes are also rational preventive measures.

Factors such as cultural deprivation, family disharmony and parental mental illness present difficult challenges, though social change in communities can lead to the lessening of psychiatric morbidity. In a classic study, Leighton (1965) described changes in a rural community over a ten-year period. Initially the community was impoverished materially, culturally and socially, with a high prevalence of broken marriages, interparental strife, and child neglect. As a result of changes in the community, notably group action and the emergence of local leadership, there were great improvements in these areas over the ten years.

Contributory factors included the activities of the official responsible for adult education and the local teacher. Some external factors, such as the arrival of electrical power in the village, seemed to help but for the most part the changes in the community came from within. Outside people and agencies did, however, act as catalysts. The role of the *consolidated school* in a town several miles away seemed important. The village children started going to this school during the course of the study. The influence of the school, through the ideas, concepts, values and standards of behaviours brought home by the children, seemed helpful.

Leighton (1965) reported a great lowering of the prevalence of psychiatric disorders over the ten-year period. By contrast, other communities which had been equally disintegrated when the study started, remained so ten years later and showed no comparable decline in the prevalence of psychiatric disorders.

Other studies, for example those by Rutter and his colleagues (1979) have confirmed the important role of the school, as an institution, in the psychosocial development of children. In many troubled communities, unfortunately, the quality of the schools is as poor as the quality of life. In many of the world's urban ghettos substandard schools, high crime rates, delinquent gangs, widespread drug abuse and prostitution combine to make the prospects for children growing up in those communities bleak indeed. The desperate situation in the gang-controlled Chicago public housing projects has been well described by Garbarino and his colleagues (1991). In such situations, the provision of child psychiatry services such as are outlined in the previous chapters seems almost irrelevant. The challenge in such areas is the promotion of social change, without which the treatment of individual children, even in the context of their families, is likely to have limited effect.

Secondary prevention

Secondary intervention involves early diagnosis and case finding, followed by intervention to bring the disorder under control as rapidly as possible. The screening of populations to detect disorders early in their development is a first step.

In most school systems the academic progress of children is assessed from time to time, either by regular administration of tests of educational attainment, or more informally by teachers' observations, supplemented by the use of tests on an *ad hoc* basis. The screening of child populations for behavioural, emotional and other psychiatric disorders is less widespread, but perceptive teachers, and those who work with pre-school children in daycare and other centres, are often able to identify children showing early signs of such disorders. Various screening questionnaires that can assist in the identification of children with early signs of disorders are available. Examples are the Bristol Social Adjustment Guide (Stott, 1966) and the Child Behaviour Checklist (Achenbach & Edelbrock, 1983).

Academic failure often accompanies psychiatric disorders in children. Not only is there an association between antisocial behaviour and school failure, but children suffering from depression, neurotic disorders, psychotic disorders and other psychiatric problems may also present with academic failure. Vigilance by school staff can pay dividends in the early detection of problems other than primary learning disorders.

When disorders are detected in their early stages, the treatment methods described elsewhere in this book are usually indicated. Many schools and school systems have psychological and remedial services which can help children with academic problems, including those that are associated with other emotional or behavioural disorders. Many schools also have school counsellors, sometimes called guidance counsellors, as members of their staff. These are usually teachers who have received special training in dealing with children's emotional and social problems. They offer support and counselling to children in difficulty and, in many cases, also to the families of such children. They are in the front line of services for disturbed children, who may seek their help themselves or may be referred by other teachers, by parents or by others – for example child welfare workers.

Most developed societies also have services which provide support and other help for families containing young, and especially preschool, children. In the UK this service is provided mainly by health visitors, specialized nurses who have statutory duties which include visiting the families of all children soon after birth, and at intervals thereafter. In North America, nurses with similar functions are usually called public health nurses. These nurses do both primary preventive work by advising parents on the care and management of their children, and secondary prevention, by detecting problems early and either intervening themselves or referring children and families for assessment and treatment.

Tertiary prevention

Tertiary prevention comprises measures taken once a disorder is established. It aims to limit the effect of the disorder, to prevent it getting worse and to give support to affected individuals and their families. It requires active involvement and usually a lot of work on the part of the professionals concerned, but it may be very important, for example in the management of families in which there has been serious abuse and/or neglect of children. Primary and secondary prevention are to be preferred, but it often happens that troubled children and families come to attention only when their disorders are fully established.

In many communities there is a variety of agencies and workers providing tertiary prevention services, usually for families in which there appears to be a high risk of deterioration. These include community services for abusive and other dysfunctional families, and hospital-based 'child abuse' programs which provide specialized assessment and treatment. Many agencies offer treatment for abused children and their families. These aim to restore families to better ways of functioning, so that abuse does not occur, or recur, and the children's healthy development is promoted.

Other points

One of the problems confronting those who seek to promote primary prevention is that, as Kessler & Albee (1977) pointed out, 'practically every effort aimed at improving child rearing, increasing effective communication, building inner control and such like – in short everything aimed at improving the human condition – may be considered to be part of the primary prevention of mental or emotional disturbance'. It is therefore important to consider the likely cost effectiveness of proposed measures, and to build into programs of prevention measures to assess their effectiveness.

What preventive measures prove feasible depends largely on community attitudes and especially the attitudes of community leaders. Extravagant claims concerning expected results, programme failures, and excessively expensive schemes do not endear professionals to the communities they serve. It is the collective motivation of communities that determines whether rational preventive programs are developed and implemented. Community education is therefore important.

Concern has been expressed by many during the latter part of this century that western societies have not been providing good conditions for the raising of emotionally healthy children. They point to rising divorce rates, increasing numbers of single parent families attempting to live on inadequate incomes, and the growth of urban ghettos with much crime, violence and drug abuse. Goldsmith (1977) expressed the view that modern urban society undermines the essential functions of the family. The family, in turn, is undermined as the basic unit of our social system. He maintained that the educative, economic, welfare and social control functions of the family have all largely been taken away by the modern industrial state. At the same time, increasing numbers of poor, dispossessed, alienated people struggle to bring up children in deteriorating inner city areas. Economic and social problems make this increasingly difficult. Goldsmith's (1977) solution is *de-urbanization*, that is the settlement of people in smaller, ecologically based societies.

Whatever the best solutions to the ills of industrial societies may be, the deterioration of many inner city areas, and of public housing schemes, seems to have continued, rather as Goldsmith suggested. In many areas it has become necessary to have police and security guards in schools and to screen children for guns and other weapons when they arrive in their schools. Bronfenbrenner (1977) suggested that, 'in recent decades the American family has been falling apart'. He asserts that children's needs are being met less and less effectively and he too sees this as due to changing social standards. He asked how it was possible to deliver men and survival systems to the moon but not health care to many neighbourhoods. He blamed the self-centredness of people in today's society, and their failure to contribute adequately to the communities in which they live, for these problems.

It seems clear that social changes such as a decline in the rate of breakup of families would be helpful (Shamsie, 1985). It is less clear what steps should be taken, and by whom, to achieve such changes. Spiritual values seem to have been changing. Bronfenbrenner (1977) suggested that a selfseeking materialism is increasingly preferred to a philosophy which puts helping others first. As he put it, 'doing your own thing [is] our undoing'. The accumulation of material possessions seems to be a main aim of many in today's society. This has its limitations as a background for family life, the rearing of children, and the creation and maintenance of a functional social system.

The above issue are philosophical, moral, social and political, rather than clinical ones. They concern the whole of society, not just those professionally concerned with mental health issues. Yet all of us who are professionally involved should be aware of them and should constantly bring them to the attention of society, especially its leaders.

As this edition is written the industrial era is becoming the post-industrial age. The day when most depended on large industrial concerns for employment and security is passing. Downsizing, redeployment, retraining and small-scale entrepreneurship are becoming the order of the day. Will this be of benefit to the family? How can we make sure that, at a time of change – indeed of a major paradigm shift – the needs of our children are taken care of? Can the family be strengthened? Is there any alternative to it? This generation and the next will be severely challenged in answering such questions. In helping to find the answers, though, those trained and working in the mental health field will need to play major roles.

Appendix

The Children Act 1989 (England and Wales)

It is preferable, when children and their families require professional help, for this to be provided without legal compulsion or the intervention of the courts. In the great majority of cases this is indeed how problems are tackled. Unfortunately, this does not invariably prove possible and intervention backed by the force of law sometimes proves necessary. It is to meet the needs of such cases that in many jurisdictions legislation exists, which aims to protect children who are neglected or abused.

In England and Wales, the Children Act of 1989 replaced previous child welfare legislation. It was implemented in 1991. The definitive publication is the Act itself (Department of Health, 1989), and there is also available a summary, *The Children Act 1989 – An Introductory Guide for the NHS* (Department of Health, 1991). In addition the Royal College of Psychiatrists has published *A Concise Guide to the Children Act 1989* (Williams, 1992). Jones (1991) discusses the particular responsibilities which the Act places upon child and adolescent psychiatrists.

This appendix outlines the main points of the Act, with emphasis on its general principles and on sections of special importance to mental health professionals. The above publications should be consulted for further information.

The 1989 Act was designed to achieve a proper balance between the protection of children and the rights of parents to challenge the State when it seeks to intervene. In drafting any child welfare legislation the challenge must be faced of providing protection for children while at the same time respecting the roles of parents. The Children Act of 1989 represents the latest attempt to meet this challenge. It takes the welfare of the child as the paramount consideration and replaces the emphasis which previous legislation placed on parental rights with that of parental responsibility.

The Courts

The three courts which normally adjudicate on matters concerned with the Children Act are the magistrates court, the county court and the High Court.

In the *magistrates court* a 'family panel' of two or three lay magistrates, sitting with a justices' clerk or a stipendiary magistrate, is empowered, under the Children Act 1989, to deal with most of the matters discussed below, including the making of 'Section 8' orders. This is designated the 'family proceedings court'.

The *county court* deals with cases considered too complex to be dealt with by the magistrates court. These are heard at a family hearing centre or at a care centre which is presided over by a judge specially trained to deal with care proceedings. The family hearing centres can deal with such matters as divorce, nullity, domestic violence and adoption, which magistrates are not empowered to hear.

The *High Court* has a Family Division which deals with complex cases under the Children Act 1989, as well as adoption and other matters, and hears appeals from the magistrates courts.

There is also a *Court of Appeal* which hears appeals from the county court and High Court. In exceptional cases, where a matter of general public importance is involved, appeal can be made to the House of Lords.

The Act contains 12 Parts:

I. *Introductory.* This makes clear, in general terms, what the responsibilities of parents, courts and local authorities are. It enables local authorities to request the help of others, including health authorities, under certain circumstances and directs such others to comply if this is compatible with their own duties and obligations and does not interfere unduly with their own functions. It also requires that children's cases be handled expeditiously, since delay is likely to be harmful to the child. This requirement applies to the making of the various orders discussed below.

This part of the Act also provides a 'welfare check-list', consisting of the matters which courts are required to take into account when considering contested applications for orders under the Act. These are:

- The child's ascertainable wishes and feelings.
- The child's physical, emotional and educational needs.
- The likely effect on the child of changes in that child's circumstances.
- The child's age, sex and background and any other factors that appear relevant.
- Harm already suffered or which there is a risk that the child may suffer.
- The ability of the parents (or other relevant persons) to meet the child's needs.
- The range of powers available to the court.

II. *Orders with respect to children in family proceedings.* This part of the Act is concerned with the various 'private law orders' which may be made in the course of family proceedings. The most important are the 'Section 8' orders:

- Residence order. This is an order specifying with whom the child is to live. Such an order cannot, other than in exceptional circumstances, have effect beyond age 16. It gives parental responsibility to the person in whose favour it is made. The order may have special conditions attached and may be for a specified time period. If the application is opposed, the 'welfare check-list' applies. A residence order may be made in a magistrates court, a county court or the High Court. It ceases to have effect if the parents live together for a continuous period of six months or when the child reaches the age of 16.

– Contact order. This is an order requiring a person with whom a child is living or will be living, to permit the child to have contact with the person named in the order. The order may specify how the contact is to occur and it may impose conditions to be complied with by the person in whose favour the order is made, or by others concerned. Again, the child's welfare is the paramount consideration, and the order may be made in any of the three courts mentioned in the previous paragraph.

– Specific issue order. This is an order dealing with a specific issue concerning parental responsibility, which has arisen or may in the future arise. Examples are the child's education, religious upbringing or medical treatment. The court may direct how the order is to be carried out and may impose specific conditions.

– Prohibiting steps order. This sets out what a person with parental responsibility may not do, for example take the child out of the country or raise the child in a particular religion.

– Family assistance order. Under certain exceptional circumstances, a court may make an order requiring a probation officer or an officer of the local authority to advise, assist and, when appropriate, befriend any person named in the order. Those who may be named include a child's guardian, anyone with whom the child is living, anyone to whom a contact order applies and the child himself or herself. These orders may be made for a maximum of six months and may be renewed.

III.   *Local authority support for children and families.* The Act places a general duty on local authorities to safeguard and promote the welfare of children in their respective areas. They must provide appropriate services for children who are disabled or who are unlikely to be properly cared for unless they receive special services.

Child welfare legislation generally allows the relevant authorities to take more intrusive action when the circumstances of a child warrant this. In the UK it is the local authority that is charged with responsibility for such action. The 1989 Act also established new criteria for this, providing for both care and supervision orders.

Various 'threshold criteria' must be met before a care or supervision order is made. This process involves a series of steps. The first is consideration of whether the child is suffering or is likely to suffer from harm; this may involve ill-treatment, impairment of health, or impairment of development.

If the child's health or development are being affected, the next question to be considered is how that child's health or development compares with that to be expected in other similar children.

Then consideration must be given to whether the harm is significant. If it is, the court must decide whether it can be attributed to the care given, or likely to be given, if an order is not made.

Consideration must next be given to whether the care given to the child is not what a parent can reasonably be expected to give.

Finally the court must decide whether making an order would be better than not making an order, taking into account the 'welfare check-list' and the criterion that the welfare of the child is paramount.

In order to make proper decisions on questions such as those above, courts may seek the expert advice of relevant health-care professionals; the advice of psychiatrists, among others, may be sought.

IV.   *Care and supervision.* The orders a court may make if the above conditions are satisfied (public law orders) are:

  – A care order (Section 31). This provides for the local authority to take the child into its care and to provide accommodation and other necessities. While the local authority acquires parental authority for the child, it shares this with the parents. There is a presumption that children will maintain contact with their parents and others who have cared for them previously. Application for a care order may be made by the local authority or an 'authorized person'. The order may remain in force until the age of 18, or it may be terminated by the making of a residence order or a supervision order, or when anyone concerned, including the child, makes a successful application to the court. It is also terminated if an adoption order is made.

  – Interim care order. This is similar in its effects to a care order, but initially it may only be made for up to a maximum of eight weeks. Extensions of up to four weeks are permitted. Such orders are made when there is a need for further investigation of the circumstances of the child's case, but there is already reason to believe that the criteria for such action may be met.

  – Contact with child in care (Section 34). This is an order which specifies who may have contact with a child in care and under what circumstances. The 'welfare check-list' applies.

  – Supervision order (Section 31). This provides for the supervision of the child by a person who will advise, assist and befriend the child. The order may specify certain actions to be carried out by child or supervisor. If the order is not complied with, or the supervisor considers that it is no longer needed, the supervisor may apply for its variation or discharge. Similar application may be made by the child or anyone with parental responsibility.

  – Interim supervision order. This has a similar effect to that of a supervision order but may be made initially for up to eight weeks, with four-week extensions if necessary, while the child's circumstances are investigated further. The further investigation may include medical or psychiatric examination.

  – Education supervision order (Section 36). This is for use when a child who is of compulsory school age is not being properly educated. Such an order can be made for a child who is in local authority care. The supervisor must advise, assist and befriend the child and give directions to child and parents with a view to ensuring that the child receives a proper education. There is provision for actions to be taken, including investigation of the care the child is receiving by the local authority, if the directions are not complied with and the child is still not being properly educated. The order lasts for one year and extensions of up to three years may be made. The order ceases to be valid when the child reaches school leaving age or if the child is taken into care.

V.   *Protection of children.* Orders under this part of the Act are concerned with the protection of children. They include:

– Child assessment order. This may be made when the local authority or an 'authorized person' has reason to suspect that the child is suffering, or is likely to suffer significant harm, and an assessment of the child's health and/or development is necessary to determine whether this is the case. The order may only be made when it is considered unlikely that such an assessment will otherwise be satisfactorily carried out – or carried out at all – if the order is not made. The order does not require that the child be kept away from home, except in so far as this is necessary to enable the assessment to be carried out. The order is valid for a period of seven days from the date specified in the order.

– Emergency protection order. This authorizes removal of the child to accommodation provided by the applicant – often the local authority, though others can apply for an emergency protection order. It also prevents removal of the child from a hospital or other place where the child was accommodated immediately before the order was made, and it assigns parental responsibility to the applicant. If necessary a warrant may be issued allowing the police to assist a person attempting to exercise powers granted by the order if that person is being prevented from exercising those powers. (There is also a provision in the Act (Section 46) that allows the police to take a child into police protection under certain circumstances.)

– Recovery order. This may be made when a child has been unlawfully taken away or kept apart from the responsible person named in an emergency protection or care order; when the child has run away or is staying away from that person; or when the child is missing. It directs anyone who can do so to produce the child to an authorized person; it allows such a person to remove the child; requires all those who have knowledge of the child's whereabouts to disclose this information when required to do so by a constable or court officer; and authorizes the police to enter premises specified in the order to search for the child.

Parts VI to XII deal with the arrangements laid down for the operation of the various institutions and services named. They are of less direct relevance to most health professionals but are listed below for completeness.

VI.   *Community homes.*
VII.   *Voluntary homes and voluntary organizations.*
VIII.   *Registered children's homes.*
IX.   *Private arrangements for fostering children.*
X.   *Child minding and day care for young children.*
XI.   *The Secretary of States supervisory functions and responsibilities.*
XII.   *Miscellaneous and general.*

References

Achenbach, T.M. and Edelbrock, C.S. (1983). *Manual for Child Behaviour Checklist and Revised Child Behaviour Profile*. Burlington: Department of Psychiatry, University of Vermont.

Adams, P.L. (1982). *A Primer of Child Psychotherapy*, 2nd edn. Boston: Little, Brown.

Ainsworth, M.D.S., Blehar, M.C., Waters, E. and Wall, S. (1978). *Patterns of Attachment: A Psychological Study of Strange Situations*. Hillsdale, NJ: Lawrence Erlbaum.

Akiskal, H.S. and Weller, E.B. (1989). 'Mood disorders and suicide in children and adolescents'. In: *Comprehensive Textbook of Psychiatry*, 5th edition, eds H.I. Kaplan and B.J. Sadock. Baltimore: Williams and Wilkins.

Allen, F.H. (1942). *Psychotherapy with Children*. New York: Norton.

Allen, R. and Wasserman, G.A. (1985). 'Origins of language delay in abused infants'. *Child Abuse and Neglect*, **9**, 335–340.

Allen, R.P., Singer, H.S., Brown, J.E. and Salam, M.M. (1992). 'Sleep disorder in Tourette syndrome: a primary or unrelated problem?' *Paediatric Neurology*, **8**, 275–280.

Aman, M.G., Kern, R.A., McGhee, D.E. and Arnold, L.E. (1993). 'Fenfluramine and methylphenidate in children with mental retardation and attention deficit disorder: laboratory effects'. *Journal of Autism and Developmental Disorders*, **23**, 491–506.

Ambrosini, P.J., Bianchi, M.D., Rabinovich, H. and Elia, J. (1993a). 'Antidepressant treatments in children and adolescents. 1. Affective disorders'. *Journal of the American Academy of Child and Adolescent Psychiatry*, **32**, 1–6.

Ambrosini, P.J., Bianchi, M.D., Rabinovich, H. and Elia, J. (1993b). 'Antidepressant treatments in children and adolescents'. *Journal of the American Academy of Child and Adolescent Psychiatry*, **32**, 483–493.

American Psychiatric Association (1980). *Diagnostic and Statistical Manual of Mental Disorders*, 3rd edn (DSM-III) Washington, DC: APA.

American Psychiatric Association (1987). *Diagnostic and Statistical Manual of Mental Disorders*, 3rd edn, revised. *(DSM-III-R)* Washington, DC: APA.

American Psychiatric Association (1994) *Diagnostic and Statistical Manual of Mental Disorders*, 4th edn. *(DSM-IV)*. Washington, DC: APA.

Amini, F., Salasnek, S. and Burke, E.L. (1976). 'Adolescent drug abuse: etiological and treatment considerations'. *Adolescence*, **11**, 381–299.

Anthony, E.J. (1957). 'An experimental approach to the psychopathology of childhood: encopresis'. *British Journal of Medical Psychology*, **30**, 146–175.

Aponte, H. (1976). 'The family-school interview'. *Family Process*, **15**, 303–311.

August, G.J., Stewart, M.A. and Tsai, L. (1981). 'The incidence of cognitive disabilities in the siblings of autistic children'. *British Journal of Psychiatry*, **138**, 416–422.

Balbernie, R. (1974). 'Unintegration, integration and level of ego functioning as the determinants of planned 'cover therapy', of unit task and of placement'. *Journal of the Association of Workers for Maladjusted Children*, **2**, 6–46.

Bandini, L.G. and Dietz, W.H. (1992). 'Myths about childhood obesity'. *Pediatric Annals*, **21**, 647–652.

Bandler, R. and Grinder, J. (1979). *Frogs into Princes*. Palo Alto: Science and Behavior Books.

Barber, J.B. (1982). 'Techniques of pain management'. In: *Psychological Approaches to the Management of Pain*, eds. J.B. Barber and C. Adrian. New York: Brunner/Mazel.

Barker, P. (1968). 'The inpatient treatment of school refusal'. *British Journal of Medical Psychology*, **41**, 381–387.

Barker, P. (1981). 'Paradoxical techniques in psychotherapy'. In: *Treating Families with Special Needs*, eds. D.S. Freeman and B. Trute. Ottowa: Canadian Association of Social Workers.

Barker, P. (1982). 'Residential treatment for disturbed children: its place in the 80s'. *Canadian Journal of Psychiatry*, **27**, 634–639.

Barker, P. (1984). 'Recognition and treatment of anxiety in children by means of psychiatric interview'. In: *Anxiety in Children*, ed. V.P. Varma. London: Croom Helm.

Barker, P. (1985). *Using Metaphors in Psychotherapy*. New York: Brunner/Mazel.

Barker, P (1988). 'The future of residential treatment for children'. In: *Children in Residential Care: Critical Issues in Treatment*, eds. C.E. Schaefer and A.J. Swanson. New York: Van Nostrand Reinhold.

Barker, P. (1990). *Clinical Interviews with Children and Adolescents*. New York: Norton.

Barker, P. (1992). *Basic Family Therapy*. 3rd edn. Oxford: Blackwell.

Barker, P. (1993a). 'The effects of physical illness'. In: *How and why Children Fail*, ed. V. Varma. London: Jessica Kingsley.

Barker, P. (1993b). 'The child from the chaotic family'. In *How and Why Children Fail*, ed. V. Varma. London: Jessica Kingsley.

Barker, P. (1993c). 'The effects of child abuse'. In: *How and Why Children Fail*, ed. V. Varma. London: Jessica Kingsley.

Barker, P. (1994). 'Reframing: The Essence of Psychotherapy?' In: *Ericksonian Methods: The Essence of the Story*, ed. J.K. Zeig. New York: Brunner/Mazel.

Barker, P., Buffe, C. and Zaretsky, R. (1978). 'Providing a family alternative for the disturbed child'. *Child Welfare*, **57**, 373–379.

Barnhill, L.H. and Longo, D. (1978). 'Fixation and regression in the family life cycle'. *Family Process*, **17**, 469–478.

Bartak, L., Rutter, M. and Cox, A. (1975). 'A comparative study of infantile autism and specific developmental receptive language disorder'. *British Journal of Psychiatry*, **126**, 127–145.

Baskin, E.J. and Hess, R.D. (1980). 'Does affective education work?' *Journal of School Psychology*, **18**, 40–50.

Beitchman, J.H. (1983). 'Childhood schizophrenia: a review and comparison with adult onset schizophrenia', *Psychiatric Journal of the University of Ottowa*, **8**, 25–37.

Bellman, M. (1966). 'Studies on encopresis'. *Acta Paediatrica Scandinavica*, Supplement, **170**.

Bender, L. and Schilder, P. (1940). 'Impulsions: a specific disorder of the behaviour of children'. *Archives of Neurology and Psychiatry*, **44**, 990–1008.

Benoit, D. (1993). 'Failure to thrive and feeding disorders'. In: *Handbook of Infant Mental Health*, ed. C.H. Zeanah. New York: Guilford.

Berecz, J.M. (1968). 'Phobias in childhood: aetiology and treatment'. *Psychological Bulletin*, **70**, 694–720.

Berg, I. (1979). 'Day wetting in children'. *Journal of Child Psychology and Psychiatry*, **20**, 167–173.

Berg, I. (1985). 'The management of truancy'. *Journal of Child Psychology and Psychiatry*, **26**, 325–331.

Berg, I., Forsythe, I., Holt, P. and Watta, J. (1983). 'A controlled trial of 'Senokot' on faecal soiling treated by behavioural methods'. *Journal of Child Psychology and Psychiatry*, **24**, 543–549.

Berger, M., Yule, W. and Rutter, M. (1975). 'Attainment and adjustment in two geographical areas'. *British Journal of Psychiatry*, **126**, 110–118.

Berney, T., Kolvin, I., Bhate, S.R., Garside, R.F., Jeans, B., Kay, B. and Scarth, L. (1981). 'School phobia: a therapeutic trial with clomipramine and short-term outcome'. *British Journal of Psychiatry*, **138**, 110–118.

Bernstein, G.A. and Garfinkel, B.D. (1986). 'School phobia: the effective overlap of effective and anxiety disorders'. *Journal of the American Academy of Child Psychiatry*, 25, 235–241.

Bicknell, J. (1975). *Pica: A Childhood Symptom*. London: Butterworth.

Billiard, M. (1989). 'The Kleine-Levin Syndrome'. In: *Principles and Practice of Sleep Medicine*, ed. T. Roth and W.C. Dement. Philadelphia: W.B. Saunders.

Bishop, D.V.M. (1993). 'Autism, executive functions and theory of mind: a neuropsychological perspective'. *Journal of Child Psychology and Psychiatry*, **34**, 279–293.

Blagg, N.R. and Yule, W. (1984). 'The behavioural treatment of school refusal: a comparative study'. *Behaviour Research and Therapy*, **22**, 119–127.

Boulos, C. and Kutcher, S.P. (1992), 'The pharmacological treatment of adolescent depression'. *Canadian Child Psychiatric Bulletin*, **1**, 52–56.

Bowlby, J. (1951). *Maternal Care and Mental Health*. Geneva: World Health Organization.

Bowlby J. (1969). *Attachment*. London: Hogarth; New York: Basic Books.

Bowlby, J. (1979). *The Making and Breaking of Affectional Bonds*. London: Tavistock.

Bowlby, J. (1980). *Attachment and Loss: III. Loss, Sadness and Depression*. London: Hogarth; New York: Basic Books.

Boyle, M.H. and Offord, D.R. (1986). 'Smoking, drinking and the use of illicit drugs among adolescents in Ontario'. *Canadian Medical Association Journal*, **135**, 1113–1121.

Boyle, M.H., Offord, D.R., Hofman, H.G., Catlin, G.P., Byles, J.A., Cadman, D.T., Crawford, J.W., Links, P.S., Rae-Grant, N.I. and Szatmari, P. (1987). 'Ontario child health study: methodology'. *Archives of General Psychiatry*, **44**, 826–831.

Bradford, J. and Dimock, J. (1986). 'A comparative study of adolescents and adults who willfully set fires'. *Psychiatric Journal of the University of Ottowa*, **11**, 228–234.

Bradley, S.J., Doering, R.W., Zucker, K.F., Finegan, J.K. and Gonda, G.M. (1980). 'Assessment of the gender-disturbed child: a comparison to sibling and psychiatric controls'. In: *Childhood and Sexuality*, ed. J. Samson. Montreal: Editions Etudes Vivantes.

Brandenburg, N.A., Friedman, R.M. and Silver S.E. (1990). 'The epidemiology of childhood psychiatric disorders: prevalence findings from recent studies'. *Journal of the American Academy of Child and Adolescent Psychiatry*, **29**, 76–83.

Brent, D.A., Kalas, R., Edelbrock, C., Costello, A.J., Dulcan, M.K. and Conover, N. (1986). 'Psychopathology and its relationship to suicidal ideating in childhood and adolescence'. *Journal of the American Academy of Child Psychiatry*, **25**, 666–673.

Bridgland, M. (1971). *Pioneer Work with Maladjusted Children*. London: Crosby Lockwood Staples.

British Medical Journal. (1977). (Editorial). **1**, 4.

Bronfenbrenner, U. (1977). 'Doing your own thing – our undoing'. *Child Psychiatry and Human Development*, **8**, 3–10.

Brown, B. and Lloyd, H. (1975). 'A controlled study of children not speaking in school'. *Journal of the Association of Workers for Maladjusted Children*, **3**, 49–63.

Brown, B.D. and Fromm, E. (1986). *Hypnosis and Hypnotherapy*. Hillsdale, NJ: Lawrence Erlbaum.

Bullard, D.M., Glaser, H.H., Hagerty, M.C. and Pivchik, E.C. (1967). 'Failure to thrive in the "neglected" child'. *American Journal of Orthopsychiatry*, **37**, 680–690.

Byrne, C.M.N. and Cadman, D. (1987). 'Prevention of the adverse effects of hospitalization in children'. *Journal of Preventive Psychiatry*, **3**, 167–190.

Cadman, D., Rosenbaum, P. and Pettinghill, P. (1987). 'Prevention of emotional, behavioural, and family problems of children with chronic medical illness'. *Journal of Preventive Psychiatry*, **3**, 147–165.

Caffey, J. (1946). 'Multiple fractures in the long bones of infants suffering from chronic subdural haematoma'. *American Journal of Roentgenology*, **56**, 163–173.

Calgary Herald (1993). Article by Bob Beaty, page A1, 27 November, 1993.

Cameron, J.R. (1977). 'Parental treatment, children's temperament and the risk of childhood behavioural problems'. *American Journal of Orthopsychiatry*, **47**, 568–576.

Cantor, S. and Kestenbaum, C. (1986). 'Psychotherapy with schizophrenic children'. *Journal of the American Academy of Child Psychiatry*, **25**, 623–630.

Cantwell, D.P. and Rutter, M. (1994). 'Classifications, conceptual issues and substantive findings'. In: *Child and Adolescent Psychiatry: Modern Approaches*, 3rd edn., edited by M. Rutter, E. Taylor and L. Hersov. Oxford: Blackwell Science Ltd.

Caplan, G. (1964). *Principles of Preventive Psychiatry*. New York: Basic Books.

Caplan, G. (1980). 'An approach to preventive intervention in child psychiatry'. *Canadian Journal of Psychiatry*, **25**, 623–630.

Carlson, G.A. (1990a). 'Child and adolescent mania – diagnostic considerations'. *Journal of Child Psychology and Psychiatry*, **31**, 331–341.

Carlson, G.A. (1990b). 'Suicidal behaviour and psychopathology in children and adolescents'. *Current Opinion In Psychiatry*, **3**, 449–452.

Carpenter, S.P.C. (1989). 'Development of a young man with Prader-Willi syndrome and secondary functional encopresis'. *Canadian Journal of Psychiatry*, **34**, 123–126.

Carter, E.A. and McGoldrick, M. (1980). *The Family Life Cycle*. New York: Gardner.

Chess, S. (1977). 'Follow-up report on autism in congenital rubella'. *Journal of Autism and Childhood Schizophrenia*, **7**, 69–81.

Chess, S. and Thomas, A. (1984). *Origins and Evolution of Behaviour Disorders from Infancy to Early Adult Life*. New York: Brunner/Mazel.

Chudley, A.E. (1991). 'Sex chromosome and autosomal aneuploidy in the fragile X syndrome'. In: *Children and Young Adults with Sex Chromosome Aneuploidy*, eds J.A. Evans, J.L. Hamerton and A. Robinson.

Clore, E.R. and Hibel, J. (1993). 'The parasomnias of childhood'. *Journal of Pediatric Health Care*, **7**, 12–16.

Coates, S. and Person, E.S. (1985). 'Extreme boyhood femininity: isolated behaviour of pervasive disorder?' *Journal of the American Academy of Child Psychiatry*, **24**, 702–709.

Cohen, P., Cohen, J. and Brook, J. (1993a). 'An epidemiological study of disorders in late childhood and adolescence'. *Journal of Child Psychology and Psychiatry*, **34**, 869–877.

Cohen, P., Cohen, J., Kasen, S., Velez, C.N., Hartmark, C., Johnson, J., Rojas, M., Brook and Streuning, E.L. (1993b). 'An epidemiological study of disorders in late childhood and adolescence – I. Age and gender-specific prevalence'. *Journal of Child Psychology and Psychiatry*, **34**, 851–867.

Conners, C.K. (1969). 'A teacher rating scale for use in drug studies with children'. *American Journal of Psychiatry*, **126**, 884–888.

Conture, A.G. (1990). *Stuttering*, 2nd edn. Englewood Cliffs, New Jersey: Prentice Hall.

Cooper, S. (1987). 'The fetal alcohol syndrome'. *Journal of Child Psychology and Psychiatry*, **28**, 223–227.

Coopersmith, S. (1967). *The Antecedents of Self-Esteem*. San Francisco: W.H. Freeman.

Coppersmith, E.I. (1981). 'Developmental reframing'. *Journal of Strategic and Systemic Therapies*, **1**, 1–8.

Coppersmith, E.I. (1985). 'Teaching trainees to think in triads'. *Journal of Marital and Family Therapy*, **11**, 61–66.

Corbett, J.A. (1979). 'Psychiatric morbidity and mental retardation'. In: *Psychiatric Illness and Mental Handicap*, eds F.E. James and R.P. Snaith. London: Gaskell Press.

Corbett, J.A., Matthews, A.M., Connell, P.H. and Shapiro, D.A. (1969). 'Tics and Gilles de la Tourette's syndrome: a follow-up study and critical review'. *British Journal of Psychiatry*, **115**, 1229–1241.

Costello, A.J. (1986). 'Assessment and diagnosis of affective disorder in children'. *Journal of Child Psychology and Psychiatry*, **27**, 565–574.

Cotton, N.S. (1983). 'The development of self-esteem and self- esteem regulation'. In: *The Development of Self-Esteem*, eds J.E. Mack and S.L. Ablon. New York: International Universities Press.

Covitz, J. (1986). *Emotional Child Abuse*. Boston: Sigo Press.

Cramer-Azima, F.J. (1991). 'Group psychotherapy for children and adolescents'. In: *Child and Adolescent Psychiatry: A Comprehensive Textbook*, ed. M. Lewis. Baltimore: Williams and Wilkins.

Crasnilneck, H.B. and Hall, J.A. (1985). *Clinical Hypnosis: Principles and Applications*, 2nd edn. Orlando, Fl: Grune and Stratton.

Crnic, K.A. and Reid, M. (1989). 'Mental retardation'. In: *Treatment of Childhood Disorders*, eds E.J. Mash and E.A. Barklay. New York: Guilford.

Cytryn, L., McKnew, D.H., Zahn-Waxler, C. and Gershon, E.S. (1986). 'Developmental issues in risk research: the offspring of affectively ill parents'. In: *Depression in Young People: Developmental and Clinical Perspectives*, eds M. Rutter, C.E. Izard and P.B. Read. New York: Guilford.

Davie, R., Butler, N. and Goldstein, H. (1972). *From Birth to Seven*. London: Longman.

Davies, K. (1991). 'Breaking the fragile X'. *Nature*, **351**, 439–440.

Department of Health (1989). *The Children Act 1989*. London: HMSO.

Department of Health (1991). *The Children Act 1989 – An Introductory Guide for the NHS*. London: HMSO.

DeVaaugh-Geiss, J., Moroz, G., Biederman, J., Cantwell, D., Fontaine, R., Greist, J.H., Reichler, R., Katz, R. and Landau, P. (1992). 'Chlorimipramine hydrochloride in childhood and adolescent obsessive-compulsive disorder – a multicentre trial'. *Journal of the American Academy of Child and Adolescent Psychiatry*, **31**, 45–49.

Deykin, E.Y. and MacMahon, B. (1979). 'The incidence of seizures among autistic children'. *American Journal of Psychiatry*, **136**, 1310–1312.

DiLeo, J.H. (1983). *Interpreting Children's Drawings*. New York: Brunner/Mazel.

Dilts, R., Grinder, J., Bandler, R., Bandler, L.C. and DeLozier, J. (1980). *Neuro-Linguistic Programming: Volume 1*. Cupertino, CA: Meta Publications.

Dische, S., Yule, W., Corbett, J.A. and Hand, D. (1983). 'Childhood enuresis: factors associated with outcome of treatment with an enuresis alarm'. *Developmental Medicine and Child Neurology*, **25**, 67–80.

Dixon, S.D. and Stein, M.T. (1992). *Encounters with Children*. St. Louis: Mosby Year Book.

Dobson, K.S. (Ed.) (1988). *Handbook of Cognitive-Behavioural Therapies*. New York: Guilford.

Dockar-Drysdale, B. (1968). *Therapy in Child Care* (collected papers). London: Longman.

Dockar-Drysdale, B. (1973). *Consultation in Child Care*. London: Longman.

Douglas, V.I., Barr, R.G., O'Neill, M.E. and Britton, B.G. (1986). 'Short term effects of methylphenidate on the cognitive, learning and academic performance of children with attention deficit disorder in the laboratory and classroom'. *Journal of Child Psychology and Psychiatry*, **27**, 191–211.

Driscoll, J.M., Driscoll, Y.T., Steir, M.E., Stark, R.I., Dangman, B.C., Perez, A., Wung, J.T. and Kritz, P. (1982). 'Mortality and morbidity in infants less than 1000 grams birth weight'. *Pediatrics*, **69**, 21–26.

Durrant, M. (1993). *Residential Treatment: A Cooperative, Competency-Based Approach to Therapy and Program Design.* New York: Norton.

Duvall, E.M. and Miller, B.C. (1985). *Marriage and Family Development*, 6th edn. New York: Harper & Row.

Earls, F., Jacobs, G., Goldfein, R., Silbert, A., Beardslee, W. and Rivinus, T. (1982). 'Concurrent validation of a behaviour problems scale to use with three-year-olds'. *Journal of Child Psychology and Psychiatry*, **21**, 47–57.

Edwards, S.D. and van der Spuy, H.I.J. (1985). 'Hypnotherapy as a treatment for enuresis'. *Journal of Child Psychology and Psychiatry*, **26**, 161–170.

Egger, J., Carter, C.M.N., Graham, P.J., Gumley, D. and Soothill, J.F. (1985). 'Controlled trial of oligoantigenic diet in the hyperkinetic syndrome'. *Lancet*, **1**, 540–545.

Elmer, E. (1986). 'Outcome of residential treatment for abused and high-risk infants. Child Abuse and Neglect, **10**, 351–360.

Emde, R.N. (1985). 'Assessment of infancy disorders'. In: *Child and Adolescent Psychiatry: Modern Approaches*, 2nd edn, eds M. Rutter and L. Hersov. Oxford: Blackwell.

Emler, N., Reichler, S. and Ross, A. (1987). 'The social context of delinquent conduct'. *Journal of Child Psychology and Psychiatry*, **28**, 99–109.

Epstein, N.B., Bishop, D.S. and Levin, S. (1978). 'The McMaster model of family functioning'. *Journal of Marriage and Family Counselling*, **4**, 19–31.

Erikson, E.H. (1965) *Childhood and Society*. London: Penguin.

Erikson, E.H. (1968). *Identity and the Life Cycle.* London: Faber.

Erickson, M.H., Hershman, S. and Secter, I.I. (1961). *The Practical Application of Medical and Dental Hypnosis.* Chicago: Seminars on Hypnosis Publishing Co.

Evans, J.A., Hamerton, J.L. and Robinson, A. (eds) (1991). *Children and Young Adults with Sex Chromosome Aneuploidy.* New York: Wiley-Liss.

Eysenck, H.J. (1959). 'Learning theory and behaviour therapy', *Journal of Mental Science*, **105**, 61–95.

Farber, E.D., Kinast, C., McCoard, W.D. and Falkner, D. (1984). 'Violence in families of adolescent runaways'. *Child Abuse and Neglect*, **8**, 295–299.

Farrington, D.P. (1978). 'The family background of aggressive youths'. In: *Aggression and Anti-social Behaviour in Childhood and Adolescence*, eds L. Hersov, M. Berger and D. Shaffer. Oxford: Pergamon.

Ferguson, B.G. (1986). 'Kleine-Levin syndrome: a case report'. *Journal of Child Psychology and Psychiatry*, **27**, 275–278.

Ferrari, M. (1986). 'Fear and phobias in childhood: some clinical and developmental considerations'. *Child Psychiatry and Human Development*, **17**, 75–87.

Fish, B. (1986). 'Antecedents of an acute schizophrenic break'. *Journal of the American Academy of Child Psychiatry*, **25**, 595–600.

Fisher, G.C. and Mitchell, I. (1992). 'Munchausen's syndrome by proxy (factitious illness by proxy)'. *Current Opinion in Psychiatry*, **5**, 224–227.

Flavell, J.H. (1963). *The Developmental Psychology of Jean Piaget*. Princeton: van Norstrand.

Flint, J. and Yule, W. (1994). 'Behavioural prototypes'. In: *Child and Adolescent Psychiatry: Modern Approaches*, 3rd edn., edited by M. Rutter, E. Taylor and L. Hersov. Oxford: Blackwell Science Ltd.

Folstein, S. and Rutter, M, (1977). 'Genetic influences and autism'. *Nature*, **265**, 726–728.

Fossen, A., Knibbs, J., Bryant-Waugh, R. and Lask, B. (1987). 'Early onset anorexia nervosa'. *Archives of Disease in Childhood*, **62**, 114–118.

Frankl, V.E. (1960). 'Paradoxical intention: a logotherapeutic technique'. *American Journal of Psychotherapy*, **14**, 520–535.

Freud, A. (1966). *Normality and Pathology in Childhood*. New York: International Universities Press; and London: Hogarth.

Freud, A. (1972). *A Short History of Child Analysis*. London: Hogarth.

Freud, S. (1905). 'Three essays on the theory of sexuality'. *Standard Edition*, **7**. London: Hogarth (1953).

Fundudis, T. (1986). 'Anorexia nervosa in a pre-adolescent girl: a multimodal behaviour therapy approach'. *Journal of Child Psychology and Psychiatry*, **27**, 261–273.

Gabel, S. and Hsu, L.K.G. (1986). 'Routine laboratory tests in adolescent inpatients'. *Journal of the American Academy of Child and Adolescent Psychiatry*, **25**, 113–119.

Gadow, K.D. (1992). 'Pediatric psychopharmacology: a review of recent research'. *Journal of Child Psychology and Psychiatry*, **33**, 153–195.

Gaensbauer, T.J. and Harmon, R.J. (1981). 'Clinical assessment in infancy utilizing structured playroom situations'. *Journal of the American Academy of Child Psychiatry*, **20**, 264–280.

Garbarino, J., Guttman, E. and Seeley, J.W. (1986). *The Psychologically Battered Child*. San Francisco: Jossey-Bass.

Garbarino, J., Kostelny, K. and Dubrow, N. (1991). *No Place to be a Child: Growing Up in a War Zone*. Lexington, Mass: Lexington Books.

Gardner, G.G. and Olness, K. (1981). *Hypnosis and Hypnotherapy with Children*. New York: Grune and Stratton.

Garfinkel, P.E. and Garner, D.M. (1982). *Anorexia Nervosa: A Multidimensional Perspective*. New York: Brunner/Mazel.

Garner, D.M. and Garfinkel, P.E. (1980). 'Sociocultural factors in the development of anorexia nervosa'. *Psychological Medicine*, **10**, 647–656.

Garrison, C.Z., Addy, C.L., Jackson, K., McKeown, R.E. and Waller, J.L. (1991) 'A longitudinal study of suicidal ideation in young adolescents'. *Journal of the American Academy of Child and Adolescent Psychiatry*, **30**, 597–603.

Gaynor, J. and Hatch, C. (1987). *The Psychology of Firesetting*. New York: Brunner/Mazel.

German, G.A. (1972). 'Aspects of clinical psychiatry in Sub-Saharan Africa'. *British Journal of Psychiatry*, **121**, 461–479.

Ghent, W.R., Da Sylva, N.P. and Farren, M.E. (1985). 'Family violence: guidelines for recognition and management'. *Canadian Medical Association Journal*, **132**, 541–548.

Gillberg, I.C. and Gillberg, C. (1989). 'Asperger Syndrome – some epidemiological considerations: a research note'. *Journal of Child Psychology and Psychiatry*, **30**, 631–638.

Gittelman, R. (1986). *Anxiety Disorders in Childhood*. New York: Guilford.

Goldsmith, E. (1977). 'The future of an affluent society: the case of Canada'. *Ecologist*, **7**, 160–194.

Goodman, R. and Stevenson, J. (1989). 'A twin study of hyperactivity – II. The aetiological role of genes, family relationships and perinatal adversity'. *Journal of Child Psychology and Psychiatry*, **30**, 691–709.

Goodyer, I.M. (1985). 'Epileptic and pseudoepileptic seizures in childhood and adolescence'. *Journal of the American Academy of Child Psychiatry*, **24**, 3–9.

Goswami, U. (1992). 'Phonological factors in spelling development'. *Journal of Child Psychology and Psychiatry*, **33**, 967–975.

Goodman, R. (1994). 'Brain disorders'. In: *Child and Adolescent Psychiatry: Modern Approaches*, 3rd edn., edited by M. Rutter, E. Taylor and L. Hersov. Oxford: Blackwell Science Ltd.

Gould, M.S., Wunsch-Hitzig, R. and Dohrenwend, B.P. (1980). 'Formulation of hypotheses about the prevalence, treatment and prognostic significance of psychiatric disorders in children in the United States'. In: *Mental Illness in the United States*, eds B.P. Dohrenwend, B.S. Dohrenwend, M.S. Gould, B. Link, R. Neugebauer and R. Wunsch-Hitzig. New York: Praeger.

Government of Alberta (1984). *Child Welfare Act*. Edmonton: Queen's Printer.

Graham, P.J. (1985). 'Psychosomatic relationship'. In: *Child and Adolescent Psychiatry: Modern Approaches*, 2nd edn, eds M. Rutter and L. Hersov. Oxford: Blackwell.

Green, R. (1985). 'Atypical psychosexual development'. In: *Child and Adolescent Psychiatry: Modern Approaches*, 2nd edn, eds, M. Rutter and L. Hersov. Oxford: Blackwell.

Green, R., Roberts, C.W., Williams, K., Goodman, M. and Mixon, A. (1987). 'Specific cross-gender behaviour in boyhood and later homosexual orientation'. *British Journal of Psychiatry*, **151**, 84–88.

Green, W.H. (1991). *Child and Adolescent Clinical Psychopharmacology*. Baltimore: Williams and Wilkins.

Green, W.H., Campbell, M., Hardesty, A.S., Grega, D.M., Padron-Gayol, M., Shell, J. and Erlenmeyer-Kimling, L. (1984). 'A comparison of schizophrenic and autistic children'. *Journal of the American Academy of Child Psychiatry*, **23**, 399–409.

Greiner, J.R., Fitzgerald, H.E., Cooke, P.A. and Djurdjic, S.D. (1985). 'Assessment of sensitivity to interpersonal stress in stutterers and non-stutterers'. *Journal of Communication Disorders*, **18**, 215–225.

Group for the Advancement of Psychiatry (1968). *Normal Adolescence: Its Dynamics and Impact*. New York: GAP. (Also London: Crosby, Lockwood, Staples, 1974).

Gualtieri, C.T., Wargin, W., Kanoy, P., Patrick, K., Shen, C.D., Youngblood, W., Mueller, R.A. and Breese, G.R. (1982). 'Clinical studies of methylphenidate levels in children and adults.' *Journal of the American Academy of Child Psychiatry*, **21**, 19–26.

Gubbay, S.S. (1975) *The Clumsy Child*. London: Saunders.

Guilleminault, C., Eldridge, F.L., Simmons, F.B. and Dement, W.C. (1976). 'Sleep apnoea in eight children'. *Pediatrics*, **58**, 23–30.

Guiness, E. (1986). 'Social origins of a neurosis: the African brain fag syndrome'. Paper presented at a meeting of the African Psychiatric Association, Nairobi, Kenya, 1986.

Hagerman, R.J. (1992). 'Fragile X syndrome: advances and controversy'. *Journal of Child Psychology and Psychiatry*, **33**, 1127–1139.

Hagerman, R.J. and Sobesky, W.E. (1989). 'Psychopathology in fragile X syndrome'. *American Journal of Orthopsychiatry*, **59**, 142–152.

Haley, J. (1973). *Uncommon Therapy: The Psychiatric Techniques of Milton H. Erickson, M.D.* New York: Norton.

Hall, B.D. and Smith, D.W. (1972). 'Prader-Willi syndrome'. *Journal of Pediatrics*, **81**, 286–293.

Halliday, S., Meadow, S.R. and Berg, I. (1987).'Successful management of daytime enuresis using alarm procedures: a randomly controlled trial'. *Archives of Disease in Childhood*, **62**, 132–137.

Hassanyeh, F. and Davidson, K. (1980). 'Bipolar affective psychosis with onset before age 16 years: report of 10 cases'. *British Journal of Psychiatry*, **137**, 530–537.

Hawton, K., O'Grady, J., Osborn, M. and Cole, D. (1982). 'Adolescents who take overdoses: their characteristics, problems and contacts with helping agencies'. *British Journal of Psychiatry*, **140**, 118–123.

Hayden, T.L. (1980). 'Classification of elective mutism'. *Journal of the American Academy of Child Psychiatry*, **19**, 118–133.

Hazel, N. (1977). 'How family placements can combat delinquency'. *Social Work Today*, **8**, 6–7.

Heard, D. (1982). 'Family systems and the attachment dynamic'. *Journal of Family Therapy*, **4**, 99–116.

Hensey, O., Williams, J.K. and Rosenbloom, L. (1983). 'Intervention in child abuse: experience in Liverpool'. *Developmental Medicine and Child Neurology*, **25**, 606–611.

Hersov, L. (1980). 'Hospital inpatient and daypatient treatment of school refusal'. In: *Out of School – Modern Perspectives in School Refusal and Truancy*, eds. L. Hersov, and I. Berg. Chichester: Wiley.

Hetherington, E.M., Cox, M. and Cox, R. (1982). 'Family interaction and the social, emotional and cognitive development of children following divorce'. In: *The Family: Setting Priorities*, eds V. Vaughan and T. Brazelton. New York: Science and Medicine.

Hirshberg, L.M. (1993). 'Clinical interviews with infants and their families'. In: *Handbook of Infant Mental Health*, ed. C.H. Zeanah. New York: Guilford.

Hoberman, H.M. and Kroll-Mensing, D. (1992). 'Adolescent eating disorders'. *Current Opinion in Psychiatry*, **5**, 523–534.

Hobson, R.P. (1985). 'Piaget: on ways of knowing in childhood'. in: *Child and Adolescent Psychiatry*, 2nd edn, eds M. Rutter and L. Hersov. Oxford: Blackwell.

Hong, K. (1978). 'The transitional phenomena'. *Psychoanalytic Study of the Child*, **3**, 47–49.

Hunt, R.D. (1987). 'Treatment effects of oral and transdermal clonidine in relation to methylphenidate'. *Psychopharmacology Bulletin*, **23**, 111–114.

Hunt, R.D., Capper, L., and O'Connell, P. (1990). 'Clonidine in child and adolescent psychiatry'. *Journal of Child and Adolescent Psychopharmacology*, **1**, 87–102.

Imber-Black, E., Roberts, J. and Whiting, R. (1988). *Rituals in Families and Family Therapy*. New York: Norton.

Jacobson, R.R. (1985a). 'Child firesetters: a clinical investigation'. *Journal of Child Psychology and Psychiatry*, **26**, 759–768.

Jacobson, R.R. (1985b). 'The subclassification of firesetters'. *Journal of Child Psychology and Psychiatry*, **26**, 769–775.

Jankovic, J., Caskey, T.C., Stout, J.T. and Butler, I.J. (1988). 'Lesch-Nyhan syndrome: a study of motor behaviour and cerebrospinal fluid transmitters.' *Annals of Neurology*, **23**, 466–469.

Jarvelin, M.R., Vikevainen-Tervonen, L., Moilanen, I. and Huttunen, N.P. (1988). 'Enuresis in seven-year-old children'. *Acta Paediatrica Scandinavica*, **77**, 148–153.

Jenson, J.B. and Saunders, S.M. (1991). 'Childhood depression'. *Current Opinion in Psychiatry*, **4**, 535–541.

Jones, D.P.H. (1986). 'Individual psychotherapy for the sexually abused child'. *Child Abuse and Neglect*, **10**, 377–385.

Jones, D.P.H. (1991). 'Working with the Children Act: Tasks and responsibilities of the child and adolescent psychiatrist'. In: *Proceedings of the Children Act 1989 Course (OP12)*. Ed. C. Lindsey. London: Royal College of Psychiatrists.

Kandel, D.B. and Logan, J.A. (1984). 'Patterns of drug use from adolescence to young adulthood: I. Periods of risk for initiation, continued use and discontinuation'. *American Journal of Public Health*, **74**, 660–666.

Kanner, L. (1943). 'Autistic disturbance of affective contact'. *Nervous Child*, **2**, 217–250.

Kanner, L. (1944). 'Early infantile autism'. *Journal of Pediatrics*, **25**, 211–217.

Karpel, M.A. and Strauss, E.S. (1983). *Family Evaluation*. New York: Gardner Press.

Kashani, J.H., McGee, R.D., Clarkson, S.E., Anderson, J.C., Walton, L.A., Williams, S., Silva, P.A., Robins, A.L., Cytryn, L. and McKnew, D.H. (1983). 'Depression in a sample of nine year old children'. *Archives of General Psychiatry*, **40**, 1217–1227.

Kaufman, J. and Zigler, W. (1987). 'Do abused children become abusive parents?' *American Journal of Orthopsychiatry*, **57**, 186–192.

Kazdin, A.E. (1991). 'Aggressive behaviour and conduct disorder'. In: *The Practice of Child Therapy*, 2nd edn, eds T.R. Kratochwill and R.J. Morris. New York: Pergamon.

Kempe, C.H., Silverman, F.N., Steele, B.F., Droegemueller, W. and Silver, H.K. (1962). 'The battered child syndrome'. *Journal of the American Medical Association*, **191**, 17–23.

Kendall, P.C. and Braswell, L. (1985). *Cognitive-Behavioural Therapy for Impulsive Children*. New York: Guilford.

Kessler, M. and Albee, G.W. (1977). 'An overview of the literature of primary prevention'. In: *Primary Prevention of Psychopathology Volume 1*, ed. W. Ablee and J.M. Jolle. Hanover, New Hampshire: University Press of New England.

King, R.D., Raynes, N.V. and Tizard, J. (1971). *Patterns of Residential Care*. London: Routledge and Kegan Paul.

Klein, D.F., Gittelman, R., Quitkin, F. and Rifkin, A. (1980). *Diagnosis and Drug Treatment of Psychiatric Disorders: Adults and Children*. Baltimore: Williams and Wilkins.

Klein, M. (1932). *The Psychoanalysis of Children*. London: Hogarth.

Klein, M. (1948). *Contributions to Psychoanalysis 1921–1945*. London: Hogarth.

Kolvin *et al.* (1971). 'Studies in the childhood psychoses'. *British Journal of Psychiatry*, **118**, 381–419.

Kolvin, I. and Fundudis, T. (1981). 'Electively mute children: psychological development and background factors'. *Journal of Child Psychology and Psychiatry*, **22**, 219–232.

Kolvin, I., Garside, R.F., Nicol, A.R., MacMillan, A., Wolstenholme, F. and Leitch, I.M. (1981). *Help Starts Here: The Maladjusted Child in the Ordinary School*. London: Tavistock.

Kovach, J.A. and Glickman, N.W. (1986). 'Levels and social correlates of adolescent drug use.' *Journal of Youth and Adolescence*, **15**, 61–77.

Kraemer, S. (1987). 'Working with parents: casework or psychotherapy?' *Journal of Child Psychology and Psychiatry*, **28**, 207–213.

Lamb, D. (1986). *Psychotherapy with Adolescent Girls*, 2nd edn. New York: Plenum.

Landreth, G.L. (ed.) (1982). *Play Therapy*. Springfield, Ill: Charles C. Thomas.

Lask, B. and Bryant-Waugh, R. (1992). 'Early onset anorexia nervosa and related disorders'. *Journal of Child Psychology and Psychiatry*, **33**, 281–300.

Latz, S.R. and McCracken, J.T. (1992). 'Neuroleptic malignant syndrome (NMS) in children and adolescents'. *Journal of Child and Adolescent Psychopharmacology*, 2, 123–129.

Leckman, J.F. and Cohen, D.J. (1994). 'Tic disorders'. In: *Child and Adolescent Psychiatry: Modern Approaches*, 3rd edn., edited by M. Rutter, E. Taylor and L. Hersov. Oxford: Blackwell Science Ltd.

Ledoux, S., Choquet, M. and Flament, M. (1991). 'Eating disorders among adolescents in an unselected French population'. *International Journal of Eating Disorders*, 10, 81–89.

Leff, J.P. and Vaughn, C. (1985). *Expressed Emotion in Families*. New York: Guilford.

Leighton, A. (1965). 'Poverty and social change'. *Scientific American*, **212** (5), 21–27.

Leissner, A., Powley, T. and Evans, D. (1977). *Intermediate Treatment*. London: National Children's Bureau.

Leonard, H., Goldberg, B., Rapoport, J., Cheslow, D. and Swedos, S. (1990). 'Childhood rituals: normal development or obsessive-compulsive symptoms?' *Journal of the American Academy of Child and Adolescent Psychiatry*, **29**, 17–23.

Lerner, J.A., Inui, T.S., Turpin, E.W. and Douglas, E. (1985). 'Preschool behaviour can predict future psychiatric disorders'. *Journal of the American Academy of Child Psychiatry*, **24**, 42–48.

Lesch, K.G. and Nyhan, W.L. (1964). 'A familial disorder of uric acid metabolism and central nervous system function'. *American Journal of Medicine*, **36**, 561–570.

Levin, S., Rubenstein, J.S. and Streiner, D.C. (1976). 'The parent-therapist program: an innovative approach to treating emotionally disturbed children'. *Hospital and Community Psychiatry*, **27**, 407–410.

Lewis, D.O. (1991). 'Conduct disorder'. In: *Child and Adolescent Psychiatry: A Comprehensive Textbook*, ed. M. Lewis. Baltimore: Williams and Wilkins.

Lewis, D.O., Lovely, R., Yeager, C., Ferguson, G., Friedman, M., Sloan, G., Friedman, H. and Pincus, J.H. (1988a). 'Intrinsic and environmental characteristics of juvenile murderers'. *Journal of the American Academy of Child and Adolescent Psychiatry*, **27**, 582–587.

Lewis, D.O., Pincus, J.H., Bard, B., Richardson, E., Prichep, L.S., Feldman, M. and Yeager, C. (1988b). 'Neuropsychiatric, psychoeducational and family characteristics of 14 juveniles condemned to death in the United States'. *American Journal of Psychiatry*, **145**, 584–589.

Lewis, D.O. and Shanok, S. (1980). 'The use of a correctional setting for follow up care of psychiatrically disturbed adolescents'. *American Journal of Psychiatry*, **137**, 953–955.

Lewis, M. (ed.) (1991). *Child and Adolescent Psychiatry: A Comprehensive Textbook*. Baltimore: Williams and Wilkins.

Lewis, M. and Summerville, J.W. (1991). 'Residential treatment'. In: *Child and Adolescent Psychiatry: A Comprehensive Textbook*, ed. M. Lewis. Baltimore: Williams and Wilkins.

Little, R.E. and Streissgarth, A.P. (1981). 'The effects of alcohol on the fetus'. *Canadian Medical Association Journal*, **125**, 159–163.

Livingstone, S. (1972). 'Epilepsy in infancy, childhood and adolescence'. In: *Manual of Child Psychopathology*, ed. B.J. Wolman. New York: McGraw-Hill.

Lord, C. and Rutter, M. (1994). 'Autism and pervasive developmental disorders'. In: *Child and Adolescent Psychiatry: Modern Approaches*, 3rd edn., edited by M. Rutter, E. Taylor and L. Hersov. Oxford: Blackwell Science Ltd.

Lord, C., Schopler, E. and Revick, D. (1982). 'Sex differences in autism'. *Journal of Autism and Developmental Disorders*, **12**, 317–330.

Lotter, V. (1978). 'Follow-up studies'. In: *Autism: A Reappraisal of Concepts and Treatment*, eds M. Rutter and E. Schopler. New York: Plenum.

Lucas, C.P. (1992). 'Attention deficit disorders and hyperactivity'. *Current Opinion in Psychiatry*, **5**, 518–522.

Luthar, S.S. (1993). 'Methodological and conceptual issues in research on childhood resilience'. *Journal of Child Psychology and Psychiatry*, **34**, 441–453.

Lynch, M.A. (1978). 'The prognosis of child abuse'. *Journal of Child Psychology and Psychiatry*, **19**, 175–180.

Lynch, M.A. (1985). 'Child abuse before Kempe: an historical literature review'. *Child Abuse and Neglect*, **9**, 7–15.

MacFarlane, K. and Waterman, J. (1986). *Sexual Abuse of Young Children*. New York: Guilford.

Mack, J.E. and Ablon, S.L. (1983). *The Development of Self-Esteem in Childhood*. New York: International Universities Press.

Maclay, D. (1970). *Treatment for Children in Child Guidance*. New York: Science House.

Main, M. and Solomon, J. (1990). 'Procedures for identifying infants as disorganized/disoriented during the Ainsworth Strange Situation'. In: *Attachment in the Preschool Years*, eds M.T. Greenberg, D. Cicchetti and E.M. Cummings. Chicago: University of Chicago Press.

Manning, D.J. and Rosenbloom, L. (1987). 'Non-convulsive status epilepticus'. *Archives of Disease in Childhood*, **62**, 37–40.

Marriage, K., Fine, S., Moretti, M. and Haley, G. (1986). 'Relationship between depression and conduct disorder in children and adolescents'. *Journal of the American Academy of Child Psychiatry*, **25**, 687–691.

Martin, H.P. and Beezley, P. (1977). 'The emotional development of abused children'. *Developmental Medicine and Child Neurology*, **19**, 373–387.

Maughan, B., Gray, G. and Rutter, M. (1985). 'Reading retardation and antisocial behaviour'. *Journal of Child Psychology and Psychiatry*, **26**, 741–758.

McCormack, A., Janus, M.D. and Burgess, A.W. (1986). 'Runaway youths and sexual victimization: gender differences in an adolescent runaway population'. *Child Abuse and Neglect*, **10**, 281–285.

McFarlane, W.R. (1983). 'Introduction'. In: *Family Therapy in Schizophrenia*, ed. W.R. McFarlane. New York: Guilford.

McGee, R., Williams, S., Share, D.L., Anderson, J. and Silva, P.A. (1986). 'The relationship between specific reading retardation, general reading backwardness and behavioural problems in a large sample of Dunedin boys'. *Journal of Child Psychology and Psychiatry*, **27**, 597–610.

McGoldrick, M. and Carter, E.A. (1982). 'The family life cycle'. In: *Normal Family Processes*, ed. F. Walsh. New York: Guilford.

McGoldrick, M. and Gerson, R. (1985). *Genograms in Family Assessment*. New York: Norton.

McGuire, J. and Richman, N. (1986). 'Screening for behaviour problems in nurseries: the reliability and validity of the preschool behaviour checklist'. *Journal of Child Psychology and Psychiatry*, **27**, 7–32.

Meadow, R. (1991). 'Neurological and developmental variants of Munchausen syndrome by proxy'. *Developmental Medicine and Child Neurology*, **33**, 270–272.

Mian, M., Wehrspan, W., Klajner-Diamond, H., LeBaron, D. and Winder, C. (1986). 'Review of 125 children 6 years of age and under who were sexually abused'. *Child Abuse and Neglect*, **10**, 223–229.

Mikkleson, M. (1981). 'Epidemiology of trisomy 21'. In: *Trisomy 21*, ed. G. Burgio, M. Fraccaro, L. Tiepolo and U. Wolf. Berlin: Springer-Verlag.

Mills, J.C. and Crowley, R.J. (1986). *Therapeutic Metaphors for Children and the Child Within*. New York: Brunner/Mazel.

Minuchin, S. (1974). *Families and Family Therapy*. Cambridge, Mass: Harvard University Press.

Minuchin, S., Baker, L., Rosman, B.L., Liebman, R., Milman, L. and Todd, T.C.

(1975). 'A conceptual model of psychosomatic illness in children'. *Archives of General Psychiatry*, **32**, 1031–1038.

Mrazek, D.A. (1986). 'Childhood asthma: two central questions for child psychiatry'. *Journal of Child Psychology and Psychiatry*, **27**, 1–5.

Mulvey, E.P.O. and LaRosa, J.F. (1986). 'Delinquency cessation and adolescent development'. *American Journal of Orthopsychiatry*, **56**, 211–224.

Mundy, P., Sigman, M., Ungerer, J. and Sherman, T. (1986). 'Defining the social deficits of autism'. *Journal of Child Psychology and Psychiatry*, **27**, 657–669.

Murdoch, D. and Barker, P. (1991). *Basic Behaviour Therapy*. Oxford: Blackwell.

Myers, K.M., Burke, P. and McCauley, E. (1985). 'Suicidal behaviour by hospitalized preadolescent children on a psychiatric unit'. *Journal of the American Academy of Child Psychiatry*, **24**, 474–480.

Ney, P.G. and Mulvihill, D.L. (1985). *Child Psychiatric Treatment: A Practical Guide*. Beckenham, Kent: Croom Helm.

Nuechterlein, K.H. (1986) 'Childhood precursors of adult schizophrenia'. *Journal of Child Psychology and Psychiatry*, **27**, 133–144.

Oates, R.K. (1984). 'Personality development after physical abuse'. *Archives of Disease in Childhood*, **59**, 147–150.

Oates, R.K. and Forrest, D. (1985). 'Self-esteem and early background of abusive mothers'. *Child Abuse and Neglect*, **9**, 89–93.

Oates, R.K., Forrest, D. and Peacock, A. (1985). 'Self-esteem of abused children'. *Child Abuse and Neglect*, **9**, 159–163.

O'Connor, D.J. (1979). 'A profile of solvent abuse in school children'. *Journal of Child Psychology and Psychiatry*, **20**, 365–368.

Offord, D.R. (1987). 'Prevention of behavioural and emotional disorders in children'. *Journal of Child Psychology and Psychiatry*, **28**, 9–19.

Offord, D.R., Boyle, M.H., Szatmari, P., Rae-Grant, N.I., Links, P.S., Cadman, D.T., Byles, J.A., Crawford, J.W., Blum, H.M., Byrne, C., Thomas, H. and Woodward, C.A. (1987). 'Ontario child health study: prevalence of disorders and rates of service utilization'. *Archives of General Psychiatry*, **44**, 832–836.

O'Hanlon, W.H. and Hexum, A.L. (1990). *An Uncommon Casebook: The Complete Clinical Work of Milton H. Erickson, M.D.* New York: Norton.

Oliver, J.E. (1988). 'Successive generations of child maltreatment: the children'. *British Journal of Psychiatry*, **153**, 543–553.

Oliver, J.E. and Buchanan, A.H. (1979). 'Generations of maltreated children and multiagency care in one kindred'. *British Journal of Psychiatry*, **135**, 289–303.

Palazzoli, M.S., Boscolo, L., Cecchin, G. and Prata, G. (1978). *Paradox and Counterparadox*. New York: Jason Aronson.

Palazzoli, M.S., Boscolo, L., Cecchin, G. and Prata, G. (1980). 'Hypothesizing – circularity – neutrality: three guidelines for the conduct of the session'. *Family Process*, **19**, 3–12.

Papp, P. (1980). 'The Greek chorus and other techniques of paradoxical therapy'. *Family Process*, **19**, 45–57.

Parker, F.L., Piotrkowski, C.S. and Peay, L. (1987). 'Head start as a social support for mothers'. *American Journal of Orthopsychiatry*, **57**, 220–233.

Parkinson, C.E., Scrivener, R., Graves, L., Bunton, J. and Harvey, D. (1986).

'Behavioural differences of school-age children who were small-for-dates babies'. *Developmental Medicine and Child Neurology*, **28**, 498–505.

Patterson, D.R., Everett, J.J., Burns, G.L. and Marvin, J.A. (1992). 'Hypnosis for the treatment of burn pain'. *Journal of Consulting and Clinical Psychology*, **60**, 713–717.

Patterson, G.R. (1976). 'The aggressive child: victim or architect of a coercive system'. In: *Behaviour Modification and Families*, eds E.J. Mash, L.A. Hamerlynck and L.C. Handy. New York: Brunner/Mazel.

Patterson, G.R. (1982). *Coercive Family Process*. Eugene, Oregon: Castalia.

Pauls, D.L. and Leckman, J.F. (1986). 'The inheritance of Gilles de la Tourette's syndrome and associated behaviours'. *New England Journal of Medicine*, **315**, 993–997.

Pfeffer, C.R. (1991). 'Attempted suicide in children and adolescents: causes and management'. In: *Child and Adolescent Psychiatry: A Comprehensive Textbook*, ed. M. Lewis. Baltimore: Williams and Wilkins.

Philipp, R. (1979). 'Conducting parent training groups: approaches and strategies'. In: *New Directions in Children's Mental Health*, ed. S.J. Shamsie. New York: SP Medical and Scientific Books.

Pinkerton, P (1958). 'Psychogenic megacolon in children: the implications of bowel negativism'. *Archives of Disease in Childhood*, **33**, 371–380.

Prader, A., Labhart, A., Willi, H. (1956). 'A syndrome of obesity, short stature, cryptorchodism, and oligophrenia in the newborn period'. *Schwizersche Medizinische Wochenschrift*, **86**, 1260–1261.

Preskorn, S.H., Bupp, S.J., Weller, E.B. and Weller, R.A. (1989). 'Plasma levels of imipramine and metabolites in 68 hospitalized children'. *Journal of the American Academy of Child and Adolescent Psychiatry*, **28**, 373–375.

Price, R.A., Leckman, J.F., Pauls, D.L., Cohen, D.J. and Kidd, K.K. (1986). 'Gilles de la Tourette's syndrome: tics and central nervous stimulants in twins and non-twins with Tourette syndrome'. *Neurology*, **36**, 232–237.

Prince, R. (1960). 'The 'brain-fag syndrome in Nigerian students'. *Journal of Mental Science*, **106**, 559–570.

Pruitt, D.B. and Kiser, L.J. (1991). 'Day treatment: past, present and future'. In: *Child and Adolescent Psychiatry: a Comprehensive Textbook*, ed M. Lewis. Baltimore: Williams and Wilkins.

Puig-Antich, J. (1980). 'Affective disorders in childhood'. *Psychiatric Clinics of North America*, **3**, 403–424.

Puig-Antich, J. (1982). 'Major depression and conduct disorder in prepuberty'. *Journal of the American Academy of Child Psychiatry*, **21**, 118–128.

Puig-Antich, J. (1986). 'Psychobiological markers: effects of age and puberty'. In: *Depression in Young People: Developmental and Clinical Perspectives*, eds M. Rutter, C.E. Izard and P.B. Read. New York: Guilford.

Quinn, D.M.P. (1986). 'Prevalence of psychoactive medications in children and adolescents'. *Canadian Journal of Psychiatry*, **31**, 575–580.

Rapoport, J., Buchsbaum, M.S., Zahm, T.P., Weingartener, H., Ludlow, C. and Mikklesen, E.J. (1978). 'Dextramphetamine: cognitive and behavioural effects in normal prepubertal boys'. *Science*, **199**, 560–563.

Ratcliffe, S., Bancroft, J., Axworthy, D. and McLaren, W. (1982). 'Klinefelter's syndrome in adolescence'. *Archives of Disease in Childhood*, **57**, 6–12.

Ratcliffe, S.G., Butler, G.E. and Jones, M. (1990). 'Edinburgh study of growth and development of children with sex chromosome abnormalities'. In *Children and Young Adults with Sex Chromosome Aneuploidy*, eds J.A. Evans, J.L. Hamerton and A. Robinson. New York: Wiley-Liss.

Reid, K. (1985). *Truancy and School Absenteeism*. London: Hodder & Stoughton.

Reid, K. (1986). 'Truancy and school absenteeism: the state of the art'. *Maladjustment and Therapeutic Education*, **4**(3), 4–17.

Richman, N. (1985). 'A double-blind drug trial of treatment of sleep disorders – a pilot study'. *Journal of Child Psychology and Psychiatry*, **26**, 591–598.

Richman, N. and Graham, P.J. (1971). 'A behavioural screening questionnaire for use with 3-year-old children: preliminary findings'. *Journal of Child Psychology and Psychiatry*, **12**, 5–33.

Richman, N., Douglas, J., Hunt, H., Lansdown, R. and Levere, R. (1985). 'Behavioural methods in the treatment of sleep disorders – a pilot study'. *Journal of Child Psychology and Psychiatry*, **26**, 581–590.

Richman, N., Stevenson, J.E. and Graham, P.J. (1975). 'Prevalence of behaviour problems in 3-year-old children: an epidemiological study in a London Borough'. *Journal of Child Psychology and Psychiatry*, **16**, 277–287.

Robins, L.N. (1966). *Deviant Children Grown Up*. Baltimore: Williams and Wilkins.

Robins, L. (1978). 'Sturdy childhood predictors of adult antisocial behaviour: replications from longitudinal studies'. *Psychological Medicine*, **8**, 611–622.

Robinson, A., Bender, B.G. and Linden, M.G. (1991). 'Summary of clinical findings in children and young adults with sex chromosome abnormalities'. In: *Children and Young Adults with Sex Chromosome Aneuploidy*, eds J.A. Evans, J.L. Hamerton and A. Robinson. New York: Wiley-Liss.

Rosen, S. (ed.) (1982). *My Voice Will Go With You: The Teaching Tales of Milton H. Erickson, M.D.* New York: Norton.

Rossi, E. (1986a). *The Psychobiology of Mind-Body Healing*. New York: Norton.

Rossi, E. (1986b). 'The state-dependent memory and learning theory of therapeutic hypnosis'. In: *Mind-Body Communication in Hypnosis*, by M.H. Erickson, ed E.L. Rossi and M.O. Ryan. New York: Irvington.

Rossman, P.G. (1985). 'The aftermath of abuse and abandonment: a treatment approach for ego disturbance in female adolescence'. *Journal of the American Academy of Child Psychiatry*, **24**, 345–352.

Rumsey, J.M., Rapoport, J.L. and Sceery, W.R. (1985). 'Autistic children as adults'. *Journal of the American Academy of Child Psychiatry*, **24**, 465–473.

Russell, A.T., Bott, L. and Sammons, C. (1989). 'The phenomenology of schizophrenia occurring in childhood'. *Journal of the American Academy of Child and Adolescent Psychiatry*, **28**, 399–407.

Russell, D.H. (1981). 'On running away'. In: *Self-Destructive Behaviour in Children and Adolescents*, eds C.F. Wells and L.R. Stuart. New York: Van Nostrand Reinhold.

Rutter, M. (1979). 'Invulnerability or why some children are not damaged by stress'. In: *New Directions in Children's Mental Health,* ed. S.J. Shamsie. New York: SP Medical and Scientific Books.

Rutter, M. (1980a). 'School influences on children's behaviour and development'. *Pediatrics,* **65**, 208–220.

Rutter, M. (1980b). *Changing Youth in a Changing Society.* Cambridge, MA: Harvard University Press.

Rutter, M. (1981). 'The city and the child'. *American Journal of Orthopsychiatry,* **24**, 610–625.

Rutter, M. (1983). 'Cognitive defects in the pathogenesis of autism'. *Journal of Child Psychology and Psychiatry,* **24**, 513–531.

Rutter, M. (1986). 'The developmental psychopathology of depression: issues and perspectives'. In: *Depression in Young People: Developmental and Clinical Perspectives,* eds M. Rutler, C.E. Izard and P.B. Read. New York: Guilford.

Rutter, M., Cox, A., Tupling, G., Berger, M., and Yule, W. (1975a). 'Attainment and adjustment in two geographical areas. I. The prevalence of psychiatric disorder.' *British Journal of Psychiatry,* **126**, 493–501.

Rutter, M. and Garmezy, N. (1983). 'Developmental psychopathology'. In: *Socialization, Personality and Social Development, Vol. 4. Handbook of Child Psychology,* 4th edn, ed. E.M. Hetherington. New York: Wiley.

Rutter, M., Graham, P. and Yule, W.A. (1970a). *A Neuropsychiatric Study in Childhood.* London: Heinemann.

Rutter, M., Taylor, E. and Hersov, L. (1994). *Child and Adolescent Psychiatry,* 3rd edn. Oxford: Blackwell.

Rutter, M., Izard, C.E. and Read, P.B. (eds) (1986). *Depression in Young People: Developmental and Clinical Perspectives.* New York: Guilford.

Rutter, M., Maughan, N., Mortimore, P. and Ouston, J. (1979). *Fifteen Thousand Hours.* London: Open Books.

Rutter, M. and Rutter, M. (1993). *Developing Minds.* New York: Basic Books.

Rutter, M., Shaffer, D. and Sturge, C. (1975b). *A Guide to a Multi-Axial Classification Scheme for Psychiatric Disorders in Childhood and Adolescence.* Dept. of Child and Adolescent Psychiatry, Institute of Psychiatry, London, SE8 8AF.

Rutter, M. and Schopler, E. (1992) 'Classification of pervasive developmental disorders: some concepts and practical considerations'. *Journal of Autism and Developmental Disorders,* **22**, 459–482.

Rutter, M., Tizard, J., and Whitmore, K. (1970b). *Education, Health and Behaviour.* London: Longman.

Sadeh, A. and Anders, T.F. (1993). 'Sleep disorders'. In: *Handbook of Infant Mental Health,* ed. C.H. Zeanah, New York: Guilford.

Savicki, C.E. and Brown, R. (1981). *Working with Troubled Children.* New York: Human Sciences Press.

Schachar, R. (1991). 'Childhood hyperactivity'. *Journal of Child Psychology and Psychiatry,* **32**, 155–191.

Schachar, R. and Wachsmuth, R. (1990). 'Hyperactivity and parental psychopathology'. *Journal of Child Psychology and Psychiatry,* **31**, 381–392.

Schaefer, C.E. and Swanson, A.J. (eds.) (1988). *Children in Residential Care: Critical Issues in Treatment.* New York: Van Nostrand Reinhold.

Scheinberg, M. (1985). 'The debate: a strategic technique'. *Family Process*, **24**, 259–271.

Schmidt, E. and Eldridge, A. (1986). 'The attachment relationship and child maltreatment'. *Infant Mental Health Journal*, **7**, 264–273.

Scott, P.D. (1977). 'Non-accidental injury in children'. *British Journal of Psychiatry*, **131**, 366–380.

Scott, S. (1994). 'Mental retardation'. In: *Child and Adolescent Psychiatry: Modern Approaches*, 3rd edn., edited by M. Rutter, E. Taylor and L. Hersov. Oxford: Blackwell Science Ltd.

Seligman, M.E.O. and Peterson, C. (1986). 'A learned helplessness perspective in childhood depression'. In: *Depression in Young People: Developmental and Clinical Perspectives*, eds M. Rutter, C.E. Izard and P.B. Read. New York: Guilford.

Shachnow, J. (1987). 'Preventive intervention with children of hospitalized psychiatric patients'. *American Journal of Orthopsychiatry*, **57**, 275–291.

Shaffer, D. (1985). 'Brain damage'. In: *Child and Adolescent Psychiatry: Modern Approaches*, eds M. Rutter and L. Hersov. Oxford: Blackwell.

Shaffer, D. and Fisher, P. (1981). 'The epidemiology of suicide in children and adolescents'. *Journal of the American Academy of Child Psychiatry*, **20**, 513–565.

Shaffer, D., Gardner, A. and Hodge, B. (1984). 'Behaviour and bladder disturbance of enuretic children: a rational classification of a common disorder'. *Developmental Medicine and Child Neurology*, **26**, 781–792.

Shafii, T. (1986). 'The prevalence and use of transitional objects'. *Journal of the American Academy of Child Psychiatry*, **25**, 805–808.

Shamsie, S.J. (1985). 'Family breakdown and its effects on emotional disorders in children', *Canadian Journal of Psychiatry*, **30**, 281–287.

Shamsie, S.J. (1992). 'Conduct disordered youth: good responders and poor responders'. *Canadian Child Psychiatric Bulletin*, **1**, 35–37.

Shapland, L.M. (1978). 'Self-reported delinquency in boys aged 11 to 14'. *British Journal of Delinquency*, **18**, 255–266.

Silva, P.A., McGee, R. and Williams, S. (1985). 'Some characteristics of 9-year-old boys with general reading backwardness or specific reading retardation'. *Journal of Child Psychology and Psychiatry*, **26**, 407–421.

Simonoff, E., McGuffin, P. and Gottesman, I.I. (1994). 'Genetic influences on normal and abnormal development'. In: *Child and Adolescent Psychiatry: Modern Approaches*, 3rd edn., (eds) M. Rutter, E. Taylor and L. Hersov. Oxford: Blackwell Science Ltd.

Singer, H.S. and Walkup, J.T. (1991). 'Tourette syndrome and other tic disorders: diagnosis, pathophysiology and treatment'. *Medicine*, **70**, 15–32.

Singer, M.Y., Wynne, L.C. and Toohey, M. (1978). 'Communication deviance and the families of schizophrenics'. In: *The Nature of Schizophrenia*, ed. L.C. Wynne, R.L. Cromwell and S. Matthysse. New York: Wiley.

Skynner, A.C.R. (1975). *One Flesh: Separate Persons*. London: Constable. (Published in the USA as *Systems of Family and Marital Psychotherapy*. New York: Brunner/Mazel.)

Smith, C.J. (1990). 'The management of children with emotional and behavioural difficulties in ordinary and special schools'. In: *The Management of Children with Emotional and Behavioural Difficulties*, ed. V. Varma. London: Routledge.

Spencer, T., Biederman, J., Kerman, K., Steingard, R. and Wilens, T. (1993a). 'Desipramine treatment of children with attention-deficit hyperactivity disorder and tic disorder or Tourette's syndrome'. *Journal of the American Academy of Child and Adolescent Psychiatry*, **32**, 354–360.

Spencer, T., Biederman, J., Wilens, T., Steingard, R. and Geist, D. (1993b). 'Nortriptyline treatment of children with attention-deficit hyperactivity disorder and tic disorder or Tourette's syndrome'. *Journal of the American Academy of Child and Adolescent Psychiatry*, **32**, 205–210.

Spitz, R.A. (1946). 'Anaclitic depression'. *Psychoanalytic Study of the Child*, **2**, 113–117.

Sreenivasan, U. (1985). 'Effeminate boys in a child psychiatric clinic: prevalence and associated factors'. *Journal of the American Academy of Child Psychiatry*, **24**, 689–694.

Stanley, L. (1980). 'Treatment of ritualistic behaviour in an eight-year-old boy by response prevention'. *Journal of Child Psychology and Psychiatry*, **21**, 85–90.

Starfield, B. (1967). 'Functional bladder capacity in enuretic and non-enuretic children'. *Journal of Pediatrics*, **70**, 777–781.

Steinberg, D. (1987). *Basic Adolescent Psychiatry*. Oxford: Blackwell.

Steinhauer, P.D. (1984). 'The management of children admitted to child welfare services in Ontario'. *Canadian Journal of Psychiatry*, **29**, 77–88.

Steinhauer, P.D. (1991). *The Least Detrimental Alternative: A Systematic Guide to Case Planning and Decision Making for Children in Care*. Toronto: University of Toronto Press.

Steinhauer, P.D., Santa-Barbara, J. and Skinner, H. (1984). 'The process model of family functioning'. *Canadian Journal of Psychiatry*, **29**, 77–88.

Stevenson, J., Richman, N. and Graham, P. (1985). 'Behaviour problems and language abilities at 3 years and behavioural deviance of 8 years'. *Journal of Child Psychology and Psychiatry*, **26**, 215–230.

Stevenson, J., Graham, P., Fredman, G. and McLoughlin, V. (1987). 'A twin study of genetic influences on reading and spelling ability and disability.' *Journal of Child Psychology and Psychiatry*, **28**, 229–247.

Stores, G. (1985). 'Clinical and EEG evaluation of seizures and seizure-like disorders'. *Journal of the American Academy of Child Psychiatry*, **24**, 10–16.

Stores, G. (1987). 'Pitfalls in the management of epilepsy.' *Archives of Disease in Childhood*, **62**, 88–90.

Stott, D.H. (1966). *The Social Adjustment of Children*, 3rd edn. University of London Press.

Stubbs, E.G., Ritvo, E.R. and Mason-Brothers, A. (1985). 'Autism and shared parental HLA antigens'. *Journal of the American Academy of Child Psychiatry*, **24**, 182–185.

Sudbury, P.R. and Ghodse, A.H. (1990) 'Solvent misuse'. *Current Opinion in Psychiatry*, **3**, 388–392.

Sutcliffe, P., Lovell, J. and Walters, M. (1985). 'New directions for family therapy: rubbish removal as a task of choice'. *Journal of Family Therapy*, **7**, 175–182.

Swirsky-Sacchetti, T. and Margolis, C.G. (1986). 'The effect of a comprehensive self-hypnosis training program on the use of factor VIII in severe haemophilia'. *International Journal of Clinical and Experimental Hypnosis*, **34**, 71–83.

Szapocznik, J., Perez-Vidal, A., Brickman, A.L., Foote, F.H., Santisteban, D. Hervis, O. and Kurtines, W.M. (1988). 'Engaging adolescent drug abusers and their families in treatment: a strategic structural systems approach'. *Journal of Consulting and Clinical Psychology*, **56**, 552–557.

Tanguay, P.E. and Cantor, S.L. (1986). 'Schizophrenia in children: introduction'. *Journal of the American Academy of Child Psychiatry*, **25**, 591–594.

Taylor, E. (1985). 'Drug treatment'. In: *Child and Adolescent Psychiatry: Modern Approaches*, 2nd edn, eds M. Rutter and L. Hersov. Oxford: Blackwell.

Taylor, E.A. (1986a). *The Overactive Child* (Clinics in Developmental Medicine, No. 97). Oxford: Blackwell; Philadelphia: Lippincott.

Taylor, E.A. (1986b). 'The basis of drug treatment'. In: *The Overactive Child* (Clinics in Developmental Medicine, No. 97), ed. E.A. Taylor. Oxford: Blackwell; Philadelphia: Lippincott.

Terr, L.C. (1991). 'Acute responses to external events and posttraumatic stress disorders'. In: *Child and Adolescent Psychiatry: A Comprehensive Textbook*, ed. M. Lewis. New York: Williams and Wilkins.

Thomas, A. and Chess, S. (1977). *Temperament and Development*. New York: Brunner/Mazel.

Thompson, T.R. (1987). 'Childhood and adolescent suicide in Manitoba: a demographic study'. *Canadian Journal of Psychiatry*, **32**, 264–269.

Tizard, B. and Hodges, J. (1978). 'The effect of early institutional rearing on the development of eight year old children'. *Journal of Child Psychology and Psychiatry*, **19**, 99–118.

Tsai, L.Y. (1992). 'Is Rett Syndrome a subtype of pervasive developmental disorders?'. *Journal of Autism and Developmental Disorders*, **22**, 551–561.

Turgay, A. (1980). 'Conversion reactions in children'. *Psychiatric Journal of the University of Ottawa*, **5**, 287–294.

Vandenberg, S.G., Singer, S.M. and Pauls, D.L. (1986). *The Heredity of Behaviour Disorders in Adults and Children*. New York: Plenum.

Varma, V. (ed.) (1993). *The Management of Behaviour in Schools*. London: Longman.

Verhulst, J.H.L., Akkerhuis, G.W., Sanders-Woudstra, J.A.R., Timmer, F.C. and Donkhorst, I.D. (1985). 'The prevalence of enuresis'. *Journal of Child Psychology and Psychiatry*, **26**, 989–993.

Vicary, J.R. and Lerner, J.V. (1986). 'Parental attributes and adolescent drug use'. *Journal of Adolescence*, **9**, 115–122.

Vorrath, H.H. and Brendthro, L.K. (1985). *Positive Peer Culture*, 2nd edn. New York: Aldine.

Walker, L.G. (1992). 'Hypnosis with cancer patients'. *American Journal of Preventative Psychiatry and Neurology*, **3**, 42–49.

Wallas, L. (1985). *Stories for the Third Ear*. New York: Norton.

Wallerstein, J.S. (1983). 'Children of divorce: stress and developmental tasks'. In: *Stress, Coping and Development in Children*, ed. N. Garmezy and M. Rutter.

Wallerstein, J.S. and Corbin, S.B. (1991). 'The child and the vicissitudes of divorce'.

In: *Child and Adolescent Psychiatry: A Comprehensive Textbook*, ed. M. Lewis. Baltimore: Williams and Wilkins.

Walton, J.N., Ellis, E. and Court, S.D.M. (1962). 'Clumsy children: developmental apraxia and agnosia'. *Brain*, **85**, 603–612.

Walzer, S. (1985). 'X chromosome abnormalities and cognitive development'. *Journal of Child Psychology and Psychiatry*, **26**, 177–184.

Watkins, J.G. (1987). *Hypnotherapeutic Techniques*. New York: Irvington.

Weeks, G.R. and L'Abate, L. (1982). *Paradoxical Psychotherapy*. New York: Brunner/ Mazel.

Weiss, G. and Hechtman, L.T. (1986). *Hyperactive Children Grown Up*. New York: Guilford.

Weiner, I.B. (1982). *Child and Adolescent Psychopathology*. New York: Wiley.

Werner, E.E. and Smith, R.S. (1982). *Vulnerable but Invincible: A Longitudinal Study of Resilient Children and Youth*. New York: McGraw-Hill.

Whitaker, A., Johnson, J., Shaffer, D., Rapoport, J.L., Kalikow, K., Walsh, B.T., Davies, M., Braiaman, S. and Dolinsky, A. (1990). 'Uncommon troubles in young people'. *Archives of General Psychiatry*, **47**, 487–496.

White, R., Benedict, M.I., Wulff, L. and Kelley, M. (1987). 'Physical disabilities as risk factors for child maltreatment'. *American Journal of Orthopsychiatry*, **57**, 93–101.

White, S., Strom, G.A., Santilli, G. and Halpin, B.M. (1986). 'Interviewing young sexual abuse victims with anatomically correct dolls'. *Child Abuse and Neglect*, **10**, 519–529.

Williams, K., Goodman, M. and Green, R. (1985). 'Parent-child factors in gender role socialization in girls'. *Journal of the American Academy of Child Psychiatry*, **20**, 720–731.

Williams, R. (ed.) (1992). *A Concise Guide to the Children Act 1989*. London: Gaskell.

Wilson, H. (1980). 'Parental supervision: a neglected aspect of delinquency'. *British Journal of Criminology*, **20**, 203–235.

Winnicott, D. (1960). *The Maturational Process and the Facilitating Environment*. London: Hogarth,

Wolff, S. (1991). ' "Schizoid" personality in childhood and adult life I: the vagaries of diagnostic labelling'. *British Journal of Psychiatry*, **159**, 615–620.

Wolff, S. and Barlow, A. (1979). 'Schizoid personality in childhood: a controlled follow-up study'. *Journal of Child Psychology and Psychiatry*, **20**, 29–46.

Wolkind, S. (1981). 'Depression in mothers of young children'. *Archives of Disease in Childhood*, **56**, 1–3.

Wolkind, S. and Rutter, M. (1973). 'Children who have been 'in care' – an epidemiological study'. *Journal of Child Psychology Psychiatry*, **14**, 97–105.

World Health Organization (1977a). *International Classification of Diseases*, 1975 Revision. Geneva: WHO.

World Health Organization (1977b). *Child Mental Health and Psychosocial Development*. Geneva: WHO.

World Health Organization (1992). *The ICD-10 Classification of Mental and Behavioural Disorders: Clinical Descriptions and Diagnostic Guidelines*. Geneva: WHO.

Wright, H.H., Miller, M.D., Cook, M.A. and Littman, J.T. (1985). 'Early identification and intervention with children who refuse to speak'. *Journal of the American Academy of Child Psychiatry*, **24**, 739–746.

Wynn, A (1974). 'Health care systems for pre-school children'. *Proceedings of the Royal Society of Medicine*, **67**, 340–343.

Wynne, L.C. (1981). 'Current concepts about schizophrenia and family relationships'. *Journal of Nervous and Mental Disease*, **167**, 144–158.

Yule, W. and Carr, J. (eds) (1980). *Behaviour Modification for the Mentally Handicapped*. London: Croom Helm.

Zahner, G.E.P. and Pauls, D.L. (1987) 'Epidemiological survey of infantile autism'. In: *Handbook of Autism and Pervasive Developmental Disorders*, eds D. Cohen and A. Donnellan. New York: Wiley.

Zahner, G.E.P., Clubb, M.M., Leckman, J.F. *et al.* (1988). 'The epidemiology of Tourette's syndrome'. In: *Tourette's Syndrome and Tic Disorders*, eds D.J. Cohen, R.D. Bruun and J.F. Leckman. New York: Wiley.

Zeanah, C.H. (1993). *Handbook of Infant Mental Health*. New York: Guilford.

Zeanah, C.H., Mammen, O.K. and Lieberman, A.F. (1993). 'Disorders of attachment'. In: *Handbook of Infant Mental Health*, ed, C.H. Zeanah. New York: Guilford.

Zeig, J.K. and Munion, W.M. (eds) (1990). *What Is Psychotherapy?* San Francisco: Jossey-Bass.

Zeitlin, H. (1990). 'Current interests in child-adult psychopathological continuities'. *Journal of Child Psychology and Psychiatry*, **31**, 671–679.

Zimet, S.A.G. (1993). 'Day treatment in the year two thousand and one'. *Canadian Child Psychiatric Bulletin*, **2**, 64–68.

Zimet, S.G. and Farley, F.G.K. (1985). 'Day treatment for children in the United States'. *Journal of the American Academy of Child Psychiatry*, **24**, 732–738.

Subject Index

description, 106
drug treatment of, 295
in adolescence, 229
outcome, 113
prevalence, 93
treatment, 109
Anxiety Disorders of Childhood, 113
anxiolytics, 110
anxious-avoidant, 225
anxious personality disorder, 181
approach/withdrawal, 18
arithmetic problems, 151
Asperger's syndrome, 139–140, 145, 181
asthma, 17, 199, 202–4
attachment, 3, 212, 215
anxious, 225
anxious-avoidant, 225
behaviour, 4, 97, 224–6
disorders of, 214, 224
disorganized/disoriented, 225
secure, 224
theory, 97, 106
attention-deficit (hyperactivity) disorders, 27, 62, 74, 80, 83–90, 120, 123, 127
causes, 84
description, 87
drug treatment of, 289–91
in adolescence, 231
outcome, 89
prevalence, 86
treatment, 88, 291
attention span, 18
autism, 15, 224, 302
autism/autistic disorders, 131–145, 197
atypical, 137–8
behavioural abnormalities in, 136
causes, 132
cognitive abnormalities in, 137
communication in, 136
description, 134
genetic factors in, 132
in adolescence, 230
outcome, 144
prevalence, 132
ritualistic behaviour in, 137
self-destructive behaviour in, 137
social interaction in, 135
treatment, 141–4
twin studies in, 132
autistic aloneness, 135
autonomy, 3
avoidant disorder of childhood, 99
avoidant personality disorder, 181

Bader, Douglas, 200
barbiturate abuse, 236
barbiturates, 123, 238
Basic Adolescent Psychiatry, 245
Basic Behaviour Therapy, 286
Basic Family Therapy, 11, 21, 35, 41, 43, 45, 67, 278, 282, 283
basic tasks, 278
trust, 3, 8
battered child syndrome, 258
Bayley Infant Scales of Mental and Motor Development, 56, 216
behavioural analysis, 110
behavioural screening questionnaire, 217
behaviour disorders
drug treatment for, 296–297
see also conduct disorders
behaviour therapy, 77, 109, 253, 270, 284–7
in attention-deficit hyperactivity disorders, 89
management, 79
benzhexol, 292
benzodiazepine drugs/
benzodiazepines, 162, 238, 292, 295, 297, 298
bereavement, 121
bipolar affective disorder(s), 118, 128
birth injury, 12, 16, 64
trauma, 310
blindness, 17
body dysmorphic disorder, 91
bomb-in-the-room syndrome, 128
bonding, 3, 212
borderline personality disorder, 181
brain damage, 17
brain fag syndrome, 106, 161
brain tumours, 200
breath-holding spells, 223–224
brief psychotic disorders, 160
Bristol Social Adjustment Guide, 318
bulimia, 204, 205–209
atypical, 206
drug treatment in, 295
treatment, 209
burns, 17
buspirone, 143

cancer(s), 202
cannabis products, 238
carbamazepine, 197, 198
care order, 325
caretaker-selves, 180
casework, 275, 276, 277

Author Index